Frontiers in Anti-Infective Drug Discovery

(Volume 7)

Edited by

Atta-ur-Rahman, *FRS*

Honorary Life Fellow, Kings College, University of Cambridge, Cambridge, UK

&

M. Iqbal Choudhary

H.E.J. Research Institute of Chemistry, International Center for Chemical and Biological Sciences, University of Karachi, Karachi, Pakistan

Frontiers in Anti-Infective Drug Discovery

Volume # 7

Editors: Atta-ur-Rahman and M. Iqbal Choudhary

ISSN (Online): 1879-663X

ISSN (Print): 2451-9162

ISBN (Online): 978-1-68108-562-3

ISBN (Print): 978-1-68108-563-0

General:

1. Any dispute or claim arising out of or in connection with this License Agreement or the Work (including non-contractual disputes or claims) will be governed by and construed in accordance with the laws of the U.A.E. as applied in the Emirate of Dubai. Each party agrees that the courts of the Emirate of Dubai shall have exclusive jurisdiction to settle any dispute or claim arising out of or in connection with this License Agreement or the Work (including non-contractual disputes or claims).
2. Your rights under this License Agreement will automatically terminate without notice and without the need for a court order if at any point you breach any terms of this License Agreement. In no event will any delay or failure by Bentham Science Publishers in enforcing your compliance with this License Agreement constitute a waiver of any of its rights.
3. You acknowledge that you have read this License Agreement, and agree to be bound by its terms and conditions. To the extent that any other terms and conditions presented on any website of Bentham Science Publishers conflict with, or are inconsistent with, the terms and conditions set out in this License Agreement, you acknowledge that the terms and conditions set out in this License Agreement shall prevail.

Bentham Science Publishers Ltd.
Executive Suite Y - 2
PO Box 7917, Saif Zone
Sharjah, U.A.E.
Email: subscriptions@benthamscience.org

**BENTHAM
SCIENCE**

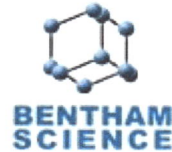

CONTENTS

PREFACE

The 7th volume of the book series entitled, *"Frontiers in Anti-infective Drug Discovery"* comprises seven comprehensively written reviews on therapeutic advances against bacterial, fungal, and viral infections and cancers, and on study of the mechanism of action of various drugs, and drug candidates, including natural products.

Amedei and Russo have reviewed the role of gut microbiota in the on-set and progression of gastrointestinal (GI) cancers in chapter 1. GI cancers are among the most prevalent cancers with complex aetiologies and high mortality rate. Along with many other factors, human gut microbiota has been found to play an important role in GI cancers. GI cancers are multifactorial diseases influenced by genetic and environmental factors, as well as by *Helicobacter pylori* infection. Association between the gut microorganisms and GI tumours has attracted major scientific interests in recent years. Modern sequencing techniques have been used to understand various features of the complex microbial communities, as well as the mechanisms through which the gut microbiota are involved in carcinogenesis and cancer progression. The authors have provided a detailed description of how microbial dysbiosis (microbial imbalance) contributes to oncogenesis *via* multiple pathways, including tumour progression and response to the cancer treatments.

Dengue viral fever has emerged as one of the most important epidemics in recent times. Its re-emergence in tropical and sub-tropical regions of the world is causing considerable morbidity and mortality. Currently, no vaccine is available which can protect against four serotypes of the Dengue virus (DENV) which are known to use host's biological systems to propagate, and cause infections. These host biological processes include cytoplasmic and nuclear structures and components. Damonte *et al.* have reviewed the recent literature in this important area of research in chapter 2. Their emphasis has been on the identification of host factors, and processes which are involved in viral infection.

Plant products have played a key role in the treatment of diseases since antiquity, including treatment of infections in the pre-antibiotics era. With the discovery of natural products and their synthetic analogues with good antibiotic activity, the importance of phytochemicals had diminished. However, with the emergence of antibiotic resistance, the search of new antibiotics including resistance reversal agents from the plant kingdom against novel targets, was globally initiated. Hazra *et al.* in chapter 3 discuss various classes of plant secondary metabolites which have the capacity to serve as resistance modifying agents (RMA), thus helping conventional antibiotics to function again. The authors have discussed various screening approaches protocols which have been successfully used for the discovery of RMAs, as well as approaches to study their possible mechanism of actions. The discovery of plant-based RMAs is thus a powerful new approach for the treatment infections caused by multi-drug resistant bacteria.

Computer-aided drug design (CADD) has emerged as an important tool in the modern drug discovery and development process. CADD approach plays a key role in drug target identification, study of mechanism of action, as well as in the prediction of drug candidates in the initial drug discovery process. However, CADD-predicted compounds are often found to be ineffective in biochemical and cellular assays. Kaczor and his colleagues have reviewed the application and limitations of CADD approach in chapter 4. They critically analyse the strengths and weaknesses of CADD based lead identification in the context of antibacterial drug discovery and emphasize the need to further improve the CADD based methods, as well the need for experimental verification of computational results at an early phase of drug discovery process.

Since the FDA approval of first aptamer-based drug for the treatment of age-related macular degeneration in 2004, interest in therapeutic uses of aptamers has increased substantially. These molecules are capable of specifically binding with proteins, and inhibiting targets such as vascular endothelial growth factor (VEGF), thrombin and other cellular disease targets. These oligonucleotide aptamers are essentially the small molecular equivalent of antibodies, and thus have the advantage of being highly specific and non-immunogenic. Evran *et al.* present a comprehensive review on the applications of small single-stranded RNA and DNA (oligonucleotide aptamers) as targeted therapies against virulence factors of drug resistance microorganisms in chapter 5. Many aptamers have been investigated and developed for the treatment of diseases, such as cancers, HIV, and macular degeneration. The review of Evran *et al.* focuses on recent research on the use of various aptamers as specific blockers of the virulence factors of drug resistant pathogens. The authors have also reviewed the literature on the use of aptamers as biosensors of bacterial toxins.

Fungal skin infections are often difficult to treat completely due to their capacity to go in recession through spore formation. *Candida albicans* and its multidrug resistant strains are a major cause of superficial, and deep seeded infections in humans and livestock. The review by Hameed *et al.* in chapter 6 addresses the approaches to overcome fungal infections by using natural products, that can act by blocking or modulating the functions of drug efflux pumps in MDR fungal pathogens. These natural products thus provide an excellent opportunity to treat MDR fungal infections, including *Candida* infections effectively.

Hydrogen sulfide (H_2S) is an endogenous gaseous transmitter whose role in the pathophysiology of several diseases has been extensively studied. It has been linked to many important physiological functions and is known to play a significant role in various diseases involving inflammation, fibrosis, and vascular responses. Recent studies indicate the vasoactive, cytoprotective and anti-inflammatory role of hydrogen sulfide. It can regulate viral, bacterial, parasitic, and fungal infections through its function as signalling molecule. Bhatia et. al. has reviewed state-of-the-art understanding about the mechanisms underlying H_2S-mediated regulation of different infectious diseases in chapter 7. This can help in developing H_2S- releasing drugs as therapeutic molecules. In the absence of effective treatment for many infections, the H_2S based therapeutic agents provide a new approach for infection treatment.

The above articles by prominent researchers in chosen fields have made this volume another important treatise for scientists and research scholars. We are grateful to all the authors for their excellent and scholarly contributions for the 7th volume of this internationally recognized eBook series. We hope that like the previous volumes of this internationally reputed book series, the current compilation will also receive a wide readership and appreciation.

The editorial team of Bentham Science Publishers is greatly appreciated for efficient processing and timely management of this publication. The coordination and liaison by Ms Fariya Zulfiqar (Assistant Manager Publications), and leadership of Mr. Mahmood Alam (Director Publications) are duly acknowledged.

Atta-ur-Rahman, *FRS*   **M. Iqbal Choudhary**
Kings College   H.E.J. Research Institute of Chemistry
University of Cambridge   International Center for Chemical and Biological Sciences
UK   University of Karachi, Karachi
                                                                                                           Pakistan

List of Contributors

Agnieszka A. Kaczor
Department of Synthesis and Chemical Technology of Pharmaceutical Substances with Computer Modelling Lab, Faculty of Pharmacy with Division for Medical Analytics, Lublin, Poland
School of Pharmacy, University of Eastern Finland, Kuopio, Finland

Amedeo Amedei
Department of Experimental and Clinical Medicine, Viale Pieraccini 6, University of Florence, Florence, Italy

Antti Poso
School of Pharmacy, University of Eastern Finland, Kuopio, Finland

Banasri Hazra
Department of Pharmaceutical Technology, Jadavpur University, Kolkata 700032, India

Burhan Bora
Faculty of Science, Department of Biochemistry, Ege University, Bornova-Izmir, Turkey

Canan Ozyurt
Faculty of Science, Department of Biochemistry, Ege University, Bornova-Izmir, Turkey

Cybele C. García
Laboratorio de Virología, Departamento de Química Biológica, Facultad de Ciencias Exactas y Naturales, Universidad de Buenos Aires (UBA), Buenos Aires, Argentina
IQUIBICEN, Consejo Nacional de Investigaciones Científicas y Técnicas (CONICET)-UBA, Buenos Aires, Argentina

Damian Bartuzi
Department of Synthesis and Chemical Technology of Pharmaceutical Substances with Computer Modelling Lab, Faculty of Pharmacy with Division for Medical Analytics, Lublin, Poland

Dariusz Matosiuk
Department of Synthesis and Chemical Technology of Pharmaceutical Substances with Computer Modelling Lab, Faculty of Pharmacy with Division for Medical Analytics, Lublin, Poland

Dhruti Avlani
Division of Pharmaceutics, NSHM Knowledge Campus, Kolkata-Group of Institutions, Kolkata 700053, India

Edda Russo
Department of Experimental and Clinical Medicine, Viale Pieraccini 6, University of Florence, Florence, Italy

Elsa B. Damonte
Laboratorio de Virología, Departamento de Química Biológica, Facultad de Ciencias Exactas y Naturales, Universidad de Buenos Aires (UBA), Buenos Aires, Argentina
IQUIBICEN, Consejo Nacional de Investigaciones Científicas y Técnicas (CONICET)-UBA, Buenos Aires, Argentina

Madhav Bhatia
Department of Pathology and Biomedical Science, University of Otago-Christchurch, Christchurch, New Zealand

Magdalena Kondej
Department of Synthesis and Chemical Technology of Pharmaceutical Substances with Computer Modelling Lab, Faculty of Pharmacy with Division for Medical Analytics, Lublin, Poland

Ozge Ugurlu
Faculty of Science, Department of Biochemistry, Ege University, Bornova-Izmir, Turkey

Piyush Jha	Department of Pathology and Biomedical Science, University of Otago-Christchurch, Christchurch, New Zealand
Prasanthi Medarametla	School of Pharmacy, University of Eastern Finland, Kuopio, Finland
Ravinder R. Gaddam	Department of Pathology and Biomedical Science, University of Otago-Christchurch, Christchurch, New Zealand
Saif Hameed	Amity Institute of Biotechnology, Amity University Haryana, Gurugram (Manesar), India
Sandeep Hans	Amity Institute of Biotechnology, Amity University Haryana, Gurugram (Manesar), India
Serap Evran	Faculty of Science, Department of Biochemistry, Ege University, Bornova-Izmir, Turkey
Shweta Singh	Amity Institute of Biotechnology, Amity University Haryana, Gurugram (Manesar), India
Subhalakshmi Ghosh	Department of Pharmaceutical Technology, Jadavpur University, Kolkata 700032, India
Sutapa Biswas Majee	Division of Pharmaceutics, NSHM Knowledge Campus, Kolkata-Group of Institutions, Kolkata 700053, India
Verónica M. Quintana	Laboratorio de Virología, Departamento de Química Biológica, Facultad de Ciencias Exactas y Naturales, Universidad de Buenos Aires (UBA), Buenos Aires, Argentina
Viviana Castilla	Laboratorio de Virología, Departamento de Química Biológica, Facultad de Ciencias Exactas y Naturales, Universidad de Buenos Aires (UBA), Buenos Aires, Argentina
Zeeshan Fatima	Amity Institute of Biotechnology, Amity University Haryana, Gurugram (Manesar), India

CHAPTER 1

The Role of the Microbiota in the Genesis of Gastrointestinal Cancers

Edda Russo and **Amedeo Amedei**[*]

Department of Experimental and Clinical Medicine, Viale Pieraccini 6, University of Florence, Florence, Italy

Abstract: The term "Gastro-Intestinal (GI) cancer" indicates a group of tumors that affect the digestive system. Despite progress in treatment, these widespread types of malignant condition represent a serious health problem in the world. GI cancer is a multi-factorial and multi-stage involved disorder, its progression is influenced by environmental and genetic elements and the involvement of microbial population has also recently been recognized in many studies. Today, Next Generation Sequencing (NGS) approach has been used to elucidate the involvement of microorganisms in initiating and facilitating the process of GI cancer. In this chapter, we would like to clarify the role played by the gastrointestinal microflora in the genesis of GI cancers. This chapter will draw the state of the art in the study of the GI microbiota and how the dysbiosis could affect oncogenesis, tumor progression and response to cancer.

Keywords: Cytokines, Dysbiosis, Gastro-Intestinal cancer, Gut microbiota, *Helicobacter pylori*, Immune system, Next Generation Sequencing.

1. INTRODUCTION

Gastrointestinal (GI) cancers are malignant conditions of the GI tract and accessory organs of digestion, such as esophagus, biliary system stomach, small intestine, large intestine, rectum, pancreas and anus. The symptoms can include obstruction, abnormal bleeding and different associated problems. Despite several progress in treatment, GI is one of the most common form of cancer and represents an important health problem in all the world. As of 2012, esophageal cancer is the eighth most common cancer, affecting 450,000 people worldwide [1]. Gastric cancer (GC) represents the fourth most common tumor with 1,000,000 new cases per year and 850,000 deaths [2, 3], but, GC prevalence is constantly decreasing; a possible cause could be the decrease of the *H. pylori* (HP) diffusion, a bacterium involved in the GC pathogenesis [4]. Neoplasms of the small intes-

[*] **Corresponding Authors Amedeo Amedei:** Department of Experimental and Clinical Medicine, Viale Pieraccini 6, University of Florence, Florence, Italy; Tel +39 055 2758330; Fax: +39 055 2758330; E-mail amedeo.amedei@unifi.it

Atta-ur-Rahman & M. Iqbal Choudhary (Eds.)

tine are rare, indeed the global incidence ranges from 0.3 to 2.0 per 100,000 [5]. While the Colorectal cancer (CRC) is the third most frequent tumor worldwide and the fourth most common reason of cancer death, with about 500,000 deaths per year [3]. The multi-steps mechanisms associated with GI cancer prevention and development are still largely unknown. GI cancers are considered to be a multi-factorial disease resulting from intricate relationships between genetics, epigenetics, immunity, environment (including geographical area and socioeconomic status), lifestyle and diet; all this factors could impact the GI microflora, altering its profiles and its functions during the tumor genesis and growth [4]. In healthy individuals, GI microflora acts as a symbiont offering protection from invading pathogens and preventing carcinogenesis [6]. When the fine balance of this commensal bacterial community is disrupted, the establishment of a dysbiosis state could cause pathological conditions in the host, including cancer [7, 8].

In 400 B.C, the words of Hippocrates (one of the most outstanding figures in the history of medicine) "Death sits in the bowels" [9], showed that the involvement of the intestinal metabolism in human health has been long acknowledged. In the past, most researches on the impact of bacteria colonization in the gut have been focused on gastrointestinal pathogens. While recent evidences still corroborate individual microorganisms influencing tumor genesis (*e.g.*, human papilloma virus the cervical cancer, hepatitis B and C virus the hepatocellular carcinoma, *Helicobacter pylori* the gastric cancer) [10, 11] also microbial dysbiosis could have a large impact in malignant promotion and progression.

In this chapter, we would like to revisit the state of the art of microbiota influence in the genesis of GI cancers, discussing how disequilibria (dysbiosis) could influence the mutual relationship between the host and intestinal bacteria affecting oncogenesis, tumor progression and response to cancer treatment. We will present challenging questions to be addressed in the future of microbiota research, such as how the gut microbiota may be manipulated for therapeutic strategies.

2. THE HUMAN MICROBIOTA

In the past, the human body has been considered as a self-sustaining organism that can control all of its metabolic reactions. Today, scientists have shown that the human body indeed is an ecosystem containing trillions of microorganisms. The communities of microorganisms living in coexistence with their hosts has been referred as **microbiota,** microflora or normal flora.

The human microbiota could contain approximately 1,014 bacteria, a number that is 10 times greater than the amount of the total human cells in the body. The microflora is resident in every surface of the body exposed to the external environment such as skin and mucosa (from the GI, to respiratory and urogenital tract). The gastrointestinal tract (GIT) is the organ that contains the larger fraction of bacteria producing molecules that can be used as nutrients, making it a preferred site for colonization; indeed the colon contains over 70% of all the bacteria in the body. This human GIT ecosystem results from an evolutionary process of co-existence between the microflora and the body. The microbiota significantly influences physiological functions such as food digestion and immune system stimulation [12].

The human microbiota includes microorganisms belonging to the domains of the Archaea, Bacteria, Eukarya and their viruses. The majority of bacteria are strict anaerobes, which predominate the facultative anaerobes and aerobes. The commensal bacteria are symbiotic, but they can cause a pathological state after translocation through the mucosa or in specific conditions such as immunodeficiency. In general, the composition of the human microbiota is strictly personal, but the diversity in the structure of the bacterial population among the body sites is greater than it is between individuals. This state indicates that the human microbiota is a highly variable ecosystem that embraces different microbiological components [13, 14]. It is possible to term a bacterial community "core" of a healthy microbiota that is commonly present within different body sites.

To date, although there have been over 50 bacterial phyla described, only 2 of them dominates the human gut normal flora: the *Bacteroidetes* and the *Firmicutes,* whereas *Actinobacteria, Proteobacteria, Fusobacteria*, *Verruco-microbia* and *Cyanobacteria* appear in minor proportion [15]. Estimates of the amount of bacterial species present in the human intestine vary extensively between different studies, but it has been widely accepted that it contains 500 to 1,000 species. A recent study involving multiple subjects has suggested that the total human gut microbiota is composed of over 35,000 bacterial species [16]. Interestingly, a wide proportion, about 70%, of the human microbiota is com-posed of microbes that cannot be cultivated by common microbiological methods. The traditional culture-based methods capture less than 30%, of our bacterial microflora [17]. Today, genomic Next-Generation Sequencing (NGS) analysis has been crucial to analyze the bacterial microbiota profile and the metagenome, and also these techniques give more information about the impact of microflora in host metabolic reaction, cancer progression and inflammation [18, 19].

3. THE GASTROINTESTINAL MICROBIOTA

3.1. Composition and Activities

The human digestive system is composed of distinct regions with different functions: the oral cavity, stomach, small intestine and colon. The intestinal mucosa is the largest surface of the body that is regularly exposed to bacterial and dietary antigens. The bacterial phyla present on Earth are more than 50, but the most common human gut-associated microbiota is composed of four phyla: *Firmicutes, 30.6-83% (Ruminococcus, Clostridium, Peptococcus, Eubacterium, Dorea, Lactobacillus - L, Peptostreptococcus); Bacteroidetes, 8-48% (Bacteroides); Actinobacteria, 0.7-16.7% (Bifidobacterium - BF)* and *Proteobacteria, 0.1-26.6% (Enterobacteriacee)* [15, 20].

But the intestinal microbiota organization is not homogeneous. In the human GIT, the content of bacteria increases from mouth (less than 200 species) to the colon (bacteria reaching 1010-1012/gram of luminal content, with a predominance of anaerobe bacteria) [21]. Notably, the proportion of bacterial cells resident in the mammalian gut goes from 101 to 103 bacteria x gram (g) of contents in the stomach and duodenum, progressing to 104 to 107 bacteria x g in the jejunum and ileum and ending in 1011 to 1012 cells x g in the colon [22]. Furthermore, the bacterial structure changes between these GIT sites. Various microbial strains are enriched at different sections when comparing biopsy samples of the small intestine and colon from healthy controls. *Bacilli* class of the *Firmicutes* and *Actinobacteria* are increased in the specimens of the small intestine. On the contrary, *Bacteroidetes* and the *Lachnospiraceae* families of the *Firmicutes* were more dominant in colonic samples [16]. A thick mucus layer divides the intestinal epithelium from the lumen leading to a great latitudinal heterogeneity in the bacterial composition. The microbiota assemblage of the intestinal lumen is significantly different from the microbiota embedded in this mucus layer as well as the bacterial population resident in the immediacy of the epithelium. Several bacterial strains resident in the intestinal lumen did not access the mucus layer and epithelial crypts. *Streptococcus, Bacteroides, Bifidobacterium,* members of *Enterobacteriacea, Enterococcus, Clostridium, Lactobacillus* and *Ruminococcus* were all detected in feces, whereas only *Clostridium, Lactobacillus* and *Enterococcus* were observed in the mucus layer and epithelial crypts of the small intestine [23]. Different factors could contribute to the diversifications along the length of the GI tract such as bacterial factors (enzymes, metabolic activity, adhesion capacity), host elements (bile acids, mucus pH, digestive enzymes, transit time,) and non-host aspects (medication, nutrients, environmental factors) [24].

Due to the abundance of nutrients, the human oral cavity represents the ideal habitat for microorganisms. At least six billion microorganisms take place in mouth belonging to the *Bacteroidetes (e.g. Bacteroides, Prevotella), Firmicutes* (Gram positive; *e.g., Clostridia, Bacilli,*), *Proteobacteria* (Gram negative, *e.g., Salmonella, Escherichia, Helicobacter* and *Yersinia*), *Fusobacteria* (Gram negative, *e.g., Fusobacterium*) and *Actinobacteria* (Gram positive, *e.g.,*

Streptomyces, Actinomyces) [25]. The gastric microbiota is composed mostly of *Actinobacteria* but, due to the acidic environment, *Helicobacter* (*e.g., H. pylori*) is also present [26]. The small intestine microbiota has a qualitative composition similar to the colon microbiota, but the latter contains a higher number of microorganisms. The small intestine hosts few bacteria in its proximal part, the microbiota is composed of Gram+ *Lactobacillus* and *Enterococcus faecalis*. More microorganisms occur in the distal part, *e.g., Bacteroides* and coliforms. In the colon quantitatively *Firmicutes* and *Bacteroidetes* were dominant and, at the genus level, anaerobic lactic acid bacteria, *e.g., Bifidobacterium bifidum* and anaerobic *Bacteroides*, prevailed [25].

The GI microbiota is crucial to the physiology of the human body, as it could produce molecules able to interact with the host and performs important metabolic functions. In particular, the bacteria of the gut microbiota act as a first defense against pathogen colonization and they break down indigestible dietary components [27], promote angiogenesis, support fat metabolism, synthesize vitamins, help the development of the immune system and maintain homeostasis [28]. The bacteria population is separated from the internal gut milieu by a layer of epithelial cells, which is a physical and chemical barrier that balances the crosstalk between the immune host system and the external environment. Moreover, the epithelial surfaces have evolved mechanisms to counteract the microorganism invasion. Adaptive and innate immune responses protect the mucosa and the internal environment of the human body. Almost 80% of the immunological cells are active in the mucosal-associated immune system, most of these cells are resident in the GI tract, where the level of immunogenic components of the food and the bacterial flora is at the highest respect to other districts of the body.

Usually the bacterial flora does not cause a proinflammatory response because the immune system tolerates the commensal bacteria and preserve the homeostasis but, when these mechanisms are impaired (*e.g.* use of antibiotics, immuno-deficiency and unhealthy diets) or new pathogenic bacteria are introduced into this balanced system, the immune system reacts to the microbiota triggering a pathological state, facilitating inflammation and cancer progression in the intestine [29]. Different studies suggest that an imbalance of the gut microbiota and its metabolic functions are correlated with the initiating and progression of GI pathologies, including colorectal cancer, functional dyspepsia, severe diarrhea, inflammatory bowel disease (IBD), celiac disease and irritable bowel syndrome IBS [30, 31]. It is now understood that the imbalance of gut microbial population (dysbiosis) can be activated by intrinsic (*e.g.*, stress, genetics and aging) and extrinsic factors (*e.g.*, appendectomy, diet and antibiotic use).

3.2. Gastro-Intestinal Colonization by the Microbiota and Selection

The microbiota composition is more plastic and variable than the human genome and also more readily changeable and reactive to stimuli than most human cells. The human superorganism is composed of two constituents: 1) inheritable human gene pool, surrounded by 2) evolvable and changeable bacteria gene pool, acquired after birth, whose composition varies with time, space, health and hormonal state.

Indeed, microbial colonization of the newborns commences at moment of the birth during the passage through the birth canal and is affected by the delivery mode [32]. The bacterial settling during birth impacts the development of the gut normal flora. The intestinal microbiota of infants and the mother vaginal microbiota show some similarities such as an example they are both enriched in *Prevotella, Lactobacillus or Sneathia spp* [33]. On the contrary, infants delivered through cesarean section exhibited different bacteria compositions compared with vaginally delivered newborns [34].

During the first twelvemonth of life, the microbiota structure of the infant's gut is simple and varies between different individuals and with time [35, 36] but, after 1 year of age, it looks like to young adult gut microbial assemblage [33, 35]. Experiments in mouse showed that the gut microbiota of offspring is similar to that of their mothers [36]. Other studies revealed that gut microbiota of adult monozygotic and dizygotic twins were equally similar to that of their siblings, this data suggests that the gut colonization by the microbiota from the same mother had a key role in determining the adult bacteria community composition [37]. Several other factors, as host genetics, have been found to impact the gut microbial structure. For instance, experiments in mouse revealed that the gut bacteria composition is altered in genetically obese mice *vs* genetically lean siblings [36]. Moreover, a mutation in the major component of the high density lipoprotein (apolipoprotein a-I) in mouse is associated to an altered gut bacteria assemblage [38]. Other studies in obese mouse showed the consumption of western diet can alter the gut microbiota profile [39]. Further limiting weight gain with dietary manipulations could reverse the effects of diet-induced obesity on the microbiota of murine gut.

3.3. The Human Microbiome Project

The microbial composition of a specific ecosystem and its function has been studied by several international consortium researchers such as the Human Microbiome Project (HMP; www.hmpdacc.org), launched in October 2007 by the National Institutes of Health. HMP is a global project that brought together a big number of scientists to different specific aims:

1. Characterize the microorganism communities of the major human districts (skin, mouth, nose, colon and vagina)
2. Study the functional and metabolic pathways of microbial communities
3. Determine their functional roles in health and disease

This consortium published over 350 papers [40 - 42]. The HMP estimates that the human microbiota contains between 3,500 and 35,000 Operational Taxonomic Units (OTUs). An OTU is a cluster of organisms grouped on the basis of the sequence similarity [41]. In addition, the consortium HMP discovered novel taxa at the genus level, including the *Dorea, Oscillibacter* and *Desulfovibrio* genera, which correlated with disease conditions [41, 43, 44]. Furthermore, the HMP has supported the development of new technological and Bioinformatics tools to be used in metagenomic studies [45].

3.4. Gut Enterotypes

In 2011, Arumugam *et al.* [46] identified three distinct enterotypes of the human gut microbiota (Table **1**). These enterotypes vary in functional composition, species and enzyme balance. Enterotype 1 produces enzymes associated with the biotin biosynthesis pathway, while Enterotype 2 and 3 produce those which are connected with the thiamine and heme biosynthesis pathways, respectively [42, 46]. Also, long-term diets correlated with enterotypes [47], indeed, food rich in protein and fat was associated with the *Bacteroides* enterotype, while food rich in carbohydrate and simple sugars was associated with the *Prevotella* enterotype. *Ruminococcus* enterotype did not correlate with feeding [47].

Table 1. Phylogenetic and functional variation between the three suggested human enterotypes.

	Phylogenetic Variation		Functional Variation	
	Main Contribution	**Co-occurring Genus**	**Energy Generation**	**Overrepresented Vitamin**
Enterotype 1	*Bacteroides*	*Parabacteroides*	Fermentation of carbohydrates and proteins	Biotin (vitamin B7)
Enterotype 2	*Prevotella*	*Desulfovibrio*	Degradation of mucin glycoproteins in mucosal layer	Thiamine (vitamin B1)
Enterotype 3	*Ruminococcus Clostridiales*	*Akkermansia*	Degradation of mucin	Heme (involved in vitamin B12 biosynthesis)

4. THE ROLE OF MICROBIOTA IN TUMOR DEVELOPMENT

The involvement of infectious elements in the cancer etiology has recently attracted the research attention. In 1890, the Scottish pathologist William Russell [48] reported evidence for a bacterial cause of cancer. Currently, different data have strengthened this theory suggesting a bacterial involvement in the genesis and cancer progression (often interfering with and modulating the local immune response) [49].

As previously reported, recent studies suggest that not only a single bacteria, but also global changes in the host microbiota could cause human disease [50, 51]. Different studies in germfree animals report a tumor promoting effects of the microbial community in genetically induced and spontaneous cancers as breast, lungs, skin, liver and colon tumors [52 - 54]. But, there are also conflicting data showing a central role of the gut microbiota in reducing proliferative responses that lead to cancer development in germfree animals [55].

In 1975, Reddy and colleagues for the first time, linked the gut microbiota to intestinal cancer development, establishing that only 20% of genetically modified germfree rodents develops chemically induced CRC. In contrast, the tumor incidence in rats with a normal microbiota was about 90% with several neoplasms [56]. Vannucci and colleagues confirmed these data showing that germfree rats, compared with similar animals with a normal microbiota, develop smaller tumors, as spontaneously as after chemically induced carcinogenesis [57]. In colitis-associated cancer and adenomatous polyposis coli (APC)-related colorectal cancer, germfree mice display decreased tumor formation and less oncogenic mutations [58]. In addition, antibiotics depletion of the gut microbiota in mice limits cancer growth in the colon and the liver [59 - 62] as does the eradication of specific pathogens in humans and in mice [63, 64]. All these data provide strong evidence for the microbiota role in tumor initiating and growth. Probably, the germfree rats can develop a more active anticancer immune response in the absence of the physiological inflammation induced by the gut commensal community.

4.1. Proposed Models for Microbiota-induced Carcinogenesis

Currently, researchers have proposed three mechanisms of microbiota-induced carcinogenesis:

A. The unbalanced proinflammatory signaling at the intestinal level induces an increased repair of the intestinal epithelium that can result in the tumor development
B. Some microbial species can have direct cytotoxic effects on intestinal cells.

C. Particular members of the microbiota can generate by-products that are toxic to the intestinal surface.

To better understand the microbiota's contribution in tumor growth, different "hypothesis models" have been proposed:

1. The '*alpha bugs*' (microbiota members possessing unique virulence traits) are both directly pro-oncogenic bacteria able to remold the mucosal immune response and bacteria species that protect against cancer [65]. An example of "alpha bugs" is enterotoxigenic *Bacteroides fragilis (ETBF)*,

2. The '*bacterial driver-passenger*' model describes the microbiota influence in the development of CRC. The 'driver bacteria' (indigenous intestinal bacteria), initiate the first phases of tumor progression, inducing DNA injury and driving genome instability. As a consequence of this process, the bacterial drivers (such as alpha bugs) are replaced by commensals bacteria with either tumor-promoting or tumor-suppressing properties (bacterial passengers). According to the "driver-passenger" model, the disease progression causes changes in the microenvironment resulting in a different selective pressure on the microbial population [66].

3. The '*keystone pathogen*' hypothesis. The term 'keystone' (firstly used in the ecological studies) refers to species whose effects on their communities are excessively large relative to their abundance and which are thought to form the 'keystone' of the community's structure. According to this model, some low-abundance bacterial pathogens can induce inflammatory disease by shaping a normal microbiota into a dysbiotic one [67].

Finally, inflammatory responses triggered by microbiota is able to enhance tumor progression [68]. Some microbes produce variations of mucosal permeability, inducing bacterial translocation. Different studies demonstrated the role of inflammation in creating the conditions that could change local immune responses and tissue balance. Moreover, it is well documented that the inflammatory molecules, such as TNF-α, interleukin (IL)-1), IL-8, nitric oxide, prostaglandin-2 derivatives are involved in the interplay between the immune and tissue cells undergoing transformation [69].

4.2. Antibacteria-Specific Immune Response and Cancer Promotion

As previously reported, the bacterial population is divided from the internal gut milieu by a stratum of epithelial cells, which acts as chemical and physical barrier and regulates the crosstalk between the immune host system and the external environment. This epithelial surface evolved protective mechanisms to counteract bacteria invasion. Adaptive and innate immune responses protect the mucosa and the internal environment of the human body. The normal microbiota (in eubiosis condition) does not trigger a proinflammatory reaction because commensal bacteria are usually tolerate by the immune system, but when these mechanisms are impaired, they could cause tumor development and progression [29]. So, the inflammatory and host-derived immune responses are essential actors that shape the gut microbial profile and may contribute to the dysbiosis state. Several studies demonstrated that IBD patients have an increased risk of CRC because inflammation-promoted cancerogenesis also plays an important role in CRC development [70]. Furthermore, gut microbiota has also been shown to have an impact on colitis-associated CRC progression. IL-10/ mice develop spontaneous colitis when colonized with gut microflora, but after exposure to a strong carcinogen, mice showed a very high incidence of CRC [71]. On the contrary, the contact to a carcinogen of GF IL-10/ mice did not cause a malignant neoplasia, whereas IL-10/mice mono-associated with a mildly colitogenic bacterium had a reduced incidence of CRC following exposure to a carcinogen, compared with mice colonized by the normal gut microbiota.

One of the main avenues by which the microbiota can indirectly promote tumor growth are the Th (helper) 17 cells. The bacterial flora actively shape intestinal T-cell responses to establish homeostasis. Th17 cells control microbial invasion in the gut, but specific compensatory mechanisms are required to regulate the Th17 cells. At intestinal level, the bacteria induce IL-1β production to maintain a basal level of Th17 cells in the lamina propria under physiological conditions [72], but in response to pathogenic extracellular bacterial or fungal infections, strong numbers of naive Th cells differentiate into Th17 under the influence of IL-1β, IL-6, IL-23 or TGFβ in mucosal surfaces of the intestine and respiratory tract [73]. If those mechanisms are impaired, Th17 cells become pathogenic and can induce autoimmune disease and chronic inflammation. When stimulated with IL-6 and TGF-β, the antigen-activated CD4+ T cells upregulate the transcription factor RORγt (retinoic acid receptor related orphan receptor gamma t) and secrete Th17-specific cytokines such as IL-17 and IL-22 [74]. Usually, the CD4+ T cells that express RORγt increase tight junction formation and stimulate the secretion of microbicide proteins, contributing to the barrier function of the intestinal epithelium but they can have also a protumorigenic role [74]. The functional Th17 impact in cancer is still equivocal, showing both protumorigenic and antitumorigenic activities in different cancer type [75 - 77].

Furthermore, Th17 cells can secrete IL-21, IL-17F, IL-22, granulocyte-macrophage colony-stimulating factor (GM-CSF) and interferon (IFN)-γ [78, 79]. Th17 responses and mainly the IL-17 action itself, were originally considered as a cancer growth promoters [80]. In a mouse model, Wu *et al*. demonstrate that the Th17 cells are able to promote CRC progression, induced by colon inflammation [81]. In experiments with genetically predisposed mice (APCmin/+) crossed with

IL-17A-deficient mice a drastic impairment in intestinal tumorigenesis was observed [82]. Moreover, different studies revealed that APCmin/+ mice that cannot respond to IL-17 develop fewer tumors in the colon [75].

The function of Th17 cells has been investigated in patients with different tumor types, including prostate and ovarian cancer [83 - 86]. These studies have examined Th17 cells in peripheral blood, but it is important to notice that Th17 cells may be induced in or recruited in the cancer microenvironment [87]. A more direct proof for a microbiota role in stimulating tumor growth *via* Th17 cells comes from studies of enterotoxigenic *Bacteroides fragilis (B. fragilis)*, a colonic bacterium that produces *B. fragilis* toxin (BFT). Several mouse models, predisposed to develop gut tumors, indicate that between colonization of *B. fragilis* and nontoxigenic *B. fragilis*, only the first causes colitis and produces colonic tumors [81]. Notably, *B. fragilis* induces STAT3 activation with colitis characterized by a selective Th17 response. Antibody-mediated blockade of IL-17, inhibits *B. fragilis* induced colitis, tumor formation and colonic hyperplasia. These data show that also a common human commensal bacterium could induce cancer by STAT3- and Th17-dependent pathway of inflammation, providing a new insight into CRC development.

Moreover, the Th17 response upon contact with specific microbes, stimulates neutrophil cells, required for the clearance of invading bacteria [88]. The Th17 response is important for protection against mucosal pathogens like *Klebsiella pneumonia* and *Salmonella typhimurium*. Deficient Th17 mice models show a pathological condition during infection with *Salmonella* or *C. rodentium*, with increased translocation of bacteria into lymph nodes [89]. Th17 are also activated by the segmented filamentous bacteria (SFB), belonging to nonculturable *Clostridia*-related species and flagellin-positive bacteria. These bacteria interact with the epithelial cells promoting chronic inflammation, mediated by IL-17 and IL-22 release, which favors intestinal cancer. In addition, the IL-22 has been linked to intestinal tumor in mouse models triggered by STAT3 activation and also human pancreatic cancer [90, 91]. Moreover, the conjunction of IL-22 with IFN-γ can activate inducible nitric oxide synthase (iNOS) production and procarcinogenic nitric oxygen species in human CRC cell lines [92]. Finally, the cytokine IL-23 is produced by myeloid cells in response to different bacteria molecules, such as flagellin [93]. IL-23 (able to promote Th17- type response) was increased in human colon adenocarcinoma, it promotes cancer growth through a proinflammatory response [94].

5. MICROBIOTA AND GI CANCERS

5.1. Gut Bacteria Dysbiosis Associated with GI Cancer

Dysbiosis (also called dysbacteriosis) is a term for a microbial imbalance or maladaptation on or inside the body, such as an impaired bacterial composition. It can be caused not only by pathogenic organisms and passenger commensals, but also by aging and environmental factors such as antibiotics, xenobiotics, smoking, hormones and dietary cues [29]. Of note, these are also well-established risk factors for the development of intestinal or extraintestinal neoplasms. In addition, genetic defects that affect epithelial, myeloid or lymphoid components of the intestinal immune system could favor dysbiosis because they promote inflammatory states, such as Crohn's disease, that increase the host risk of neoplastic conversion [95].

So, several factors that facilitate carcinogenesis also promote dysbiosis. Epidemiological studies linking intra-abdominal infections, antibiotic administration or both to an increased incidence of CRC [96] underscore the clinical importance of the association between dysbiosis and intestinal carcinogenesis. Abrogating or specifically altering the assemblage of the gut microbiota impacts the incidence and progression of CRC in both genetic and carcinogen-induced models of tumorigenesis [55, 97]. Moreover, several products of the gut microbiota directly target intestinal epithelial cells (IECs) and either mediate oncogenic effects (as reported for hydrogen sulfide and the *Bacteroides fragilis* toxin) or suppress tumorigenesis (as demonstrated for short-chain fatty acids, SCFA) [98].

Intestinal bugs participate in more than just colorectal carcinogenesis. Experimental alterations of the gut microbiota also influence the incidence and progression of extraintestinal cancers, including breast and hepatocellular carcinoma, presumably through inflammatory and metabolic circuitries [52, 60]. These results are compatible with the findings of epidemiological data that reveal an association between dysbiosis, its consequences or determinants (in particular the overuse of antibiotics) and an increased incidence of extracolonic neoplasms, including breast carcinoma [99, 100]. These evidences may reflect the systemic distribution of bacteria and their by-products in the course of inflammatory responses that compromise the integrity of the intestinal barrier [60]. The gut microbiota influences oncogenesis and tumor progression both locally and systemically. Although inflammatory and metabolic indications support this phenomenon, additional, uncharacterized mechanisms can contribute to the ability of dysbiosis to promote carcinogenesis (Fig. 1).

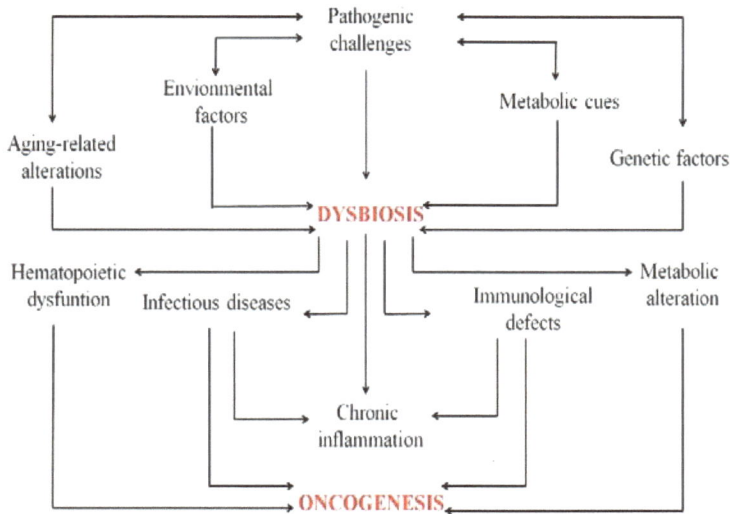

Fig. (1). Mechanisms by which dysbiosis affects oncogenesis.

5.2. Microbiota Involvement in Gastric and Esophageal Cancers, the Role of *Helicobacter pylori*

The esophagus is an organ through which food transits, aided by peristaltic contractions, from the pharynx to the stomach. The esophagus is divided into three main sections - the upper, middle and lower. Tumor can develop anywhere along the esophagus length. The mucus produced by glands in the wall of the esophagus help food slide down. The most widespread type of cancer seen in Western countries is esophagus adenocarcinoma generated by these glands.

During the past 3 decades, the amount of adenocarcinomas of distal esophagus and the gastroesophageal junction has been increasing. This data is attributed to smoking, gastroesophageal reflux and alcohol consumption [101]. On the contrary, *H. pylori* infection seems to be protective to distal esophageal cancer, leading to loss of acid secretion, hormonal deregulation or cytokine and changes in microflora composition [102, 103]. A recent Chinese research demonstrated that individuals with lower oral microbial diversity were more likely to have squamous dysplasia in the esophagus and chronic atrophic gastritis [104]. In the same study, the authors also found a correlation between esophageal squamous dysplasia with the odds ratio being significantly decreased with increasing bacterial richness. Another research performed in Northern Iran (considered part of the "esophageal cancer belt") evaluated the gastric microflora from the gastric mucosa in patients with esophageal squamous cell carcinoma [105]. An enrichment of *Erysipelotrichales* and *Clostridiales* species, belonging to the phylum *Firmicutes*, was found. These species were significantly related to early squamous dysplasia and esophageal squamous cell cancer.

Most stomach cancers develop slowly in cells that line the mucosa and are called adenocarcinoma of the stomach. As the microbiota come in close contact with gastric and esophageal linings, current studies support its influences in oncogenesis. The most important example of a cancer induced by bacteria is the *Helicobacter pylori*-mediated gastric carcinoma [106]. This bacterium takes part of the gastric microbiota [106] and its presence induces a continuous activation immune response in the human host, resulting in inflammation of stomach mucosa that leads to cancer transformations at the gastric epithelium. Different hypothesis have been suggested by which *H. pylori* influences GC development.

A. Murine models of *H. pylori* infection (infected with *H. felis*, the homologous of *H. pylori* in mouse) have shown that induction of a T cell-mediated response [107] and a Th1 cytokine environment [108] are crucial to the development of the bacterium induced pathology.
B. *H. pylori* could influence the production of reactive nitrogen compounds at the gastric mucosa [109], which could induce carcinogenic DNA damage [110].
C. *H. pylori* could affect regulators of DNA transcription [111]. *Helicobacter pylori* infection increases cell proliferation which could lead to a higher frequency of mutation and less time for DNA repair [112].

Mice deficient in secretory phospholipase A2 (sPLA2), showed increased apoptosis levels after infection with *H. felis* in mouth and the growth of aberrant gastric mucosa cell lineages [113]. Cell cycle and apoptosis are regulated by Raf-kinase inhibitor protein (RKIP) in the gastric mucosa. In infected mucosa, *H. pylori* phosphorylates RKIP, eliminating apoptotic control and increasing cell proliferation [114]. Another tumor suppressor gene, LOX, was shown to be methylated in mice infected by *H. felis* [115]. Notably, *H. pylori* derived from distinct stages of tumor progression in the same human subject, one during the chronic atrophic gastritis and the second following cancer transformation, showed different interaction with gastric epithelial stem cells [116]. Mongolian gerbils, whose gastric system is close to humans showed that 37% of animals infected by *H. pylori* developed cancer, on the contrary uninfected controls showed no tumor development [112]. A recent study suggests that long-term *H. pylori* infection disrupts the gut microbiota balance [117]. Lactobacillus species decrease *H. pylori* growth *in vitro*, suggesting a prevention of *H. pylori* infection [118].

Human studies, comparing gastric microbiota composition in cancer patients *versus* healthy subjects, indicate that also other microbes must be present to trigger the progression from healthy mucosa toward tumor development [119,

120]. Notably, there are many people *H. pylori* positive that do not develop gastric cancer [121]. GC patients showed low levels of *Porphyromonas, Meisseria* and *Streptococcus sinensis* while *Lactobacillus coleohominis, Pseudomonas* and *Lachnospiraceae* were increased [122]. *L. coleohominis* is a species initially reported to be beneficial in the gastric environment, a study showed the increase of *Lactobacilli* terminal restriction fragments (TRFs) in gastric cancer subjects, supporting the increase in the abundance of these bacteria [120].

H. pylori-associated carcinoma is one of the most preventable cancers because *H. pylori* eradication resolves the gastric inflammation and has been shown to decrease GC incidence [120]. In mice, the eradication of *Helicobacter felis*, produce a decrease in the methylation of the LOX tumor suppressor gene [115]. *H. pylori* infection was also linked with junctional tumors, those involving the esophagus and gastric cardia [121, 122]. More is known about the microbiota in precursor states to esophageal cancer like reflux esophagitis and Barrett metaplasia. In these conditions the dysbiosis plays a key role in the cancer development, indeed a shift from Gram+ bacteria to mostly Gram- has been shown [121]. Other microbes as *Streptococcus mitis*, *Treponema denticola* and *Streptococcus anginosus* induce inflammation by cytokines, possibly supporting tumor progression [119, 123].

5.3. Microbiota Involvement in Colorectal Cancer

Colorectal cancer (CRC), also referred as bowel cancer, is the third most common cancer and the fourth leading cause of cancer deaths worldwide [120]. Most bowel cancers develop from polyps in the colon or rectum but not all polyps become cancerous. Colorectal carcinogenesis is not fully understood, but it is thought to be a heterogeneous process with genetic and epigenetic alterations, influenced by diet, environment, host immunity and microbial exposures [123 - 125]. A large number of microbes is able to live in the human gut, forming complex communities which may play key roles in the CRC development [126, 127]. Interestingly, the high microbial density in the colon (*1012 cells/mL) compared to the small intestine (*102 cells/mL) is related with a *12-fold increase in tumor occurrence [128]. Furthermore, patients affected by IBD, who are more exposed to microbes because of the reduced intestinal barrier, have a*5-fold increased risk for CRC due to the abnormal inflammatory reaction to commensal bacteria [129]. Previous studies have suggested a potential dysbiosis of gut microbiota in CRC patients [130] and many other studies have been conducted to assess the possible pathogens involved in CRC progression [120]. Once they are identified, it would lead to a breakthrough in the prevention and CRC treatment, in particular for sporadic CRC that represents 85-90% of all CRC and that will be addressed in this topic. Currently, many evidences show that colonic microbiota is involved in tumorigenesis and its structure and characteristics are altered in CRC precancerous lesions [131]. However, it cannot be always clearly understood whether these variations are causally related to cancer progression or are a consequence of tumor-induced changes [132, 133].

In general, the gut microbiota could contribute to the CRC genesis *via* altered composition of its components (dysbiosis) [134], changes in the local abundance of bacteria population, harmful properties of some bacteria and change in bacterial metabolic activity [127, 132]. Many causes can influence the GI ecosystem, including physical and psychological stress, antibiotics, radiations, modified peristalsis, diet, *etc.* [9, 133].

The involvement of gut microbiota is firstly supported by the demonstration of the cytotoxicity/genotoxicity of the microflora in CRC by using fecal extracts from healthy controls (fecal water) [132]. Fecal water cytotoxicity determines mucosal cell proliferation [135, 136], possibly through secondary bile acids and produces DNA damage (genotoxicity) [137], proving that carcinogens exist in the colonic lumen. Genotoxicity has been significantly associated with fecal water from people following a diet high in fats and meat, but low in fibers (considered to be of high-risk for CRC), as compared to a diet low in fats and meat [136].

Other strong supporting data comes from mice studies: in germfree conditions, colitis and cancer genesis are significantly decreased or do not appear, compared with wild type mice [138]. *Clostridium butyricum*, *Mitsuokella multiacida* or *BF longum* have been associated with higher prevalence of colonic adenoma (68% in each case) in mice, as compared with *L acidophilus* (30%) [139, 140]. In addition, the tumor free germfree rats exhibit increased cytotoxic T lymphocytes, natural killer and B cells in peripheral blood, suggesting a better anticancer immune response. Azoxymethane-treated interleukin (IL)-10-/- mice develop colitis-associated CRC when infected with *Bacteroides vulgatus*, whereas germ-free mice do not [71]. Previous studies have indicated that different microbial species preferentially populate the cancer sites [141, 142] and the structure of gut microbiota is altered also in CRC patients [143, 144], an increase in the diversity of *Clostridium* spp. [144], as well as an enrichment of *Bifidobacterium* spp and *Bacteroides* has been observed. On the contrary, the gut microbiota composition in a group of patients at low risk for CRC progression was shown to be increased in *Eubacterium aerofaciens* and *Lactobacillus* spp, producing lactic acid [144]. Interestingly, recent data revealed that *Bacteroides fragilis*, *Bacteroides uniformis* and *Bacteroides vulgatus* were enriched in CRC patients. The genera *Escherichia/Shigella*, *Enterococcus*, *Streptococcus*, *Klebsiella* and *Peptostreptococcus* were increased in CRC patients, while the genus *Roseburia* and the family *Lachnospiraceae* were less abundant [145]. *Streptococcus bovis/gallolyticus* antigen profiles allowed the distinction between healthy controls and CRC patients [146] and were detected also in polyposis patients, indicating that the infection occurs in the first stages of carcinogenesis [147]. The gut microflora composition of patients with polyposis (which anticipate the carcinoma progression) was also altered *vs* healthy controls, but similar to the population detected in the CRC.

So these data suggest that the variation of gut microflora population paves the way to the onset of carcinogenesis, but it is still not clear if the aberrant microbiota drives the malignant progression or host and diet factors promote concurrent microflora alterations in the colonic environment.

Analyses of CRC colonic mucosa-associated microbiota have shown lower counts of total BF, especially *Bifidobacterium longum* than those with diverticulitis [148]. In contrast with fecal results [149], the composition of the mucosa-associated microbiota in adenoma patients showed significantly increased abundance of *Proteobacteria, Faecalibacterium* spp, *Dorea* spp. and decreased levels of *Bacteroidetes, Coprococcus* spp *and Bacteroides* spp. *vs* controls [150]. In addition, the mucosal district of colon adenoma had a 20-fold relative reduction of mucosa-adherent microbes compared with healthy tissue [151].

Gut microbiota influence CRC course also through interaction with the inflammatory process in the colon mucosa [152]. As previously reported, the chemically induced cell proliferation due to dextran sulfate sodium (DSS) and azoxymethane (AOM) was increased in germfree mice, which lack of protective commensal bacteria. Notably, compared to pathogen free mice, tumor development in germfree mice leads to more and larger neoplasia [55]. An inflammatory milieu in the host could disrupt the eubiosis status, indeed host inflammation could modulate microflora composition through production of particular metabolites such as nitrate, that acts as a single energy source for facultative anaerobic microbes. These conditions allow them to outcompete microbial species that cannot employ nitrates [153], disrupting eubiosis and so, promoting dysbiosis.

Pro-inflammatory host responses can also prejudice immune function and barrier to permit microbial translocation through the tight junctions of the gut and intensify the inflammatory process [154]. Several hypothetical mechanisms are suggested to explain the mutual interplay between inflammation and gut microbiota in CRC initiating and progression: 1) accordingly to the 'alpha-bug' hypothesis (previously described), keystone pathogen bacteria, such as ETBF, shape gut microflora *via* Th17and IL-17 cell-mediated inflammation. This process may be obstructed by beneficial commensal bacteria [67]. 2) the bacterial driver-passenger model proposes that 'driver' bacteria, such as ETBF, induce or exacerbate inflammation and generate genotoxins that lead to cell mutations and proliferation. In a second step, 'passenger' bacteria, such as *Fusobacterium* spp. Colonize the adenoma supporting malignant progression [66]. Following cancer generation, the gut barrier is injured by the constant inflammation and allows microbe contacts to neoplastic tissue. These microbes and their metabolites induce further inflammatory signals, including the production of IL-17 family cytokines, promoting cancer advancement [75]. Inflammatory mediators may also stimulate macrophages to generate chromosome-breaking factors, injuring DNA and causing chromosomal instability in adjacent cells [6].

When microbial population translocate beyond an injured gut epithelium, the host immune system activates multiple pattern recognition receptors (PRRs). Cytoplasmic NOD-like receptors (NLRs) and membrane Toll-like receptors (TLRs) are PRRs crucial to the CRC progression [29]. In particular, TLR4 and TLR2 were found in murine models and associations between human genetic polymorphisms in TLR4 and TLR2 and CRC risk support a role in humans [155]. Moreover, activation of nuclear factor (NF)-κB influence CRC induction enhancing both Wnt-signaling and cytokines [7], which can transform gut epithelial nonstem cells into cancer-initiating cells. NF-κB has a complex role in CRC progression and involves several signaling pathways which have recently been widely reviewed [156]. Otherwise, in colitis-associated CRC, TLR signaling in cancer-associated fibroblasts induce an inflammatory cascade *via* epiregulin (EREG), independent of NF-κB mediation. EREG stimulates the extracellular signal-regulated kinase (ERK) pathway, which promotes the proliferation of neoplastic cells [157]. Two NLRs are associated with CRC risk: NOD2, induced by the microbial muramyl dipeptide; and NLRP6 (NOD-, LRR-, and pyrin domain containing 6). In mouse models, with NOD2 deficiency, CRC development is caused by dysbiosis [158]. Conversely, recent studies reveal that NOD2- associated dysbiosis can be overcome by co-housing NOD2 mutants with wild type mice [161]. Future efforts are required to elucidate the influence of NLRP6 and NOD2 in intestinal microbial regulation. However, the hypothesis that bacterial translocation across gut epithelia could induce TLR and NLR activation and promoting inflammation process is intensely sustained [159].

5.3.1. Specific Gut Bacteria and CRC

Some members of commensal bacterial community, as potential pro-oncogenic pathogens may contribute to CRC course.

-Interesting is the *Fusobacterium* (F) *nucleatum*, a nonspore-forming, anaerobic gram-negative oral commensal. It is involved in a large spectrum of disorders, including periodontal cardiovascular and gastrointestinal diseases, respiratory tract infections, Lemierre's syndrome, rheumatoid arthritis and Alzheimer's disease [160]. Increasing evidence highlighted that members of *Fusobacterium* species, in detail *Fusobacterium nucleatum*, populate neoplastic tissues and stool samples of CRC subjects [161, 162]. In addition, a restricted number of studies have suggested a positive correlation of *F. nucleatum* with CRC invasiveness, *e.g.*, lymph node metastasis, but the finding has not been established [163, 164]. Metagenomic studies have demonstrated an abundance of *Fusobacterium nucleatum* in CRC tissue, confirmed also by qPCR of the 16S ribosomal RNA gene sequence [165]. Finally, *F. nucleatum* can activate the WNT signaling pathway in colorectal carcinoma cells, promoting colorectal tumor growth [166]. In addition, *F. nucleatum* may inhibit T cell mediated immune responses against colorectal tumors [167, 168]. A higher ratio of *F. nucleatum* DNA in tissue has been associated with advanced disease stage [163, 164, 167] and a lower density of T cells in human CRC tissue [169].

-ETBF, as previously said, is pro-oncogenic and shapes the gut microflora to induce mucosal immune responses and epithelial changes, promoting cancer process. In particular, ETBF produces fragilysin which activates the Wnt/β-catenin signaling pathway that increase cell proliferation [170]. BFT also activates NFkB to induce inflammatory mediator production. This process leads to mucosal inflammation and CRC genesis [171 - 173]. Wu *et al.* demonstrated that ETBF may promote tumorigenesis using the APC min (multiple intestinal neoplasia) model of intestinal cancer colonized with ETBF isolate from pig. They detected a strong increase in colon adenoma and tumor growth in ETBF mice compared to control [81]. The enhanced tumorigenesis by ETBF could happen *via* induction of IL-17 [174], activation of STAT3 and DNA damage [175].

-*Clostridium septicum* (*C. septicum*) infections have been clinically linked to CRC [176], indeed, gastrointestinal disease and colorectal malignancies can be found in up to 40% of infected patients [177]. Hermsen *et al.* [177] analyzed 320 cases of *C. septicum* infections, the result showed that more than 40% had a gastrointestinal origin, mainly malignant. The mechanisms of this correlation remain unknown, it is thought that acidic and hypoxic tumor microenvironment positively influence the germination of *C. septicum* spores by ingestion of contaminated food.

-*Streptococcus gallolyticus* (formerly *S. bovis*): DNA from *S. gallolyticus* was found in about 20-50% of CRC tissues compared to less than 5% in the healthy colon . *S. gallolyticus* could invade the epithelial barrier enhancing inflammation and tumorigenesis [178, 179].

-Enterococcus faecalis: promote the release of extracellular superoxide that could be converted by hydrogen peroxide inducing DNA damage [180], chromosome instability and cancer in germfree Interleukin-10 (IL-10−/−) mice [6, 181].

-Acidovorax: an acid degrading member of *Proteobacteria* phylum is associated with adenoma pathogenesis [182]. It promotes colon cancer through increased metabolism of nitro-aromatic compounds [183] in the intestine and with the induction of of inflammation by its flagellar proteins [184].

-Escherichia coli: genotoxic *E.coli* could induce DNA damage triggering CRC. Furthermore, a specific type of *E. coli* (presenting the polyketide synthase (pks) Genotoxic Island, which encodes for Colibactin), could induce CRC *via* DNA double strand breaks [185]. In mono-associated IL10−/− mice treated with azoxymethane [186] the deletion of pks in the same strain of *E.coli* reduces DNA injury, tumor numbers and invasion but not inflammation.

5.3.2. Bacteria Metabolites and CRC

Colonic microbiota produces metabolites that impact the development of CRC from adenomas. But, epidemiological studies also suggest that diet has an influence in the tumor progression [187]. The main hypothesis is that the microbial metabolic by-products, derived from dietary molecules, could exert either a cytotoxic or a cytoprotective effect on the gut mucosa [188]. Colonic epithelial cells employ short chain fatty acids (SCFAs), such as butyrate (produced by bacteria), as an energy source. CRC patients showed a decrease in butyrate-producing bacteria in fecal samples, suggesting a possible involvement of bacteria in CRC pathogenesis [145]. Furthermore, some members of the *Clostridium* cluster XI, IX and XVIa are able to process primary bile acids into secondary bile acids [189], this process could interact with host metabolism and immunity, contributing to CRC development [190, 191]. In addition, cytotoxic and carcinogenic effect is also due to the production of microbiota toxic compounds, such as hydrogen sulfide [188], through the metabolism of several amino acid, related to a high-protein diet. In fact, as previously reported, fecal water of CRC patients showed an increased number of amino acids [141]. Both patients at low and high risk for CRC showed methanogenic and nonmethanogenic bacteria composition. Methanogenic microbes release harmless methane as an end-product of the amino acid metabolism, while nonmethanogenic bacteria, enriched in sulfate-reducing microbes, result in an elaboration of toxic hydrogen sulfide [192].

5.4. Gallbladder Cancer

Gallbladder cancer (GBC) is a tumor of the biliary tract, rare in Western

Countries, but not uncommon in the other different parts of the world. It is also lethal, with a 5-year survival of approximately 12%. Unluckily, most people are diagnosed this tumor once the neoplasia is too large to be surgically removed so, only 10%-30% of people with this cancer could undergo surgery. For these patients, ineligible for surgery, chemotherapy is the main treatment but currently, no chemotherapy treatment has been shown to be effective to help people live longer.

In GBC, chronic biliary infection with *Salmonella enterica* serovar Typhi (*S. Typhi*), the causative agent of typhoid fever, has been proposed as one possible additional risk factor [193]. This hypothesis developed from a case report of a patient who showed documented typhoid fever for 30 years before GBC, with *S. Typhi* subsequently isolated from the gallbladder. The gallbladder is known to be a reservoir of *Salmonella*, leading to increases in secondary bile acid concentrations, which associated to cancer development [194]. Sharma *et al.* showed a link between GBC and the typhoid carrier state. Furthermore, bile culture-positivity is related with increase in GBC, especially positivity for the Vi antigen (antigen associated with *Salmonella*) [193].

5.5. Liver Cancer

The liver produces the bile that aids the digestion of lipids in food so, that they can be absorbed by the bowel. The liver stores glycogen, which is made from sugars and it also process drugs, alcohol, toxins and poisons. Primary liver cancer originates from liver cells that have become neoplastic, secondary liver cancers originate from tumors of other organs such as the colon or rectum. Obese mice showed gut microbiota dysbiosis, with an increased production of deoxycholic acid (DCA) which is a cause of DNA damage [60]. This metabolite could produce a senescence-associated secretory phenotype in the hepatic stellate cells, which secrete tumor-promoting and inflammatory molecules in the liver. After contact with a chemical carcinogen the obese mice showed hepatocellular carcinoma (HCC). This result points out that intestinal microbial metabolites could promote obesity-induced HCC progression in mice. In addition, in a mouse model [52], TLR4 indicted by the LPS from the gut microflora was closely associated with tumor course, but not with the HCC genesis, induced by a mix of hepatotoxin carbon tetrachloride and diethylnitrosamine. The role of gut bacterial flora was indicated by a decrease in liver cancers in germfree mice compared to pathogen-free mice. On the contrary, propionate, produced by gut microbiota, inhibit liver tumor cell proliferation in a mouse model [195]. Intratumoral IL-17 is related to poor prognoses of patients with HCC [196], possibly because of the promotion of tumor growth and angiogenesis [80]. Furthermore, most of the Th17 cells could be originated by an interaction with intestinal microflora [197]. The pathogenesis of liver cancer can be regulated by gut microflora, suggesting the opportunity of therapeutic treatment.

5.6. Pancreatic Cancer

The pancreas is gland between the stomach and spine, joined by the pancreatic duct to the first part of the duodenum. The main role of the pancreas is the production of insulin, which controls the quantity of sugar in the blood. Pancreatic cancers (PC) begin in the lining of the pancreatic duct, if early diagnosed, are removed by surgery. However, this is not always feasible as the tumor is often noticed after it has spread to outlying organs and tissues. Pancreatic cancer is the seventh cause of cancer deaths worldwide [198, 199]. Exocrine and endocrine cells of the pancreas can develop tumors, but those formed by exocrine cells are much more aggressive [200, 201]. About 95% of pancreatic cancers are adenocarcinomas, produced in gland cells [200]. Endocrine pancreas cancers are unusual, making up less than 2% of all pancreatic cancers. They are called as neuroendocrine tumors (NET) [202, 203]. Current data indicate a potential involvement for the oral and intestinal microflora in the pancreatic cancer pathogenesis and progression [204]. Germfree mouse models have been used to evaluate the influence of the microbiota in pancreatic carcinogenesis [29, 72, 205]. An epidemiological study revealed associations between specific oral bacteria assemblage and the PC risk [206]. A decline in the number of *Streptococcus mitis* and *Neisseria elongata*, with a proliferation of *Granulicatella adiacens*, has been detected, suggesting the evaluation of this specific bacterial profiling as a PC biomarker [207]. Dysbiosis of the host microbiota could induce inflammation in PC [62], leading to opportunistic infection microbes [208]. Different studies demonstrated a relation between chronic inflammation and the PC pathogenesis and progression [208, 209]. Opportunistic microbes, such as *H. pylori* [210, 211], have been associated with the development of PC. *H. pylori* infects the pancreas *via* translocation from the intestine [212], inducing upregulation of NF-κB, which can also be promoted by inflammatory cytokines including IL-1β in PC [213]. Also, bacterial LPS is a potent activator of NF-κB in PC [214] indeed, in mouse PC models, tumor development was increased by the LPS treatment, precisely recognized by TLR4 [215]. Furthermore, when matching healthy controls to PC patients, the profiling of saliva microflora showed that the bacterial composition change [206]. These validated microbial signatures were related to PC, providing a possible source of diagnostic biomarkers.

6. BENEFICIAL ACTIVITIES OF GUT MICROBIOTA

Among the beneficial activities of the gut microbiota on human, many are related to cancer protection [21]:

a. Control of the intestinal epithelial cell proliferation and differentiation;
b. Growth and progression of the epithelial wall [190];
c. Apical tightening of the tight junctions;
d. Protection against pathogenic species;
e. Development/ modulation of gut-associated lymphoid tissue (including host innate immune system, with the important roles of NOD-like receptors and Toll-like receptors - TLRs);
f. Fermentation of nondigestible carbohydrates to produce SCFA; butyrate is the most important SCFA that modulates cell differentiation and growth, impedes CRC cell proliferation induces apoptosis of CRC cells, colon adenoma and colon cell lines [216, 217]. Anticarcinogenic effects of butyrate include expression of differentiation indicators (alkaline phosphatase) [218] and of the host's glutathione-S-transferases and other stress response patterns as well as suppression of cyclooxygenase- 2 expression [219]. In addition, butyrate alters the epigenome through inhibition of histone deacetylases [220];
g. Biliary acids metabolism;
h. Xenobiotics and dietary carcinogens degradation [22];

6.1. Antitumorigenic Impact of Microbiota

Most of the studies reveal a tumor-promoting role of the microflora but antitumor properties have also been described. In the past, antitumor activity was detected in patients with sarcomas, after injection of heat killed bacteria or bacterial infections [221]. Subsequent studies assign these antitumor effects to specific bacterial components as NOD-like receptor (NLR) agonists and TLR agonists. The stimulation of innate immunity can convert cancer tolerance into an anticancer immune response [222]. Moreover, mouse models described an effective immune role in tumor surveillance and in the inhibition of proliferation and metastasis, which results in the cancer regression [76]. An anticancer microbiota-mediated effect was noted also in hematopoietic tumors, through the Th17 response. In mouse models, the alkylating agent cyclophosphamide, changes the microflora structure, causing dysbiosis in the small intestine and inducing the translocation of Gram+ bacteria into secondary lymphoid organs. Gram+ microbes activate a specific subset of 'pathogenic' Th17 cells and memory Th1 immune responses, which result in a potent cancer-suppressive Th17 response [223]. Recently, our group [86], demonstrated that Th17 cells have a specific antitumor effector function in patients with pancreatic cancer, and that there are decreased levels of these cells in cancer tissue compared to healthy mucosa. These findings propose that the intestinal microflora can help to profile the anticancer immune response. In other words, although some bacteria are able to induce Th17 cells, others could promote the control of Th17 cells, limiting cancer development. *Lactobacillus, Bifidobacteria* and *Clostridium* can induce

Foxp3+ Treg cells [224] that can modulate the production of IL-17A and the proliferation of Th17 cells, through IL-10 secretion [225]. These interactions can have an anti-tumorigenic activity in the intestine. It is still not clear if this result is due to the suppression of Th17 pro-tumorigenic activity, but Foxp3+ Treg cells can actively block intestinal tumor growth through IL-10 secretion [226, 227].

Also, the *Bacteroides* species have been shown to have immunomodulatory effects. In particular *B. fragilis* releases polysaccharide A (PSA) that seems to stop intestinal inflammation. Mice colonization with *B. fragilis* resulted in the suppression of a proinflammatory Th17 reaction and this modulation could be attributed to PSA because *B. fragilis* PSA lacking was unable to suppress Th17 response, and also failed to persistently colonize the intestine [228]. Actually, a selected mixture of *Clostridia* strains could attenuate disease in preclinical models of colitis through the induction of Tregs [229], revealing a potential antitumorigenic role. These results suggest that therapeutic colonization with specific strains of human-associated bacteria may have the potential to reduce tumorigenesis.

6.2. Manipulating the Microbiota for Cancer Therapy

The selective manipulating of gut microbiota may represent a feasible means to limit the incidence of specific tumors and to improve the activity of various anticancer agents [230]. Although the first possibility has been investigated in several models of oncogenesis with promising results, the actual oncopreventive effects of anticancer agents in humans remain to be established.

Different anticancer agents could be used to manipulate the microbiota for anti-cancer treatment:

1. Antibiotics, chemicals with a preferential cytotoxicity for one or more bacterial species;
2. Probiotics, living bacteria or other microorganisms;
3. Prebiotics, nondigestible compounds that stimulate the growth and/or functions of specific components of the intestinal microflora;
4. Postbiotics, nonviable products of the intestinal microflora that exert biological activities in the host.

It may be possible to use antibiotics to reverse the dysbiosis [230]. Recent data indicate that bacteriocins, proteinaceous antibiotics produced by some bacterial strains, may be used to deplete one or a few specific components of the gut microbiota for therapeutic purposes [29].

Although antibiotics have been shown to reduce the inflammation and consequently cancer development in mouse models, they are not considered as good players for chemotherapeutic adjuvants or chemoprevention in the clinic. The abuse of antibiotics produces antibiotic-resistant bacterial strains and furthermore, this treatment kills many symbiotic/commensal bacteria, including some that protect against carcinogenesis and promote homeostasis. In addition, not all bacteria are restored to normal levels after the antibiotic treatment [231]. It has been supposed that the antibiotics usage is altering the microbiota composition, contributing to the increased incidence of obesity, allergies, IBD, asthma and different types of tumors [231]. Therefore, instead of using antibiotics to destroy microbes indiscriminately, it would be better to maintain or restore a beneficial microbial composition. This is the basis for a potential direct microbial intervention thought probiotics, defined as live microorganisms present in foods or dietary supplements that confer a health benefit. Different experiments suggest that systematic assumption of probiotics can improve the qualitative and quantitative structure of the gut microbiota [232, 233]. Notably, some probiotics influence the commensal microbiota, either by replacing a missing part of the local bacterial flora or by modifying the composition or changing the metabolic activity. The microflora can trigger a chronic inflammation in the gut and can induce the production of carcinogenic molecules from diet or from the bile salts, endogenously generated thanks to specific enzymes. These products have genotoxic and cytotoxic activities which can induce abnormal cell growth contributing to CRC development [234]. Some particular probiotics can reduce the activity of these bacterial enzymes and they can degrade carcinogenic compounds present in the intestinal lumen or produce molecules with anticarcinogenic activity, such as SCFAs. Between SCFA, butyrate is related to CRC as it is involved in the regulation of the balance between growth and apoptosis of colon cells. Moreover butyrate can help the prevention of CRC thought the increase of mucus production that improve the intestinal barrier and also stimulates the production of anti-inflammatory cytokines inducing immunomodulation. The amount of SCFA naturally produced by the gut microbiota is not enough to inhibit CRC development, so the administration of probiotics may help the increase of quotidian production of SCFA. As previously said, probiotics could induce also immunomodulation [234], indeed bacterial products are recognized by immune and epithelial receptors such as NOD-like and Toll-like receptors, stimulating cytokines secretion [235]. The consumption of probiotics is able to increase the anti-inflammatory cytokines and decrease proinflammatory cytokines leading to a delay in the development of colon cancer cells. Furthermore, some probiotics can activate phagocytes, contributing to eliminate early cancer cells [236]. In addition, probiotics can be improved by supplementing foods also with engineered bacteria, in order to have stronger beneficial effects or to more stably colonize the human GI tract. Currently, the positive roles of probiotics in lowering the gastrointestinal inflammation and preventing colorectal cancer have been frequently demonstrated, but in the specific, their immunomodulatory effects and mechanism in suppressing the growth of tumors remain unexplored. Probiotic have been tested in animal tumor models for their ability to prevent carcinogenesis, with promising results [237]. In particular, engineered *Lactobacillus acidophilus* (with a phosphoglycerol transferase gene deletion) unable to produce lipoteichoic acid, was administrated to Apc$^{\Delta floxed}$ mice, the results showed a regression of colonic polyps [238]. Furthermore, engineered *Lactobacillus casei* and *Lactococcus lactis* synthesizing "elafin" (a protein that reduces inflammation in a mouse model of colitis [239]) when added to *ex vivo* inflamed human colitis cells, are able to reduce cytokine production and cell permeability. Also engineered *Lactobacillus gasseri* (overexpressing superoxide dismutase) reduced colitis in IL-10 knockout mice [240].

Some probiotic strains can produce antibiotic-like molecules to avoid localized evolution of potential competitors. Genetically modified probiotics have been effectively employed as vectors for the delivery of immunostimulatory molecules, tumor associated antigens or enzymes that limit the toxicity of conventional chemotherapy, at least in animal models [241].

Prebiotics have also been related to the reduction of cancer initiation and development. The most used prebiotics include inulin, fructans, xylooglio-saccharides (XOS), galactogliosaccharides (GOS) and fructooligossacharides (FOS) [242]. Different studies have demonstrated the anticarcinogenic properties of inulin oligo-fructans [243]. Inulin-type fructans are present in foods such as onion, *etc*. They can increase SCFA amount and bifidobacteria in the intestinal lumen. In addition, inulin and oligofructose could reduce the severity of 1, 2-dimethylhydrazine induced CRC in rats [45]. In general, the antitumorigenic effect of prebiotics is due to:

1. Manipulation of intestinal microflora and inhibition of the growth of pathogens
2. Production of SCFA and bifidogenic activity
3. Immunomodulation and induction of apoptosis
4. Induction of heat shock protein 25 and protein kinase C-d, down-regulation of the expression levels of NF-kB, gastrointestinal glutathione peroxidase (GI-GPx), COX-2, and iNOS [244].

The transplantation of intestinal microflora (FMT) is an alternative to the modulation of specific bacteria. FMT is the administration of a fecal solution from healthy to diseased individuals into the intestinal tract, aiming for total replacement of one microbiota by another, conferring a health benefit [245]. It was used for the first time in fourth-century China for the treatment of a variety of intestinal disease conditions [245].

Once a donor is selected, according to specific exclusion criteria (donor without a family history of metabolic, autoimmune and malignant diseases and screening for any potential pathogens), the feces are mixed with saline and administered through a nasogastric tube, nasojejunal tube, esophagogastroduodenoscopy, colonoscopy or retention enema.

The fecal microbial transplant has been effectuated to treat diseases related to antibiotic-associated diarrhea and *Clostridium difficile* infection [246] but currently the potential use for other diseases like inflammatory bowel disease, irritable bowel syndrome and metabolic and cardiovascular disorders is under investigation [247].

7. CONCLUSION

The gut homeostasis is obtained by symbiotic interactions between resident microflora and the cells of the digestive tract. Changes to the microbiota composition caused by environmental changes (*e.g.*, diet, infection and/or lifestyle) can disrupt this symbiotic interplay and induce diseases, such as cancer, a plague of our century. NGS technologies improved the characterization of microbiota composition in organic samples. So, the growing importance of the role of the intestinal microbiota in health and diseases and the acknowledgement of the host-microbe mutualism at the metabolic and immunological levels became crucial for a better understanding of tumor dynamics.

Different possible relations between GI cancerogenesis and the composition of gut microbiota have been elucidated, focusing on dysbiosis and the pro-carcinogenic effects of microbes, such as virulence factors, genotoxicity, host defenses modulation, inflammation, bacterial-derived metabolism, anti-oxidative defenses and oxidative stress modulation. Microbiota alterations could be used as prognosis markers for novel therapeutic strategies, in particular with respect to RNA sequencing and metabolomics approaches. Today, finding new methods to selectively manipulate the microbiota, in order to stop tumor initiation and progression, represents an exciting challenge. In the near future, high quality mechanistic experimental studies and interventional human studies might provide the scientific premise for the clinical use of probiotics/prebiotics (also genetically modified) for the cancer treatment and therapies for other multifactorial human diseases.

Supported by The research was funded with a grant from the regional contribution of "The Programma Attuativo Regionale (Toscana) funded by FAS (now FSC), the Italian Ministry of University and Research (MIUR) and the Foundation 'Ente Cassa di Risparmio di Firenze'.

CONSENT FOR PUBLICATION

Not applicable.

CONFLICT OF INTEREST

The author declares no conflict of interest, financial or otherwise.

ACKNOWLEDGEMENTS

We thank Dr. Giulia Nannini for the help in compiling the bibliography

REFERENCES

[1]   Pennathur A, Gibson MK, Jobe BA, Luketich JD. Oesophageal carcinoma. Lancet 2013; 381(9864): 400-12.
        [http://dx.doi.org/10.1016/S0140-6736(12)60643-6] [PMID: 23374478]

[2]   Thiel A, Ristimäki A. Gastric cancer: basic aspects. Helicobacter 2012; 17 (Suppl. 1): 26-9.
        [http://dx.doi.org/10.1111/j.1523-5378.2012.00979.x] [PMID: 22958152]

[3]   Ferlay J, Shin HR, Bray F, Forman D, Mathers C, Parkin DM. Estimates of worldwide burden of cancer in 2008: GLOBOCAN 2008. Int J Cancer 2010; 127(12): 2893-917.
        [http://dx.doi.org/10.1002/ijc.25516] [PMID: 21351269]

[4]   Correa P, Piazuelo MB. *Helicobacter pylori* infection and gastric adenocarcinoma. US Gastroenterol Hepatol Rev 2011; 7(1): 59-64.
        [PMID: 21857882]

[5]   Schottenfeld D, Beebe-Dimmer JL, Vigneau FD. The epidemiology and pathogenesis of neoplasia in the small intestine. Ann Epidemiol 2009; 19(1): 58-69.
        [http://dx.doi.org/10.1016/j.annepidem.2008.10.004] [PMID: 19064190]

[6]   Yang Y, Wang X, Huycke T, Moore DR, Lightfoot SA, Huycke MM. Colon macrophages polarized by commensal bacteria cause colitis and cancer through the bystander effect. Transl Oncol 2013; 6(5): 596-606.
        [http://dx.doi.org/10.1593/tlo.13412] [PMID: 24151540]

[7]   Candela M, Turroni S, Biagi E, *et al.* Inflammation and colorectal cancer, when microbiota-host mutualism breaks. World J Gastroenterol 2014; 20(4): 908-22.
        [http://dx.doi.org/10.3748/wjg.v20.i4.908] [PMID: 24574765]

[8]   Sears CL, Garrett WS. Microbes, microbiota, and colon cancer. Cell Host Microbe 2014; 15(3): 317-28.
        [http://dx.doi.org/10.1016/j.chom.2014.02.007] [PMID: 24629338]

[9]   Hawrelak JA, Myers SP. The causes of intestinal dysbiosis: a review. Altern Med Rev 2004; 9(2): 180-97.
        [PMID: 15253677]

[10]   Amedei A, Munari F, Bella CD, *et al.* Helicobacter pylori secreted peptidyl prolyl cis, trans-isomerase drives Th17 inflammation in gastric adenocarcinoma. Intern Emerg Med 2014; 9(3): 303-9.

[http://dx.doi.org/10.1007/s11739-012-0867-9] [PMID: 23054412]

[11] D'Elios MM, Amedei A, Manghetti M, *et al.* Impaired T-cell regulation of B-cell growth in *Helicobacter pylori*--related gastric low-grade MALT lymphoma. Gastroenterology 1999; 117(5): 1105-12.
      [http://dx.doi.org/10.1016/S0016-5085(99)70395-1] [PMID: 10535873]

[12] Ackerman J. The ultimate social network. Sci Am 2012; 306(6): 36-43.
      [http://dx.doi.org/10.1038/scientificamerican0612-36] [PMID: 22649992]

[13] Proctor LM. The human microbiome project in 2011 and beyond. Cell Host Microbe 2011; 10(4): 287-91.
      [http://dx.doi.org/10.1016/j.chom.2011.10.001] [PMID: 22018227]

[14] Ursell LK, Metcalf JL, Parfrey LW, Knight R. Defining the human microbiome. Nutr Rev 2012; 70 (Suppl. 1): S38-44.
      [http://dx.doi.org/10.1111/j.1753-4887.2012.00493.x] [PMID: 22861806]

[15] Eckburg PB, Bik EM, Bernstein CN, *et al.* Diversity of the human intestinal microbial flora. Science 2005; 308(5728): 1635-8.
      [http://dx.doi.org/10.1126/science.1110591] [PMID: 15831718]

[16] Frank DN, St Amand AL, Feldman RA, Boedeker EC, Harpaz N, Pace NR. Molecular-phylogenetic characterization of microbial community imbalances in human inflammatory bowel diseases. Proc Natl Acad Sci USA 2007; 104(34): 13780-5.
      [http://dx.doi.org/10.1073/pnas.0706625104] [PMID: 17699621]

[17] Fraher MH, O'Toole PW, Quigley EM. Techniques used to characterize the gut microbiota: a guide for the clinician. Nat Rev Gastroenterol Hepatol 2012; 9(6): 312-22.
      [http://dx.doi.org/10.1038/nrgastro.2012.44] [PMID: 22450307]

[18] Kau AL, Ahern PP, Griffin NW, Goodman AL, Gordon JI. Human nutrition, the gut microbiome and the immune system. Nature 2011; 474(7351): 327-36.
      [http://dx.doi.org/10.1038/nature10213] [PMID: 21677749]

[19] Human Microbiome Project Consortium. Structure, function and diversity of the healthy human microbiome. Nature 2012; 486(7402): 207-14.
      [http://dx.doi.org/10.1038/nature11234] [PMID: 22699609]

[20] Mahowald MA, Rey FE, Seedorf H, *et al.* Characterizing a model human gut microbiota composed of members of its two dominant bacterial phyla. Proc Natl Acad Sci USA 2009; 106(14): 5859-64.
      [http://dx.doi.org/10.1073/pnas.0901529106] [PMID: 19321416]

[21] Ottman N, Smidt H, de Vos WM, Belzer C. The function of our microbiota: who is out there and what do they do? Front Cell Infect Microbiol 2012; 2: 104.
      [http://dx.doi.org/10.3389/fcimb.2012.00104] [PMID: 22919693]

[22] O'Hara AM, Shanahan F. The gut flora as a forgotten organ. EMBO Rep 2006; 7(7): 688-93.
      [http://dx.doi.org/10.1038/sj.embor.7400731] [PMID: 16819463]

[23] Swidsinski A, Loening-Baucke V, Lochs H, Hale LP. Spatial organization of bacterial flora in normal and inflamed intestine: a fluorescence *in situ* hybridization study in mice. World J Gastroenterol 2005; 11(8): 1131-40.
      [http://dx.doi.org/10.3748/wjg.v11.i8.1131] [PMID: 15754393]

[24] McConnell EL, Fadda HM, Basit AW. Gut instincts: explorations in intestinal physiology and drug delivery. Int J Pharm 2008; 364(2): 213-26.
      [http://dx.doi.org/10.1016/j.ijpharm.2008.05.012] [PMID: 18602774]

[25] Dave M, Higgins PD, Middha S, Rioux KP. The human gut microbiome: current knowledge, challenges, and future directions. Transl Res 2012; 160(4): 246-57.
      [http://dx.doi.org/10.1016/j.trsl.2012.05.003] [PMID: 22683238]

[26] Bik EM, Eckburg PB, Gill SR, *et al.* Molecular analysis of the bacterial microbiota in the human stomach. Proc Natl Acad Sci USA 2006; 103(3): 732-7.
[http://dx.doi.org/10.1073/pnas.0506655103] [PMID: 16407106]

[27] Sonnenburg JL, Angenent LT, Gordon JI. Getting a grip on things: how do communities of bacterial symbionts become established in our intestine? Nat Immunol 2004; 5(6): 569-73.
[http://dx.doi.org/10.1038/ni1079] [PMID: 15164016]

[28] Holmes E, Li JV, Athanasiou T, Ashrafian H, Nicholson JK. Understanding the role of gut microbiome-host metabolic signal disruption in health and disease. Trends Microbiol 2011; 19(7): 349-59.
[http://dx.doi.org/10.1016/j.tim.2011.05.006] [PMID: 21684749]

[29] Schwabe RF, Jobin C. The microbiome and cancer. Nat Rev Cancer 2013; 13(11): 800-12.
[http://dx.doi.org/10.1038/nrc3610] [PMID: 24132111]

[30] Mukherjee PK, Sendid B, Hoarau G, Colombel JF, Poulain D, Ghannoum MA. Mycobiota in gastrointestinal diseases. Nat Rev Gastroenterol Hepatol 2015; 12(2): 77-87.
[http://dx.doi.org/10.1038/nrgastro.2014.188] [PMID: 25385227]

[31] Rautava S, Luoto R, Salminen S, Isolauri E. Microbial contact during pregnancy, intestinal colonization and human disease. Nat Rev Gastroenterol Hepatol 2012; 9(10): 565-76.
[http://dx.doi.org/10.1038/nrgastro.2012.144] [PMID: 22890113]

[32] Redondo-Lopez V, Cook RL, Sobel JD. Emerging role of lactobacilli in the control and maintenance of the vaginal bacterial microflora. Rev Infect Dis 1990; 12(5): 856-72.
[http://dx.doi.org/10.1093/clinids/12.5.856] [PMID: 2237129]

[33] Mändar R, Mikelsaar M. Transmission of mother's microflora to the newborn at birth. Biol Neonate 1996; 69(1): 30-5.
[http://dx.doi.org/10.1159/000244275] [PMID: 8777246]

[34] Huurre A, Kalliomäki M, Rautava S, Rinne M, Salminen S, Isolauri E. Mode of delivery - effects on gut microbiota and humoral immunity. Neonatology 2008; 93(4): 236-40.
[http://dx.doi.org/10.1159/000111102] [PMID: 18025796]

[35] Mackie RI, Sghir A, Gaskins HR. Developmental microbial ecology of the neonatal gastrointestinal tract. Am J Clin Nutr 1999; 69(5): 1035S-45S.
[PMID: 10232646]

[36] Ley RE, Bäckhed F, Turnbaugh P, Lozupone CA, Knight RD, Gordon JI. Obesity alters gut microbial ecology. Proc Natl Acad Sci USA 2005; 102(31): 11070-5.
[http://dx.doi.org/10.1073/pnas.0504978102] [PMID: 16033867]

[37] Zoetendal EG, Akkermans AD, Akkermans-van Vliet WM, de Visser JA, de Vos WM. The host genotype affects the bacterial community in the human gastrointestinal tract. Microb Ecol Health Dis 2001; 13: 129-34.
[http://dx.doi.org/10.1080/089106001750462669]

[38] Zhang C, Zhang M, Wang S, *et al.* Interactions between gut microbiota, host genetics and diet relevant to development of metabolic syndromes in mice. ISME J 2010; 4(2): 232-41.
[http://dx.doi.org/10.1038/ismej.2009.112] [PMID: 19865183]

[39] Turnbaugh PJ, Bäckhed F, Fulton L, Gordon JI. Diet-induced obesity is linked to marked but reversible alterations in the mouse distal gut microbiome. Cell Host Microbe 2008; 3(4): 213-23.
[http://dx.doi.org/10.1016/j.chom.2008.02.015] [PMID: 18407065]

[40] Gevers D, Knight R, Petrosino JF, *et al.* The Human Microbiome Project: a community resource for the healthy human microbiome. PLoS Biol 2012; 10(8): e1001377.
[http://dx.doi.org/10.1371/journal.pbio.1001377] [PMID: 22904687]

[41] Human Microbiome Project Consortium. A framework for human microbiome research. Nature 2012;

486(7402): 215-21.
[http://dx.doi.org/10.1038/nature11209] [PMID: 22699610]

[42]   Koren O, Knights D, Gonzalez A, *et al.* A guide to enterotypes across the human body: meta-analysis of microbial community structures in human microbiome datasets. PLOS Comput Biol 2013; 9(1): e1002863.
[http://dx.doi.org/10.1371/journal.pcbi.1002863] [PMID: 23326225]

[43]   Morgan XC, Segata N, Huttenhower C. Biodiversity and functional genomics in the human microbiome. Trends Genet 2013; 29(1): 51-8.
[http://dx.doi.org/10.1016/j.tig.2012.09.005] [PMID: 23140990]

[44]   Wylie KM, Truty RM, Sharpton TJ, *et al.* Novel bacterial taxa in the human microbiome. PLoS One 2012; 7(6): e35294.
[http://dx.doi.org/10.1371/journal.pone.0035294] [PMID: 22719826]

[45]   Ravel J, Blaser MJ, Braun J, Brown E, Bushman FD, Chang EB, *et al.* Human microbiome science: vision for the future. Bethesda MD Microbiome. 2-16.
[http://dx.doi.org/10.1186/2049-2618-2-16]

[46]   Arumugam M, Raes J, Pelletier E, *et al.* MetaHIT Consortium. Enterotypes of the human gut microbiome. Nature 2011; 473(7346): 174-80.
[http://dx.doi.org/10.1038/nature09944] [PMID: 21508958]

[47]   Wu GD, Chen J, Hoffmann C, *et al.* Linking long-term dietary patterns with gut microbial enterotypes. Science 2011; 334(6052): 105-8.
[http://dx.doi.org/10.1126/science.1208344] [PMID: 21885731]

[48]   Russell W. An address on a characteristic organism of cancer. BMJ 1890; 2(1563): 1356-60.
[http://dx.doi.org/10.1136/bmj.2.1563.1356] [PMID: 20753194]

[49]   Shahanavaj K, Gil-Bazo I, Castiglia M, *et al.* Cancer and the microbiome: potential applications as new tumor biomarker. Expert Rev Anticancer Ther 2015; 15(3): 317-30.
[http://dx.doi.org/10.1586/14737140.2015.992785] [PMID: 25495037]

[50]   Turnbaugh PJ1. Ley RE, Mahowald MA, Magrini V, Mardis ER, Gordon JI. An obesityassociated gut microbiome with increased capacity for energy harvest. Nature 2006; 444(7122): 1027-31.
[http://dx.doi.org/10.1038/nature05414] [PMID: 17183312]

[51]   Smith MI, Yatsunenko T, Manary MJ, *et al.* Gut microbiomes of Malawian twin pairs discordant for kwashiorkor. Science 2013; 339(6119): 548-54.
[http://dx.doi.org/10.1126/science.1229000] [PMID: 23363771]

[52]   Tao X, Wang N, Qin W. Gut microbiota and hepatocellular carcinoma. Gastrointest Tumors 2015; 2(1): 33-40.
[http://dx.doi.org/10.1159/000380895] [PMID: 26673641]

[53]   Sacksteder MR. Occurrence of spontaneous tumors in the germfree F344 rat. J Natl Cancer Inst 1976; 57(6): 1371-3.
[http://dx.doi.org/10.1093/jnci/57.6.1371] [PMID: 1069860]

[54]   Dove WF, Clipson L, Gould KA, *et al.* Intestinal neoplasia in the ApcMin mouse: independence from the microbial and natural killer (beige locus) status. Cancer Res 1997; 57(5): 812-4.
[PMID: 9041176]

[55]   Zhan Y, Chen PJ, Sadler WD, *et al.* Gut microbiota protects against gastrointestinal tumorigenesis caused by epithelial injury. Cancer Res 2013; 73(24): 7199-210.
[http://dx.doi.org/10.1158/0008-5472.CAN-13-0827] [PMID: 24165160]

[56]   Reddy BS, Narisawa T, Maronpot R, Weisburger JH, Wynder EL. Animal models for the study of dietary factors and cancer of the large bowel. Cancer Res 1975; 35(11 Pt. 2): 3421-6.
[PMID: 1192409]

[57] Vannucci L, Stepankova R, Kozakova H, Fiserova A, Rossmann P, Tlaskalova-Hogenova H. Colorectal carcinogenesis in germ-free and conventionally reared rats: different intestinal environments affect the systemic immunity. Int J Oncol 2008; 32(3): 609-17. [PMID: 18292938]

[58] Rakoff-Nahoum S, Medzhitov R. Role of toll-like receptors in tissue repair and tumorigenesis. Biochemistry (Mosc) 2008; 73(5): 555-61. [http://dx.doi.org/10.1134/S0006297908050088] [PMID: 18605980]

[59] Dapito DH, Mencin A, Gwak GY, *et al.* Promotion of hepatocellular carcinoma by the intestinal microbiota and TLR4. Cancer Cell 2012; 21(4): 504-16. [http://dx.doi.org/10.1016/j.ccr.2012.02.007] [PMID: 22516259]

[60] Yoshimoto S, Loo TM, Atarashi K, *et al.* Obesity-induced gut microbial metabolite promotes liver cancer through senescence secretome. Nature 2013; 499(7456): 97-101. [http://dx.doi.org/10.1038/nature12347] [PMID: 23803760]

[61] Chen GY, Shaw MH, Redondo G, Núñez G. The innate immune receptor Nod1 protects the intestine from inflammation-induced tumorigenesis. Cancer Res 2008; 68(24): 10060-7. [http://dx.doi.org/10.1158/0008-5472.CAN-08-2061] [PMID: 19074871]

[62] Klimesova K, Kverka M, Zakostelska Z, *et al.* Altered gut microbiota promotes colitis-associated cancer in IL-1 receptor-associated kinase M-deficient mice. Inflamm Bowel Dis 2013; 19(6): 1266-77. [http://dx.doi.org/10.1097/MIB.0b013e318281330a] [PMID: 23567778]

[63] Lee CW, Rickman B, Rogers AB, Ge Z, Wang TC, Fox JG. *Helicobacter pylori* eradication prevents progression of gastric cancer in hypergastrinemic INS-GAS mice. Cancer Res 2008; 68(9): 3540-8. [http://dx.doi.org/10.1158/0008-5472.CAN-07-6786] [PMID: 18441088]

[64] Wong BC, Lam SK, Wong WM, *et al.* China Gastric Cancer Study Group. *Helicobacter pylori* eradication to prevent gastric cancer in a high-risk region of China: a randomized controlled trial. JAMA 2004; 291(2): 187-94. [http://dx.doi.org/10.1001/jama.291.2.187] [PMID: 14722144]

[65] Sears CL, Pardoll DM. Perspective: alpha-bugs, their microbial partners, and the link to colon cancer. J Infect Dis 2011; 203(3): 306-11. [http://dx.doi.org/10.1093/jinfdis/jiq061] [PMID: 21208921]

[66] Tjalsma H, Boleij A, Marchesi JR, Dutilh BE. A bacterial driver-passenger model for colorectal cancer: beyond the usual suspects. Nat Rev Microbiol 2012; 10(8): 575-82. [http://dx.doi.org/10.1038/nrmicro2819] [PMID: 22728587]

[67] Hajishengallis G, Darveau RP, Curtis MA. The keystone-pathogen hypothesis. Nat Rev Microbiol 2012; 10(10): 717-25. [http://dx.doi.org/10.1038/nrmicro2873] [PMID: 22941505]

[68] Fukata M, Abreu MT. Role of Toll-like receptors in gastrointestinal malignancies. Oncogene 2008; 27(2): 234-43. [http://dx.doi.org/10.1038/sj.onc.1210908] [PMID: 18176605]

[69] Mantovani A, Allavena P, Sica A, Balkwill F. Cancer-related inflammation. Nature 2008; 454(7203): 436-44. [http://dx.doi.org/10.1038/nature07205] [PMID: 18650914]

[70] Mantovani A. Cancer: inflammation by remote control. Nature 2005; 435(7043): 752-3. [http://dx.doi.org/10.1038/435752a] [PMID: 15944689]

[71] Uronis JM, Mühlbauer M, Herfarth HH, Rubinas TC, Jones GS, Jobin C. Modulation of the intestinal microbiota alters colitis-associated colorectal cancer susceptibility. PLoS One 2009; 4(6): e6026. [http://dx.doi.org/10.1371/journal.pone.0006026] [PMID: 19551144]

[72] Shaw MH, Kamada N, Kim YG, Núñez G. Microbiota-induced IL-1β, but not IL-6, is critical for the

development of steady-state TH17 cells in the intestine. J Exp Med 2012; 209(2): 251-8.
[http://dx.doi.org/10.1084/jem.20111703] [PMID: 22291094]

[73]   Ouyang W, Kolls JK, Zheng Y. The biological functions of T helper 17 cell effector cytokines in inflammation. Immunity 2008; 28(4): 454-67.
[http://dx.doi.org/10.1016/j.immuni.2008.03.004] [PMID: 18400188]

[74]   Korn T, Bettelli E, Oukka M, Kuchroo VK. IL-17 and Th17 Cells. Annu Rev Immunol 2009; 27: 485-517.
[http://dx.doi.org/10.1146/annurev.immunol.021908.132710] [PMID: 19132915]

[75]   Grivennikov SI, Wang K, Mucida D, *et al*. Adenoma-linked barrier defects and microbial products drive IL-23/IL-17-mediated tumour growth. Nature 2012; 491(7423): 254-8.
[PMID: 23034650]

[76]   Muranski P, Boni A, Antony PA, *et al*. Tumor-specific Th17-polarized cells eradicate large established melanoma. Blood 2008; 112(2): 362-73.
[http://dx.doi.org/10.1182/blood-2007-11-120998] [PMID: 18354038]

[77]   Murugaiyan G, Saha B. Protumor vs antitumor functions of IL-17. J Immunol 2009; 183(7): 4169-75.
[http://dx.doi.org/10.4049/jimmunol.0901017] [PMID: 19767566]

[78]   Zheng Y, Valdez PA, Danilenko DM, *et al*. Interleukin-22 mediates early host defense against attaching and effacing bacterial pathogens. Nat Med 2008; 14(3): 282-9.
[http://dx.doi.org/10.1038/nm1720] [PMID: 18264109]

[79]   Mitsdoerffer M, Lee Y, Jäger A, *et al*. Proinflammatory T helper type 17 cells are effective B-cell helpers. Proc Natl Acad Sci USA 2010; 107(32): 14292-7.
[http://dx.doi.org/10.1073/pnas.1009234107] [PMID: 20660725]

[80]   Numasaki M, Fukushi J, Ono M, *et al*. Interleukin-17 promotes angiogenesis and tumor growth. Blood 2003; 101(7): 2620-7.
[http://dx.doi.org/10.1182/blood-2002-05-1461] [PMID: 12411307]

[81]   Wu S, Rhee KJ, Albesiano E, *et al*. A human colonic commensal promotes colon tumorigenesis *via* activation of T helper type 17 T cell responses. Nat Med 2009; 15(9): 1016-22.
[http://dx.doi.org/10.1038/nm.2015] [PMID: 19701202]

[82]   Chae WJ, Gibson TF, Zelterman D, Hao L, Henegariu O, Bothwell AL. Ablation of IL-17A abrogates progression of spontaneous intestinal tumorigenesis. Proc Natl Acad Sci USA 2010; 107(12): 5540-4.
[http://dx.doi.org/10.1073/pnas.0912675107] [PMID: 20212110]

[83]   Charles KA, Kulbe H, Soper R, *et al*. The tumor-promoting actions of TNF-α involve TNFR1 and IL-17 in ovarian cancer in mice and humans. J Clin Invest 2009; 119(10): 3011-23.
[http://dx.doi.org/10.1172/JCI39065] [PMID: 19741298]

[84]   Dhodapkar KM, Barbuto S, Matthews P, *et al*. Dendritic cells mediate the induction of polyfunctional human IL17-producing cells (Th17-1 cells) enriched in the bone marrow of patients with myeloma. Blood 2008; 112(7): 2878-85.
[http://dx.doi.org/10.1182/blood-2008-03-143222] [PMID: 18669891]

[85]   Koyama K, Kagamu H, Miura S, *et al*. Reciprocal CD4+ T-cell balance of effector CD62Llow CD4+ and CD62LhighCD25+ CD4+ regulatory T cells in small cell lung cancer reflects disease stage. Clin Cancer Res 2008; 14(21): 6770-9.
[http://dx.doi.org/10.1158/1078-0432.CCR-08-1156] [PMID: 18980970]

[86]   Amedei A, Niccolai E, Benagiano M, *et al*. *Ex vivo* analysis of pancreatic cancer-infiltrating T lymphocytes reveals that ENO-specific Tregs accumulate in tumor tissue and inhibit Th1/Th17 effector cell functions. Cancer Immunol Immunother 2013; 62(7): 1249-60.
[http://dx.doi.org/10.1007/s00262-013-1429-3] [PMID: 23640603]

[87]   Kryczek I, Wei S, Zou L, *et al*. Cutting edge: Th17 and regulatory T cell dynamics and the regulation by IL-2 in the tumor microenvironment. J Immunol 2007; 178(11): 6730-3.

[http://dx.doi.org/10.4049/jimmunol.178.11.6730] [PMID: 17513719]

[88]   Aujla SJ, Dubin PJ, Kolls JK. Th17 cells and mucosal host defense. Semin Immunol 2007; 19(6): 377-82.
       [http://dx.doi.org/10.1016/j.smim.2007.10.009] [PMID: 18054248]

[89]   Raffatellu M, Santos RL, Verhoeven DE, *et al.* Simian immunodeficiency virus-induced mucosal
       interleukin-17 deficiency promotes Salmonella dissemination from the gut. Nat Med 2008; 14(4): 421-8.
       [http://dx.doi.org/10.1038/nm1743] [PMID: 18376406]

[90]   Kirchberger S, Royston DJ, Boulard O, *et al.* Innate lymphoid cells sustain colon cancer through
       production of interleukin-22 in a mouse model. J Exp Med 2013; 210(5): 917-31.
       [http://dx.doi.org/10.1084/jem.20122308] [PMID: 23589566]

[91]   Niccolai E, Cappello P, Taddei A, *et al.* Peripheral ENO1-specific T cells mirror the intratumoral
       immune response and their presence is a potential prognostic factor for pancreatic adenocarcinoma. Int
       J Oncol 2016; 49(1): 393-401.
       [http://dx.doi.org/10.3892/ijo.2016.3524] [PMID: 27210467]

[92]   Ziesché E, Bachmann M, Kleinert H, Pfeilschifter J, Mühl H. The interleukin-22/STAT3 pathway
       potentiates expression of inducible nitric-oxide synthase in human colon carcinoma cells. J Biol Chem
       2007; 282(22): 16006-15.
       [http://dx.doi.org/10.1074/jbc.M611040200] [PMID: 17438334]

[93]   Kinnebrew MA, Buffie CG, Diehl GE, *et al.* Interleukin 23 production by intestinal
       CD103(+)CD11b(+) dendritic cells in response to bacterial flagellin enhances mucosal innate immune
       defense. Immunity 2012; 36(2): 276-87.
       [http://dx.doi.org/10.1016/j.immuni.2011.12.011] [PMID: 22306017]

[94]   Langowski JL, Zhang X, Wu L, *et al.* IL-23 promotes tumour incidence and growth. Nature 2006;
       442(7101): 461-5.
       [http://dx.doi.org/10.1038/nature04808] [PMID: 16688182]

[95]   Kamada N, Seo SU, Chen GY, Núñez G. Role of the gut microbiota in immunity and inflammatory
       disease. Nat Rev Immunol 2013; 13(5): 321-35.
       [http://dx.doi.org/10.1038/nri3430] [PMID: 23618829]

[96]   Wang JL, Chang CH, Lin JW, Wu LC, Chuang LM, Lai MS. Infection, antibiotic therapy and risk of
       colorectal cancer: a nationwide nested case-control study in patients with Type 2 diabetes mellitus. Int
       J Cancer 2014; 135(4): 956-67.
       [http://dx.doi.org/10.1002/ijc.28738] [PMID: 24470385]

[97]   Bonnet M, Buc E, Sauvanet P, *et al.* Colonization of the human gut by *E. coli* and colorectal cancer
       risk. Clin Cancer Res 2014; 20(4): 859-67.
       [http://dx.doi.org/10.1158/1078-0432.CCR-13-1343] [PMID: 24334760]

[98]   Louis P, Hold GL, Flint HJ. The gut microbiota, bacterial metabolites and colorectal cancer. Nat Rev
       Microbiol 2014; 12(10): 661-72.
       [http://dx.doi.org/10.1038/nrmicro3344] [PMID: 25198138]

[99]   Xuan C, Shamonki JM, Chung A, *et al.* Microbial dysbiosis is associated with human breast cancer.
       PLoS One 2014; 9(1): e83744.
       [http://dx.doi.org/10.1371/journal.pone.0083744] [PMID: 24421902]

[100] Velicer CM, Heckbert SR, Lampe JW, Potter JD, Robertson CA, Taplin SH. Antibiotic use in relation
       to the risk of breast cancer. JAMA 2004; 291(7): 827-35.
       [http://dx.doi.org/10.1001/jama.291.7.827] [PMID: 14970061]

[101] Correa P, Houghton J. Carcinogenesis of *Helicobacter pylori.* Gastroenterology 2007; 133(2): 659-72.
       [http://dx.doi.org/10.1053/j.gastro.2007.06.026] [PMID: 17681184]

[102] Roth KA, Kapadia SB, Martin SM, Lorenz RG. Cellular immune responses are essential for the

development of *Helicobacter felis*-associated gastric pathology. J Immunol 1999; 163(3): 1490-7. [PMID: 10415051]

[103] Mohammadi M, Czinn S, Redline R, Nedrud J. Helicobacter-specific cell-mediated immune responses display a predominant Th1 phenotype and promote a delayed-type hypersensitivity response in the stomachs of mice. J Immunol 1996; 156(12): 4729-38. [PMID: 8648119]

[104] Mannick EE, Bravo LE, Zarama G, *et al.* Inducible nitric oxide synthase, nitrotyrosine, and apoptosis in *Helicobacter pylori* gastritis: effect of antibiotics and antioxidants. Cancer Res 1996; 56(14): 3238-43. [PMID: 8764115]

[105] Bartsch H, Nair J. Chronic inflammation and oxidative stress in the genesis and perpetuation of cancer: role of lipid peroxidation, DNA damage, and repair. Langenbecks Arch Surg 2006; 391(5): 499-510. [http://dx.doi.org/10.1007/s00423-006-0073-1] [PMID: 16909291]

[106] Manzo BA, Crabtree JE, Fiona Campbell M, *et al. Helicobacter pylori* regulates the expression of inhibitors of DNA binding (Id) proteins by gastric epithelial cells. Microbes Infect 2006; 8(4): 1064-74. [http://dx.doi.org/10.1016/j.micinf.2005.11.003] [PMID: 16473539]

[107] Watanabe T, Tada M, Nagai H, Sasaki S, Nakao M. *Helicobacter pylori* infection induces gastric cancer in mongolian gerbils. Gastroenterology 1998; 115(3): 642-8. [http://dx.doi.org/10.1016/S0016-5085(98)70143-X] [PMID: 9721161]

[108] Wang TC, Goldenring JR, Dangler C, *et al.* Mice lacking secretory phospholipase A2 show altered apoptosis and differentiation with *Helicobacter felis* infection. Gastroenterology 1998; 114(4): 675-89. [http://dx.doi.org/10.1016/S0016-5085(98)70581-5] [PMID: 9516388]

[109] Moen EL, Wen S, Anwar T, *et al.* Regulation of RKIP function by *Helicobacter pylori* in gastric cancer. PLoS One 2012; 7(5): e37819. [http://dx.doi.org/10.1371/journal.pone.0037819] [PMID: 22662230]

[110] Shin CM, Kim N, Lee HS, *et al.* Changes in aberrant DNA methylation after *Helicobacter pylori* eradication: a long-term follow-up study. Int J Cancer 2013; 133(9): 2034-42. [http://dx.doi.org/10.1002/ijc.28219] [PMID: 23595635]

[111] Giannakis M, Chen SL, Karam SM, Engstrand L, Gordon JI. *Helicobacter pylori* evolution during progression from chronic atrophic gastritis to gastric cancer and its impact on gastric stem cells. Proc Natl Acad Sci USA 2008; 105(11): 4358-63. [http://dx.doi.org/10.1073/pnas.0800668105] [PMID: 18332421]

[112] Osaki T, Matsuki T, Asahara T, *et al.* Comparative analysis of gastric bacterial microbiota in Mongolian gerbils after long-term infection with *Helicobacter pylori.* Microb Pathog 2012; 53(1): 12-8. [http://dx.doi.org/10.1016/j.micpath.2012.03.008] [PMID: 22783557]

[113] Zaman C, Osaki T, Hanawa T, Yonezawa H, Kurata S, Kamiya S. Analysis of the microbial ecology between *Helicobacter pylori* and the gastric microbiota of Mongolian gerbils. J Med Microbiol 2014; 63(Pt 1): 129-37. [http://dx.doi.org/10.1099/jmm.0.061135-0] [PMID: 24164959]

[114] Aviles-Jimenez F, Vazquez-Jimenez F, Medrano-Guzman R, Mantilla A, Torres J. Stomach microbiota composition varies between patients with non-atrophic gastritis and patients with intestinal type of gastric cancer. Sci Rep 2014; 4: 4202. [http://dx.doi.org/10.1038/srep04202] [PMID: 24569566]

[115] Dicksved J, Lindberg M, Rosenquist M, Enroth H, Jansson JK, Engstrand L. Molecular characterization of the stomach microbiota in patients with gastric cancer and in controls. J Med Microbiol 2009; 58(Pt 4): 509-16.

[http://dx.doi.org/10.1099/jmm.0.007302-0] [PMID: 19273648]

[116]   Yang L, Chaudhary N, Baghdadi J, Pei Z. Microbiome in reflux disorders and esophageal adenocarcinoma. Cancer J 2014; 20(3): 207-10.
        [http://dx.doi.org/10.1097/PPO.0000000000000044] [PMID: 24855009]

[117]   Anderson LA, Murphy SJ, Johnston BT, *et al.* Relationship between *Helicobacter pylori* infection and gastric atrophy and the stages of the oesophageal inflammation, metaplasia, adenocarcinoma sequence: results from the FINBAR case-control study. Gut 2008; 57(6): 734-9.
        [http://dx.doi.org/10.1136/gut.2007.132662] [PMID: 18025067]

[118]   Enany S, Abdalla S. *In vitro* antagonistic activity of Lactobacillus casei against Helicobacter pylori. Braz J Microbiol 2015; 46(4): 1201-6.
        [http://dx.doi.org/10.1590/S1517-838246420140675] [PMID: 26691482]

[119]   Narikiyo M, Tanabe C, Yamada Y, *et al.* Frequent and preferential infection of *Treponema denticola, Streptococcus mitis*, and *Streptococcus anginosus* in esophageal cancers. Cancer Sci 2004; 95(7): 569-74.
        [http://dx.doi.org/10.1111/j.1349-7006.2004.tb02488.x] [PMID: 15245592]

[120]   Rowland IR. The role of the gastrointestinal microbiota in colorectal cancer. Curr Pharm Des 2009; 15(13): 1524-7.
        [http://dx.doi.org/10.2174/138161209788168191] [PMID: 19442169]

[121]   Polk DB, Peek RM Jr. *Helicobacter pylori*: gastric cancer and beyond. Nat Rev Cancer 2010; 10(6): 403-14.
        [http://dx.doi.org/10.1038/nrc2857] [PMID: 20495574]

[122]   Aviles-Jimenez F, Vazquez-Jimenez F, Medrano-Guzman R, Mantilla A, Torres J. Stomach microbiota composition varies between patients with non-atrophic gastritis and patients with intestinal type of gastric cancer. Sci Rep 2014; 4: 4202.
        [http://dx.doi.org/10.1038/srep04202] [PMID: 24569566]

[123]   Russo E, Taddei A, Ringressi MN, Ricci F, Amedei A. The interplay between the microbiome and the adaptive immune response in cancer development. Therap Adv Gastroenterol 2016; 9(4): 594-605.
        [http://dx.doi.org/10.1177/1756283X16635082] [PMID: 27366226]

[124]   Dejea CM, Wick EC, Hechenbleikner EM, *et al.* Microbiota organization is a distinct feature of proximal colorectal cancers. Proc Natl Acad Sci USA 2014; 111(51): 18321-6.
        [http://dx.doi.org/10.1073/pnas.1406199111] [PMID: 25489084]

[125]   Ogino S, Galon J, Fuchs CS, Dranoff G. Cancer immunology--analysis of host and tumor factors for personalized medicine. Nat Rev Clin Oncol 2011; 8(12): 711-9.
        [http://dx.doi.org/10.1038/nrclinonc.2011.122] [PMID: 21826083]

[126]   Warren RL, Freeman DJ, Pleasance S, *et al.* Co-occurrence of anaerobic bacteria in colorectal carcinomas. Microbiome 2013; 1(1): 16.
        [http://dx.doi.org/10.1186/2049-2618-1-16] [PMID: 24450771]

[127]   Parkin DM. The global health burden of infection-associated cancers in the year 2002. Int J Cancer 2006; 118(12): 3030-44.
        [http://dx.doi.org/10.1002/ijc.21731] [PMID: 16404738]

[128]   Jemal A, Siegel R, Ward E, Hao Y, Xu J, Thun MJ. Cancer statistics, 2009. CA Cancer J Clin 2009; 59(4): 225-49.
        [http://dx.doi.org/10.3322/caac.20006] [PMID: 19474385]

[129]   Rutter M, Saunders B, Wilkinson K, *et al.* Severity of inflammation is a risk factor for colorectal neoplasia in ulcerative colitis. Gastroenterology 2004; 126(2): 451-9.
        [http://dx.doi.org/10.1053/j.gastro.2003.11.010] [PMID: 14762782]

[130]   Akin H, Tözün N. Diet, microbiota, and colorectal cancer. J Clin Gastroenterol 2014; 48 (Suppl. 1): S67-9.

[http://dx.doi.org/10.1097/MCG.0000000000000252] [PMID: 25291132]

[131] Zhang MM, Cheng JQ, Xia L, Lu YR, Wu XT. Monitoring intestinal microbiota profile: a promising method for the ultraearly detection of colorectal cancer. Med Hypotheses 2011; 76(5): 670-2.
       [http://dx.doi.org/10.1016/j.mehy.2011.01.028] [PMID: 21310543]

[132] Serban DE. The gut microbiota in the metagenomics era: sometimes a friend, sometimes a foe. Roum Arch Microbiol Immunol 2011; 70(3): 134-40.
       [PMID: 22570928]

[133] Thomas LV, Ockhuizen T. New insights into the impact of the intestinal microbiota on health and disease: a symposium report. Br J Nutr 2012; 107 (Suppl. 1): S1-S13.
       [http://dx.doi.org/10.1017/S0007114511006970] [PMID: 22260731]

[134] Marchesi JR, Dutilh BE, Hall N, *et al.* Towards the human colorectal cancer microbiome. PLoS One 2011; 6(5): e20447.
       [http://dx.doi.org/10.1371/journal.pone.0020447] [PMID: 21647227]

[135] Rafter JJ, Child P, Anderson AM, Alder R, Eng V, Bruce WR. Cellular toxicity of fecal water depends on diet. Am J Clin Nutr 1987; 45(3): 559-63.
       [PMID: 3030089]

[136] de Kok TM, van Faassen A, Glinghammar B, *et al.* Bile acid concentrations, cytotoxicity, and pH of fecal water from patients with colorectal adenomas. Dig Dis Sci 1999; 44(11): 2218-25.
       [http://dx.doi.org/10.1023/A:1026644418142] [PMID: 10573365]

[137] Venturi M, Hambly RJ, Glinghammar B, Rafter JJ, Rowland IR. Genotoxic activity in human faecal water and the role of bile acids: a study using the alkaline comet assay. Carcinogenesis 1997; 18(12): 2353-9.
       [http://dx.doi.org/10.1093/carcin/18.12.2353] [PMID: 9450481]

[138] Garrett WS, Punit S, Gallini CA, *et al.* Colitis-associated colorectal cancer driven by T-bet deficiency in dendritic cells. Cancer Cell 2009; 16(3): 208-19.
       [http://dx.doi.org/10.1016/j.ccr.2009.07.015] [PMID: 19732721]

[139] Horie H, Kanazawa K, Okada M, Narushima S, Itoh K, Terada A. Effects of intestinal bacteria on the development of colonic neoplasm: an experimental study. Eur J Cancer Prev 1999; 8(3): 237-45.
       [http://dx.doi.org/10.1097/00008469-199906000-00012] [PMID: 10443953]

[140] Kado S, Uchida K, Funabashi H, *et al.* Intestinal microflora are necessary for development of spontaneous adenocarcinoma of the large intestine in T-cell receptor beta chain and p53 double-knockout mice. Cancer Res 2001; 61(6): 2395-8.
       [PMID: 11289103]

[141] Gao Z, Guo B, Gao R, Zhu Q, Qin H. Microbiota disbiosis is associated with colorectal cancer. Front Microbiol 2015; 6: 20.
       [http://dx.doi.org/10.3389/fmicb.2015.00020] [PMID: 25699023]

[142] Hope ME, Hold GL, Kain R, El-Omar EM. Sporadic colorectal cancer--role of the commensal microbiota. FEMS Microbiol Lett 2005; 244(1): 1-7.
       [http://dx.doi.org/10.1016/j.femsle.2005.01.029] [PMID: 15727814]

[143] Moore WE, Moore LH. Intestinal floras of populations that have a high risk of colon cancer. Appl Environ Microbiol 1995; 61(9): 3202-7.
       [PMID: 7574628]

[144] Scanlan PD, Shanahan F, Clune Y, *et al.* Culture-independent analysis of the gut microbiota in colorectal cancer and polyposis. Environ Microbiol 2008; 10(3): 789-98.
       [http://dx.doi.org/10.1111/j.1462-2920.2007.01503.x] [PMID: 18237311]

[145] Wang T, Cai G, Qiu Y, *et al.* Structural segregation of gut microbiota between colorectal cancer patients and healthy volunteers. ISME J 2012; 6(2): 320-9.
       [http://dx.doi.org/10.1038/ismej.2011.109] [PMID: 21850056]

[146] Abdulamir AS, Hafidh RR, Abu Bakar F. The association of *Streptococcus bovis/gallolyticus* with colorectal tumors: the nature and the underlying mechanisms of its etiological role. J Exp Clin Cancer Res 2011; 30: 11.
[http://dx.doi.org/10.1186/1756-9966-30-11] [PMID: 21247505]

[147] Tjalsma H, Schöller-Guinard M, Lasonder E, Ruers TJ, Willems HL, Swinkels DW. Profiling the humoral immune response in colon cancer patients: diagnostic antigens from *Streptococcus bovis*. Int J Cancer 2006; 119(9): 2127-35.
[http://dx.doi.org/10.1002/ijc.22116] [PMID: 16841330]

[148] Gueimonde M, Ouwehand A, Huhtinen H, Salminen E, Salminen S. Qualitative and quantitative analyses of the bifidobacterial microbiota in the colonic mucosa of patients with colorectal cancer, diverticulitis and inflammatory bowel disease. World J Gastroenterol 2007; 13(29): 3985-9.
[http://dx.doi.org/10.3748/wjg.v13.i29.3985] [PMID: 17663515]

[149] Sobhani I, Tap J, Roudot-Thoraval F, *et al.* Microbial dysbiosis in colorectal cancer (CRC) patients. PLoS One 2011; 6(1): e16393.
[http://dx.doi.org/10.1371/journal.pone.0016393] [PMID: 21297998]

[150] Shen XJ, Rawls JF, Randall T, *et al.* Molecular characterization of mucosal adherent bacteria and associations with colorectal adenomas. Gut Microbes 2010; 1(3): 138-47.
[http://dx.doi.org/10.4161/gmic.1.3.12360] [PMID: 20740058]

[151] Pagnini C, Corleto VD, Mangoni ML, *et al.* Alteration of local microflora and α-defensins hyper-production in colonic adenoma mucosa. J Clin Gastroenterol 2011; 45(7): 602-10.
[http://dx.doi.org/10.1097/MCG.0b013e31820abf29] [PMID: 21346603]

[152] Jobin C. Colorectal cancer: looking for answers in the microbiota. Cancer Discov 2013; 3(4): 384-7.
[http://dx.doi.org/10.1158/2159-8290.CD-13-0042] [PMID: 23580283]

[153] Winter SE, Winter MG, Xavier MN, *et al.* Host-derived nitrate boosts growth of *E. coli* in the inflamed gut. Science 2013; 339(6120): 708-11.
[http://dx.doi.org/10.1126/science.1232467] [PMID: 23393266]

[154] Brenchley JM, Douek DC. Microbial translocation across the GI tract. Annu Rev Immunol 2012; 30: 149-73.
[http://dx.doi.org/10.1146/annurev-immunol-020711-075001] [PMID: 22224779]

[155] Pimentel-Nunes P, Teixeira AL, Pereira C, *et al.* Functional polymorphisms of Toll-like receptors 2 and 4 alter the risk for colorectal carcinoma in Europeans. Dig Liver Dis 2013; 45(1): 63-9.
[http://dx.doi.org/10.1016/j.dld.2012.08.006] [PMID: 22999059]

[156] Zubair A, Frieri M. Role of nuclear factor-κB in breast and colorectal cancer. Curr Allergy Asthma Rep 2013; 13(1): 44-9.
[http://dx.doi.org/10.1007/s11882-012-0300-5] [PMID: 22956391]

[157] Neufert C, Becker C, Türeci Ö, *et al.* Tumor fibroblast-derived epiregulin promotes growth of colitis-associated neoplasms through ERK. J Clin Invest 2013; 123(4): 1428-43.
[http://dx.doi.org/10.1172/JCI63748] [PMID: 23549083]

[158] Couturier-Maillard A, Secher T, Rehman A, *et al.* NOD2-mediated dysbiosis predisposes mice to transmissible colitis and colorectal cancer. J Clin Invest 2013; 123(2): 700-11.
[PMID: 23281400]

[159] Shanahan MT, Carroll IM, Grossniklaus E, White A, von Furstenberg RJ, Barner R, *et al.* Mouse Paneth cell antimicrobial function is independent of Nod2. Gut 2013.
[PMID: 23512834]

[160] Nagi RS, Bhat AS, Kumar H. Cancer: a tale of aberrant PRR response. Front Immunol 2014; 5: 161.
[http://dx.doi.org/10.3389/fimmu.2014.00161] [PMID: 24782866]

[161] Han YW. *Fusobacterium nucleatum*: a commensal-turned pathogen. Curr Opin Microbiol 2015; 23:

141-7.
[http://dx.doi.org/10.1016/j.mib.2014.11.013] [PMID: 25576662]

[162] McCoy AN, Araújo-Pérez F, Azcárate-Peril A, Yeh JJ, Sandler RS, Keku TO. *Fusobacterium* is associated with colorectal adenomas. PLoS One 2013; 8(1): e53653.
[http://dx.doi.org/10.1371/journal.pone.0053653] [PMID: 23335968]

[163] Ito M, Kanno S, Nosho K, *et al.* Association of *Fusobacterium nucleatum* with clinical and molecular features in colorectal serrated pathway. Int J Cancer 2015; 137(6): 1258-68.
[http://dx.doi.org/10.1002/ijc.29488] [PMID: 25703934]

[164] Flanagan L, Schmid J, Ebert M, *et al. Fusobacterium nucleatum* associates with stages of colorectal neoplasia development, colorectal cancer and disease outcome. Eur J Clin Microbiol Infect Dis 2014; 33(8): 1381-90.
[http://dx.doi.org/10.1007/s10096-014-2081-3] [PMID: 24599709]

[165] Castellarin M, Warren RL, Freeman JD, *et al. Fusobacterium nucleatum* infection is prevalent in human colorectal carcinoma. Genome Res 2012; 22(2): 299-306.
[http://dx.doi.org/10.1101/gr.126516.111] [PMID: 22009989]

[166] Kostic AD, Gevers D, Pedamallu CS, *et al.* Genomic analysis identifies association of *Fusobacterium* with colorectal carcinoma. Genome Res 2012; 22(2): 292-8.
[http://dx.doi.org/10.1101/gr.126573.111] [PMID: 22009990]

[167] Rubinstein MR, Wang X, Liu W, Hao Y, Cai G, Han YW. *Fusobacterium nucleatum* promotes colorectal carcinogenesis by modulating E-cadherin/β-catenin signaling *via* its FadA adhesin. Cell Host Microbe 2013; 14(2): 195-206.
[http://dx.doi.org/10.1016/j.chom.2013.07.012] [PMID: 23954158]

[168] Kostic AD, Chun E, Robertson L, *et al. Fusobacterium nucleatum* potentiates intestinal tumorigenesis and modulates the tumor-immune microenvironment. Cell Host Microbe 2013; 14(2): 207-15.
[http://dx.doi.org/10.1016/j.chom.2013.07.007] [PMID: 23954159]

[169] Gur C, Ibrahim Y, Isaacson B, *et al.* Binding of the Fap2 protein of *Fusobacterium nucleatum* to human inhibitory receptor TIGIT protects tumors from immune cell attack. Immunity 2015; 42(2): 344-55.
[http://dx.doi.org/10.1016/j.immuni.2015.01.010] [PMID: 25680274]

[170] Garrett WS. Cancer and the microbiota. Science 2015; 348(6230): 80-6.
[http://dx.doi.org/10.1126/science.aaa4972] [PMID: 25838377]

[171] Sokol SY. Wnt signaling and dorso-ventral axis specification in vertebrates. Curr Opin Genet Dev 1999; 9(4): 405-10.
[http://dx.doi.org/10.1016/S0959-437X(99)80061-6] [PMID: 10449345]

[172] Sears CL. Enterotoxigenic *Bacteroides fragilis*: a rogue among symbiotes. Clin Microbiol Rev 2009; 22(2): 349-69.
[http://dx.doi.org/10.1128/CMR.00053-08] [PMID: 19366918]

[173] Shiryaev SA, Remacle AG, Chernov AV, *et al.* Substrate cleavage profiling suggests a distinct function of *Bacteroides fragilis* metalloproteinases (fragilysin and metalloproteinase II) at the microbiome-inflammation-cancer interface. J Biol Chem 2013; 288(48): 34956-67.
[http://dx.doi.org/10.1074/jbc.M113.516153] [PMID: 24145028]

[174] Tosolini M, Kirilovsky A, Mlecnik B, *et al.* Clinical impact of different classes of infiltrating T cytotoxic and helper cells (Th1, th2, treg, th17) in patients with colorectal cancer. Cancer Res 2011; 71(4): 1263-71.
[http://dx.doi.org/10.1158/0008-5472.CAN-10-2907] [PMID: 21303976]

[175] Goodwin AC, Destefano Shields CE, Wu S, *et al.* Polyamine catabolism contributes to enterotoxigenic *Bacteroides fragilis*-induced colon tumorigenesis. Proc Natl Acad Sci USA 2011; 108(37): 15354-9.
[http://dx.doi.org/10.1073/pnas.1010203108] [PMID: 21876161]

[176] Mirza NN, McCloud JM, Cheetham MJ. *Clostridium septicum* sepsis and colorectal cancer - a reminder. World J Surg Oncol 2009; 7: 73.
[http://dx.doi.org/10.1186/1477-7819-7-73] [PMID: 19807912]

[177] Hermsen JL, Schurr MJ, Kudsk KA, Faucher LD. Phenotyping *Clostridium septicum* infection: a surgeon's infectious disease. J Surg Res 2008; 148(1): 67-76.
[http://dx.doi.org/10.1016/j.jss.2008.02.027] [PMID: 18570933]

[178] Abdulamir AS, Hafidh RR, Bakar FA. Molecular detection, quantification, and isolation of Streptococcus gallolyticus bacteria colonizing colorectal tumors: inflammation-driven potential of carcinogenesis *via* IL-1, COX-2, and IL-8. Mol Cancer 2010; 9: 249.
[http://dx.doi.org/10.1186/1476-4598-9-249] [PMID: 20846456]

[179] Boleij A, van Gelder MM, Swinkels DW, Tjalsma H. Clinical Importance of *Streptococcus gallolyticus* infection among colorectal cancer patients: systematic review and meta-analysis. Clin Infect Dis 2011; 53(9): 870-8.
[http://dx.doi.org/10.1093/cid/cir609] [PMID: 21960713]

[180] Huycke MM, Abrams V, Moore DR. *Enterococcus faecalis* produces extracellular superoxide and hydrogen peroxide that damages colonic epithelial cell DNA. Carcinogenesis 2002; 23(3): 529-36.
[http://dx.doi.org/10.1093/carcin/23.3.529] [PMID: 11895869]

[181] Wang X, Huycke MM. Extracellular superoxide production by *Enterococcus faecalis* promotes chromosomal instability in mammalian cells. Gastroenterology 2007; 132(2): 551-61.
[http://dx.doi.org/10.1053/j.gastro.2006.11.040] [PMID: 17258726]

[182] Sanapareddy N, Legge RM, Jovov B, *et al.* Increased rectal microbial richness is associated with the presence of colorectal adenomas in humans. ISME J 2012; 6(10): 1858-68.
[http://dx.doi.org/10.1038/ismej.2012.43] [PMID: 22622349]

[183] Tanaka N, Che FS, Watanabe N, Fujiwara S, Takayama S, Isogai A. Flagellin from an incompatible strain of *Acidovorax avenae* mediates H2O2 generation accompanying hypersensitive cell death and expression of PAL, Cht-1, and PBZ1, but not of Lox in rice. Mol Plant Microbe Interact 2003; 16(5): 422-8.
[http://dx.doi.org/10.1094/MPMI.2003.16.5.422] [PMID: 12744513]

[184] Takakura Y, Che FS, Ishida Y, *et al.* Expression of a bacterial flagellin gene triggers plant immune responses and confers disease resistance in transgenic rice plants. Mol Plant Pathol 2008; 9(4): 525-9.
[http://dx.doi.org/10.1111/j.1364-3703.2008.00477.x] [PMID: 18705865]

[185] Cuevas-Ramos G, Petit CR, Marcq I, Boury M, Oswald E, Nougayrède JP. *Escherichia coli* induces DNA damage *in vivo* and triggers genomic instability in mammalian cells. Proc Natl Acad Sci USA 2010; 107(25): 11537-42.
[http://dx.doi.org/10.1073/pnas.1001261107] [PMID: 20534522]

[186] Arthur JC, Perez-Chanona E, Mühlbauer M, *et al.* Intestinal inflammation targets cancer-inducing activity of the microbiota. Science 2012; 338(6103): 120-3.
[http://dx.doi.org/10.1126/science.1224820] [PMID: 22903521]

[187] Bingham SA. Diet and colorectal cancer prevention. Biochem Soc Trans 2000; 28(2): 12-6.
[http://dx.doi.org/10.1042/bst0280012] [PMID: 10816091]

[188] O'Keefe SJ. Nutrition and colonic health: the critical role of the microbiota. Curr Opin Gastroenterol 2008; 24(1): 51-8.
[http://dx.doi.org/10.1097/MOG.0b013e3282f323f3] [PMID: 18043233]

[189] Ridlon JM, Kang DJ, Hylemon PB, Bajaj JS. Bile acids and the gut microbiome. Curr Opin Gastroenterol 2014; 30(3): 332-8.
[http://dx.doi.org/10.1097/MOG.0000000000000057] [PMID: 24625896]

[190] Barrasa JI, Olmo N, Lizarbe MA, Turnay J. Bile acids in the colon, from healthy to cytotoxic molecules. Toxicol In vitro 2013; 27(2): 964-77.

[http://dx.doi.org/10.1016/j.tiv.2012.12.020] [PMID: 23274766]

[191]   Bernstein C, Holubec H, Bhattacharyya AK, *et al.* Carcinogenicity of deoxycholate, a secondary bile acid. Arch Toxicol 2011; 85(8): 863-71.
        [http://dx.doi.org/10.1007/s00204-011-0648-7] [PMID: 21267546]

[192]   Gibson GR, Macfarlane GT, Cummings JH. Sulphate reducing bacteria and hydrogen metabolism in the human large intestine. Gut 1993; 34(4): 437-9.
        [http://dx.doi.org/10.1136/gut.34.4.437] [PMID: 8491386]

[193]   Sharma C. Young, M. Mshvildadze, J. Neu, Intestinal microbiota: does it play a role in diseases of the neonate? Neoreviews 2009; 10(4): 166-79.
        [http://dx.doi.org/10.1542/neo.10-4-e166]

[194]   Shukla VK, Tiwari SC, Roy SK. Biliary bile acids in cholelithiasis and carcinoma of the gall bladder. Eur J Cancer Prev 1993; 2(2): 155-60.
        [http://dx.doi.org/10.1097/00008469-199303000-00008] [PMID: 8461866]

[195]   Bindels LB, Porporato P, Dewulf EM, *et al.* Gut microbiota-derived propionate reduces cancer cell proliferation in the liver. Br J Cancer 2012; 107(8): 1337-44.
        [http://dx.doi.org/10.1038/bjc.2012.409] [PMID: 22976799]

[196]   Zhang JP, Yan J, Xu J, *et al.* Increased intratumoral IL-17-producing cells correlate with poor survival in hepatocellular carcinoma patients. J Hepatol 2009; 50(5): 980-9.
        [http://dx.doi.org/10.1016/j.jhep.2008.12.033] [PMID: 19329213]

[197]   Ivanov II, Atarashi K, Manel N, *et al.* Induction of intestinal Th17 cells by segmented filamentous bacteria. Cell 2009; 139(3): 485-98.
        [http://dx.doi.org/10.1016/j.cell.2009.09.033] [PMID: 19836068]

[198]   Hariharan D, Saied A, Kocher HM. Analysis of mortality rates for pancreatic cancer across the world. HPB 2008; 10(1): 58-62.
        [http://dx.doi.org/10.1080/13651820701883148] [PMID: 18695761]

[199]   Jemal A, Bray F, Center MM, Ferlay J, Ward E, Forman D. Global cancer statistics. CA Cancer J Clin 2011; 61(2): 69-90.
        [http://dx.doi.org/10.3322/caac.20107] [PMID: 21296855]

[200]   Hidalgo M, Cascinu S, Kleeff J, *et al.* Addressing the challenges of pancreatic cancer: future directions for improving outcomes. Pancreatology 2015; 15(1): 8-18.
        [http://dx.doi.org/10.1016/j.pan.2014.10.001] [PMID: 25547205]

[201]   Löhr M. Is it possible to survive pancreatic cancer? Nat Clin Pract Gastroenterol Hepatol 2006; 3(5): 236-7.
        [http://dx.doi.org/10.1038/ncpgasthep0469] [PMID: 16672986]

[202]   McKenna LR, Edil BH. Update on pancreatic neuroendocrine tumors. Gland Surg 2014; 3(4): 258-75.
        [PMID: 25493258]

[203]   Zambirinis CP, Pushalkar S, Saxena D, Miller G. Pancreatic cancer, inflammation, and microbiome. Cancer J 2014; 20(3): 195-202.
        [http://dx.doi.org/10.1097/PPO.0000000000000045] [PMID: 24855007]

[204]   Mulkeen AL, Yoo PS, Cha C. Less common neoplasms of the pancreas. World J Gastroenterol 2006; 12(20): 3180-5.
        [http://dx.doi.org/10.3748/wjg.v12.i20.3180] [PMID: 16718837]

[205]   Kondo NI, Ikeda Y. Practical management and treatment of pancreatic neuroendocrine tumors. Gland Surg 2014; 3(4): 276-83.
        [PMID: 25493259]

[206]   Farrell JJ, Zhang L, Zhou H, *et al.* Variations of oral microbiota are associated with pancreatic diseases including pancreatic cancer. Gut 2012; 61(4): 582-8.

[http://dx.doi.org/10.1136/gutjnl-2011-300784] [PMID: 21994333]

[207]   Li Y, Kundu P, Seow SW, *et al.* Gut microbiota accelerate tumor growth *via* c-jun and STAT3 phosphorylation in APCMin/+ mice. Carcinogenesis 2012; 33(6): 1231-8.
[http://dx.doi.org/10.1093/carcin/bgs137] [PMID: 22461519]

[208]   Pour PM, Pandey KK, Batra SK. What is the origin of pancreatic adenocarcinoma? Mol Cancer 2003; 2: 13.
[http://dx.doi.org/10.1186/1476-4598-2-13] [PMID: 12636873]

[209]   Lindkvist B, Johansen D, Borgström A, Manjer J. A prospective study of Helicobacter pylori in relation to the risk for pancreatic cancer. BMC Cancer 2008; 8: 321.
[http://dx.doi.org/10.1186/1471-2407-8-321] [PMID: 18986545]

[210]   Moore PS, Chang Y. Why do viruses cause cancer? Highlights of the first century of human tumour virology. Nat Rev Cancer 2010; 10(12): 878-89.
[http://dx.doi.org/10.1038/nrc2961] [PMID: 21102637]

[211]   Balkwill F, Mantovani A. Inflammation and cancer: back to Virchow? Lancet 2001; 357(9255): 539-45.
[http://dx.doi.org/10.1016/S0140-6736(00)04046-0] [PMID: 11229684]

[212]   Risch HA, Lu L, Kidd MS, *et al.* Helicobacter pylori seropositivities and risk of pancreatic carcinoma. Cancer Epidemiol Biomarkers Prev 2014; 23(1): 172-8.
[http://dx.doi.org/10.1158/1055-9965.EPI-13-0447] [PMID: 24234587]

[213]   Yamanaka N, Morisaki T, Nakashima H, *et al.* Interleukin 1beta enhances invasive ability of gastric carcinoma through nuclear factor-kappaB activation. Clin Cancer Res 2004; 10(5): 1853-9.
[http://dx.doi.org/10.1158/1078-0432.CCR-03-0300] [PMID: 15014040]

[214]   Kojima M, Morisaki T, Izuhara K, *et al.* Lipopolysaccharide increases cyclo-oxygenase-2 expression in a colon carcinoma cell line through nuclear factor-kappa B activation. Oncogene 2000; 19(9): 1225-31.
[http://dx.doi.org/10.1038/sj.onc.1203427] [PMID: 10713711]

[215]   Ochi A, Nguyen AH, Bedrosian AS, *et al.* MyD88 inhibition amplifies dendritic cell capacity to promote pancreatic carcinogenesis *via* Th2 cells. J Exp Med 2012; 209(9): 1671-87.
[http://dx.doi.org/10.1084/jem.20111706] [PMID: 22908323]

[216]   Bordonaro M, Lazarova DL, Sartorelli AC. Butyrate and Wnt signaling: a possible solution to the puzzle of dietary fiber and colon cancer risk? Cell Cycle 2008; 7(9): 1178-83.
[http://dx.doi.org/10.4161/cc.7.9.5818]

[217]   Dronamraju SS, Coxhead JM, Kelly SB, Mathers JC. Differential antineoplastic effects of butyrate in cells with and without a functioning DNA mismatch repair. Nutr Cancer 2010; 62(1): 105-15.
[http://dx.doi.org/10.1080/01635580903191486] [PMID: 20043265]

[218]   Domokos M, Jakus J, Szeker K, *et al.* Butyrate-induced cell death and differentiation are associated with distinct patterns of ROS in HT29-derived human colon cancer cells. Dig Dis Sci 2010; 55(4): 920-30.
[http://dx.doi.org/10.1007/s10620-009-0820-6] [PMID: 19434493]

[219]   Scharlau D, Borowicki A, Habermann N, *et al.* Mechanisms of primary cancer prevention by butyrate and other products formed during gut flora-mediated fermentation of dietary fibre. Mutat Res 2009; 682(1): 39-53.
[http://dx.doi.org/10.1016/j.mrrev.2009.04.001] [PMID: 19383551]

[220]   Davie JR. Inhibition of histone deacetylase activity by butyrate. J Nutr 2003; 133(7) (Suppl.): 2485S-93S.
[PMID: 12840228]

[221]   Starnes CO. Coley's toxins in perspective. Nature 1992; 357(6373): 11-2.
[http://dx.doi.org/10.1038/357011a0] [PMID: 1574121]

[222]   Garaude J, Kent A, van Rooijen N, Blander JM. Simultaneous targeting of toll- and nod-like receptors induces effective tumor-specific immune responses. Sci Transl Med 2012; 4(120): 120ra16.
[http://dx.doi.org/10.1126/scitranslmed.3002868] [PMID: 22323829]

[223]   Viaud S, Saccheri F, Mignot G, *et al.* The intestinal microbiota modulates the anticancer immune effects of cyclophosphamide. Science 2013; 342(6161): 971-6.
[http://dx.doi.org/10.1126/science.1240537] [PMID: 24264990]

[224]   Honda K, Littman DR. The microbiome in infectious disease and inflammation. Annu Rev Immunol 2012; 30: 759-95.
[http://dx.doi.org/10.1146/annurev-immunol-020711-074937] [PMID: 22224764]

[225]   Huber S, Gagliani N, Esplugues E, *et al.* Th17 cells express interleukin-10 receptor and are controlled by Foxp3⁻ and Foxp3+ regulatory CD4+ T cells in an interleukin-10-dependent manner. Immunity 2011; 34(4): 554-65.
[http://dx.doi.org/10.1016/j.immuni.2011.01.020] [PMID: 21511184]

[226]   Erdman SE, Rao VP, Poutahidis T, *et al.* CD4(+)CD25(+) regulatory lymphocytes require interleukin 10 to interrupt colon carcinogenesis in mice. Cancer Res 2003; 63(18): 6042-50.
[PMID: 14522933]

[227]   Erdman SE, Sohn JJ, Rao VP, *et al.* CD4+CD25+ regulatory lymphocytes induce regression of intestinal tumors in ApcMin/+ mice. Cancer Res 2005; 65(10): 3998-4004.
[http://dx.doi.org/10.1158/0008-5472.CAN-04-3104] [PMID: 15899788]

[228]   Round JL, Lee SM, Li J, *et al.* The Toll-like receptor 2 pathway establishes colonization by a commensal of the human microbiota. Science 2011; 332(6032): 974-7.
[http://dx.doi.org/10.1126/science.1206095] [PMID: 21512004]

[229]   Atarashi K, Nishimura J, Shima T, *et al.* ATP drives lamina propria T(H)17 cell differentiation. Nature 2008; 455(7214): 808-12.
[http://dx.doi.org/10.1038/nature07240] [PMID: 18716618]

[230]   Holmes E, Kinross J, Gibson GR, *et al.* Therapeutic modulation of microbiota-host metabolic interactions. Sci Transl Med 2012; 4(137): 137rv6.
[http://dx.doi.org/10.1126/scitranslmed.3004244] [PMID: 22674556]

[231]   Langdon A, Crook N, Dantas G. The effects of antibiotics on the microbiome throughout development and alternative approaches for therapeutic modulation. Genome Med 2016; 8(1): 39.
[http://dx.doi.org/10.1186/s13073-016-0294-z] [PMID: 27074706]

[232]   Capurso G, Marignani M, Delle Fave G. Probiotics and the incidence of colorectal cancer: when evidence is not evident. Dig Liver Dis 2006; 38 (Suppl. 2): S277-82.
[http://dx.doi.org/10.1016/S1590-8658(07)60010-3] [PMID: 17259091]

[233]   Sang LX, Chang B, Zhang WL, Wu XM, Li XH, Jiang M. Remission induction and maintenance effect of probiotics on ulcerative colitis: a meta-analysis. World J Gastroenterol 2010; 16(15): 1908-15.
[http://dx.doi.org/10.3748/wjg.v16.i15.1908] [PMID: 20397271]

[234]   Klaenhammer TR, Kleerebezem M, Kopp MV, Rescigno M. The impact of probiotics and prebiotics on the immune system. Nat Rev Immunol 2012; 12(10): 728-34.
[http://dx.doi.org/10.1038/nri3312] [PMID: 23007572]

[235]   Bermúdez-Humarán LG, Aubry C, Motta JP, *et al. Engineering lactococci* and lactobacilli for human health. Curr Opin Microbiol 2013; 16(3): 278-83.
[http://dx.doi.org/10.1016/j.mib.2013.06.002] [PMID: 23850097]

[236]   Hardy H, Harris J, Lyon E, Beal J, Foey AD. Probiotics, prebiotics and immunomodulation of gut mucosal defences: homeostasis and immunopathology. Nutrients 2013; 5(6): 1869-912.
[http://dx.doi.org/10.3390/nu5061869] [PMID: 23760057]

[237]   Zitvogel L, Galluzzi L, Viaud S, *et al.* Cancer and the gut microbiota: an unexpected link. Sci Transl Med 2015; 7(271): 271ps1.
[http://dx.doi.org/10.1126/scitranslmed.3010473] [PMID: 25609166]

[238]   Khazaie K, Zadeh M, Khan MW, *et al.* Abating colon cancer polyposis by Lactobacillus acidophilus deficient in lipoteichoic acid. Proc Natl Acad Sci USA 2012; 109(26): 10462-7.
[http://dx.doi.org/10.1073/pnas.1207230109] [PMID: 22689992]

[239]   Mathipa MG, Thantsha MS. Probiotic engineering: towards development of robust probiotic strains with enhanced functional properties and for targeted control of enteric pathogens. Gut Pathog 2017; 9: 28.
[http://dx.doi.org/10.1186/s13099-017-0178-9] [PMID: 28491143]

[240]   de Moreno de LeBlanc A, del Carmen S, Chate JM, *et al.* Current Review of Genetically Modified Lactic Acid Bacteria for the Prevention and Treatment of Colitis Using Murine Models. Gastroenterol Res Pract 2015; 2015: 146972.
[http://dx.doi.org/10.1155/2015/146972]

[241]   Paulos CM, Wrzesinski C, Kaiser A, *et al.* Microbial translocation augments the function of adoptively transferred self/tumor-specific CD8+ T cells *via* TLR4 signaling. J Clin Invest 2007; 117(8): 2197-204.
[http://dx.doi.org/10.1172/JCI32205] [PMID: 17657310]

[242]   Pandey KR, Naik SR, Vakil BV. Probiotics, prebiotics and synbiotics- a review. J Food Sci Technol 2015; 52(12): 7577-87.
[http://dx.doi.org/10.1007/s13197-015-1921-1] [PMID: 26604335]

[243]   Taper HS, Roberfroid MB. Possible adjuvant cancer therapy by two prebiotics--inulin or oligofructose. in vivo 2005; 19(1): 201-4.
[PMID: 15796175]

[244]   Dos Reis SA, da Conceição LL, Siqueira NP, Rosa DD, da Silva LL, Peluzio MD. Review of the mechanisms of probiotic actions in the prevention of colorectal cancer. Nutr Res 2017; 37: 1-19.
[http://dx.doi.org/10.1016/j.nutres.2016.11.009] [PMID: 28215310]

[245]   König J, Siebenhaar A, Högenauer C, *et al.* Consensus report: faecal microbiota transfer - clinical applications and procedures. Aliment Pharmacol Ther 2017; 45(2): 222-39.
[http://dx.doi.org/10.1111/apt.13868] [PMID: 27891639]

[246]   Fischer M, Sipe B, Cheng YW, *et al.* Fecal microbiota transplant in severe and severe-complicated *Clostridium difficile*: A promising treatment approach. Gut Microbes 2016; 1-14.
[PMID: 28001467]

[247]   Moelling K, Broecker F. Fecal microbiota transplantation to fight *Clostridium difficile* infections and other intestinal diseases. Bacteriophage 2016; 6(4): e1251380.
[http://dx.doi.org/10.1080/21597081.2016.1251380] [PMID: 28090385]

CHAPTER 2

Towards Host Cell-Targeting Therapies to Treat Dengue Virus Infections

Cybele C. García[1,2]**, Verónica M. Quintana**[1]**, Viviana Castilla**[1] **and Elsa B. Damonte**[1,2,*]

[1] *Laboratorio de Virología, Departamento de Química Biológica, Facultad de Ciencias Exactas y Naturales, Universidad de Buenos Aires (UBA), Buenos Aires, Argentina*

[2] *IQUIBICEN, Consejo Nacional de Investigaciones Científicas y Técnicas (CONICET)-UBA, Buenos Aires. Argentina*

Abstract: Dengue virus (DENV), a member of the genus *Flavivirus* in the family *Flaviviridae*, is the causative agent of the major human viral infection transmitted by mosquitoes in the world with about 390 million annual infections. Recently, a tetravalent vaccine has been licensed for use in highly endemic countries but protective efficacy is not complete and equivalent against the four DENV serotypes. Specific therapeutics is not available at present and treatment is limited to symptomatic supportive care. The reliance of DENV on several host processes and molecules for productive infection highlights the targeting of a cellular factor as an attractive antiviral approach. Since many host requirements are shared by different pathogenic flaviviruses, like Zika virus, West Nile virus, yellow fever virus, Japanese encephalitis virus, tick-borne encephalitis virus, this strategy may provide a wide range effective inhibitory agent and also reduce the possible emergence of antiviral resistant variants. In fact, the few drugs just evaluated or in evaluation at this moment in clinical trials include the host cell-directed compounds chloroquine, lovastatin, prednisolone and celgosivir. This review focuses on the antiviral potential of host cell factors directly participating in the viral cycle of infection as well as those ones involved in the innate antiviral response triggered to restrict and control viral dissemination and pathogenesis.

Keywords: Antiviral, Dengue virus, Endocytosis, Flavivirus, Host target, Innate response, Interferon, Kinases, Lipid metabolism, Nucleotide metabolism, Protein processing, Receptors, Restriction factors, Translation, Ubiquitin proteasome pathway, Unfolded protein response.

* **Corresponding author Elsa B. Damonte:** Laboratorio de Virología, Departamento de Química Biológica, Facultad de Ciencias Exactas y Naturales, Universidad de Buenos Aires, Buenos Aires, Argentina; Tel/Fax: 5411-45763342; E-mail: edamonte@qb.fcen.uba.ar

INTRODUCTION

Dengue virus (DENV) is a member of *Flavivirus*, a genus of the family *Flaviviridae* composed of nearly 70 arthropod-borne viruses that cause important human diseases, such as yellow fever virus (YFV), West Nile virus (WNV), Zika virus (ZIKV), Japanese encephalitis virus (JEV) and tick-borne encephalitis virus (TBEV). In particular, DENV is the most widespread arbovirus and has re-emerged in the last decades as an increasingly important public health threat [1]. Over 2.5 billion people are at risk of DENV infection in more than 100 countries worldwide and it is estimated that 350 million apparent and inapparent infections occur each year [2]. Infection with DENV produces a wide spectrum of manifestations including asymptomatic condition, the mild dengue fever (DF), or severe forms, such as dengue hemorrhagic fever and dengue shock syndrome (DHF/DSS) which cause 25,000 deaths annually [3].

The virion is an enveloped particle containing a single stranded, positive sense RNA included in an inner nucleocapsid. The genome codes for a single polyprotein that is cleaved into three structural proteins (the capsid protein C, a small membrane protein M that matures from the precursor prM, and the envelope glycoprotein E) and seven nonstructural (NS) polypeptides (NS1, NS2A, NS2B, NS3, NS4A, NS4B, and NS5) with varied functions. There are four antigenically related serotypes (DENV-1 to DENV-4), which cocirculate in tropical and subtropical regions between their vectors, the mosquitoes *Aedes aegypti* and *Aedes albopictus*, and the vertebrate hosts.

Recently, a tetravalent vaccine has been licensed for use in endemic countries but protective efficacy is not complete and equivalent against the four DENV serotypes [4]. Specific therapeutics is not available at present and treatment is limited to symptomatic supportive care. On this basis, the search of antiviral agents for dengue treatment is an urgent need. The reliance of DENV on several host processes and molecules for productive infection highlights the targeting of a cellular factor as an attractive antiviral approach. This strategy regained interest in recent years since it may provide a wide range agent with inhibitory effectiveness against all the circulating pathogenic flaviviruses that share similar host requirements as well as for future emergent pathogens. Another advantage in comparison to classical viral-targeted compounds is a reduced challenge of selection for antiviral resistant variants, a frequent event during chemotherapy of RNA viruses due to their high genetic variation.

This review focuses on the antiviral potential of those host cell factors either directly participating in the viral cycle of infection or in the innate antiviral response triggered to control viral dissemination and pathogenesis, with emphasis in the cellular molecules and pathways that have been successfully tested with promising inhibitors or are considered appropriate for drug inhibition. A list of the presently tested DENV inhibitors and the corresponding target is summarized in Table **1**.

Table 1. Dengue virus inhibitors targeting host factors.

DENV inhibitor	Target	Serotype	References
Heparin, suramin	Interaction DENV-heparan sulfate (HS)	DENV-2	[8, 10, 12, 13]
PI88	Interaction DENV-HS	DENV-2	[13]
Chondroitin sulfate	Interaction DENV-HS	DENV-1 to 4	[14]
Curdlan sulfate	Interaction DENV-HS	DENV-1 to 4	[15]
K5 polysaccharide from *E. coli*	Interaction DENV-HS	DENV-2	[16]
Algal sulfated polysaccharides (galactans, mannans, fucoidans, glucans, carrageenans)	Interaction DENV-HS	DENV-1 to 4 (dissimilar inhibition)	[17 - 27, 29]
Plant lectins from *Hippeastrum hybrid, Galanthus nivalis* and *Urtica dioica*	Interaction DENV-DC-SIGN	DENV-1 to 4	[35, 36]
Glycomimetic DC-SIGN ligand	Interaction DENV-DC-SIGN	DENV-2	[37]
Chloroquine*	Low pH-induced membrane fusion	DENV-2	[40, 41, 44, 45]
Prochlorperazine	Clathrin-mediated endocytosis	DENV-2	[46]
Cerulenin, C-75, orlistat	Fatty acid synthase	DENV-2, 4	[52 - 55]
Statins*	Hydroxyl methyl glutaryl-CoA reductase	DENV-2	[57, 58, 61, 62]
U18666A	Cholesterol transport	DENV-2	[59]
Methyl-β-cyclodextrin	Cholesterol extraction	DENV-1 to 4	[60]
Nordihydroguaiaretic acid	Broad spectrum lipid reduction	DENV-4	[64]
PF-429242	subtilisin kexin isozyme-1/site-1 protease	DENV-1 to 4	[65]
Lactimidomycin	Polypeptide elongation	DENV-2	[67]
4-HPR	Unfolded protein response		[70 - 72]
UBEI-41, MG132, IU1, β-lactone, bortezomib	Ubiquitin-proteasome pathway		[73 - 76]
Ribavirin, mycophenolic acid, ETAR	Inosine monophosphate dehydrogenase	DENV-1 to 4	[77 - 85]
N-allyl acridones	Inosine monophosphate dehydrogenase (Partial)	DENV-1 to 4	[86, 87]

(Table 1) contd.....

DENV inhibitor	Target	Serotype	References
Brequinar, NITD-982	Dihydroorotate dehydrogenase	DENV-2	[88, 89]
PD98059, U0126, FR180204	ERK pathway	DENV-2	[95, 96, 99-102]
SP60125	JNK pathway	DENV-2	[97, 99, 106, 107]
SB203580	p38 pathway	DENV-2	[97, 98, 110, 111, 113]
CGP57380	ERK and p38 pathways	DENV-2	[98]
Dasatinib, AZD0530	Src, Abl and Fyn kinases	DENV-1 to 4	[114-116]
GNF-2	Abl kinase	DENV-2	[117]
Imidazo[1,2-b] pyridazine-inhibitors	AAK1	DENV-2	[118]
isothiazolo[5,4-b] pyridines inhibitors	GAK	DENV-2	[118]
Sunitinib and erlotinib	AAK1 and GAK	DENV-2	[118]
AR-12	PI3K/AKT pathway, GRP78 expression	DENV-2	[120]
Castanospermine, deoxynojirimycin, Kotanol, CM-10-18, celgosivir*, UV-4*	Endoplasmic reticulum α-glucosidase	DENV-1 to 4	[122-126, 128-135]
Peptidomimetic furin inhibitors, luteolin	Furin	DENV-1 to 4	[136-138]
Cavinafungin	Endoplasmic reticulum associated signal peptidase	DENV-1 to 4	[140]
Interferon type I	Innate antiviral response	DENV-1 to 4	[143]
Human heme oxygenase 1	Innate antiviral response	DENV-1 to 4	[160-161]
Schisandrin A	Innate antiviral response	DENV-1 to 4	[167]
Celastrol	Innate antiviral response	DENV-1 to 4	[168]
Agonists of IRF3-terminal pathways	Innate antiviral response	DENV-2	[169]
Salidroside	Innate antiviral response	DENV-2	[170]
Asunaprevir	Innate antiviral response	DENV-2	[171]
Sequence-specific RIG-I agonist	Innate antiviral response	DENV-2	[172]
TRIF-dependent responses inductor	Innate antiviral response	DENV-2	[173]
Helicase with zinc finger 2	Innate antiviral response	DENV-2	[174]
Purinergic receptor P2X7	Innate antiviral response	DENV-2	[175]
Extract from *Uncaria tomentosa, N brasiliensis Choisy, Uncaria guianensis*	Innate antiviral response	DENV-2	[176-178]

(Table 1) contd.....

DENV inhibitor	Target	Serotype	References
Extract from *Cissampelos Pareira Linn*	Innate antiviral response	DENV-1 to 4	[179]
Proteins encoded by ISGs	Innate antiviral response	DENV-2	[184, 185, 190-195]
Ivermectin	Nuclear-cytoplasmic trafficking	DENV-1 to 4	[196]
Promyelocytic leukemia protein	Innate antiviral response	DENV-2	[197]
Tetherin	Innate antiviral response	DENV-2	[198]

DC-SIGN: C-type lectin dendritic cell-specific intercellular adhesion molecule 3-grabbing nonintegrin ;4-HPR: retinoid N-(4-hydroxyphenyl) retinamide; ETAR: 1-β-D-ribofuranosyl-3-ethynyl- [1, 2, 4]triazole; ERK: extracellular signal-regulated kinase; JNK: c-Jun N-terminal kinase; AAK1: AP2-associated protein kinase 1; GAK: cyclin G–associated kinase; PI3K: phosphatidylinositol 3 kinase; GRP 78: glucose-regulated protein 78; IRF3: interferon regulatory factor 3; RIG-I: RNA helicase retinoic acid-inducible gene I; TRIF: Toll/IL-1 receptor domain-containing adaptor inducing IFN- β; ISGs: interferon stimulated genes. *Compounds tested in clinical trials.

INTERACTION WITH CELL RECEPTORS

Virus entry is attractive for antiviral attack because it represents the first barrier to suppress the beginning of infection and the blockade can be often established without cell uptake of the inhibitor. The events involved in DENV entry start with the virion binding to specific components of the plasma membrane surface, followed by the internalization into the cell by receptor-mediated endocytosis. After intracellular trafficking through the endo-lysosomal vesicles, fusion between viral and endosomal membranes occurs and the nucleocapsid is released into the cell cytoplasm. These sequential steps are driven by the interaction of the envelope E glycoprotein with several cellular factors that are suitable for antiviral intervention.

Multiple molecules have been reported as putative dengue receptors for the initial binding to the host cell. It is probably due to the wide spectrum of cell types from vertebrate and invertebrate hosts that DENV can infect as well as to the complexity of the virus entry involving sequential interactions of E protein first with abundantly disseminated attachment factors and then with more restricted specific receptors in the same cell [5 - 7]. Among these reported ligands, the heparan sulfate (HS) proteoglycans in a variety of mammalian cells and the C-type lectin dendritic cell-specific intercellular adhesion molecule 3-grabbing non-integrin (DC-SIGN) in dendritic cells are at present the best characterized and druggable molecules with proved relevance for DENV binding.

HS is a member of the sulfated glycosaminoglycan family very abundant on the surface and in the extracellular matrix of most mammalian cells. Since the participation of HS as an attachment factor to recruit DENV virions in the cell surface was demonstrated and simultaneously HS-binding sites were identified in E glycoprotein [8 - 11], several HS-mimetics molecules were evaluated and found able to block DENV infection. The effective compounds included heparin [8, 10, 12], suramin [8, 13], chondroitin sulfate [14], curdlan sulfate [15], derivatives of the K5 capsular polysaccharide of *Escherichia coli* [16] and several algal derived sulfated polysaccharides of diverse classes such as galactans [17 - 19], fucoidans [20, 21], mannans [21, 22], glucans [23] and carrageenans [19, 24, 25].

Structure-activity relationship studies carried out with different HS-like polysulfates have demonstrated the influence on inhibitory activity of diverse parameters, such as molecular weight, the number of repetitive units, the sugar composition and the charge density determined by the extent of sulfation and the position of the sulfate groups [15, 26, 27]. Most of these sulfated compounds have no detrimental effects on cell viability or growth neither present significant anticoagulant properties, resulting very selective and safe antiviral agents. However, a disadvantage exhibited by these compounds is the dependence of their antiviral activity with the DENV serotype: DENV-2 and DENV-3 infections are very efficiently inhibited in a broad range of mammalian cells whereas DENV-1 and DENV-4 require much higher compound concentration to achieve inhibition [15, 19, 21]. Furthermore, sulfated polysaccharides are less active in mosquito cells. Recently, it has been demonstrated that the cell type used to obtain DENV-2 stocks, mammalian or mosquito cells, can also affect the antiviral activity of HS-mimicking compounds [28]. All these differences may be ascribed to host-cell dependent variations in the entry mode of different serotypes [7].

Mechanistic studies demonstrated that carrageenans, galactans and curdlan sulfate act by preventing not only DENV-2 adsorption to the host cell but also they blocked the complete process of penetration and release of viral genome into cytoplasm [15, 24, 29]. The carrageenan was shown to prevent fusion of envelope-endosome membranes and uncoating without affecting the endosomal pH, but targeting the E glycoprotein. This was corroborated by analysis of carrageenan-resistant variants of DENV-2 that presented the mutation K126E, reducing the positive charge of the protein domain [30]. Furthermore, curdlan sulfate was able to prevent antibody-dependent enhancement (ADE)-mediated DENV infection in the human monocytic cell line THP-1 expressing Fc receptor [15], a very interesting property given the proposal of ADE as a main cause of the severe forms of dengue in patients sequentially infected with two DENV serotypes [31].

The antiviral activity of HS-mimetics against DENV was also demonstrated *in vivo*. The oligosaccharide PI-88, a mixture of highly sulfated mannose-containing di- to hexasaccharides, was assayed *in vitro* and in murine models of flavivirus infection. This low molecular weight compound did not show *in vitro* effectiveness but ameliorated disease in DENV-2 infected mice, providing a note of caution about the predictive accuracy of *in vitro* assays for the *in vivo* therapeutic activity [13].

Respect to DC-SIGN, it is a transmembrane protein highly expressed in immature dendritic cells (DC) that is able to bind diverse pathogens. Immature DC in the skin are believed to be the primary target cells during DENV infection, and after virus binding DC are activated to stimulate naïve T-cells and trigger the production of cytokines and chemokines. The presence of DC-SIGN is essential for DENV productive infection of DC [32]. It was shown that the high mannose N-glycan groups located at Asn67 on DENV E glycoprotein are responsible for the binding to the C-terminal carbohydrate recognition domain present in DC-SIGN [33, 34]. Thus, several carbohydrate-binding agents, such as the plant lectins from *Hippeastrum hybrid, Galanthus nivalis* and *Urtica dioica*, were found strong inhibitors of DENV infection in DC-SIGN-transfected cells and in monocyte-derived DC [35, 36]. These compounds prevented the attachment of the four DENV serotypes by interfering the interaction between DENV and DC-SIGN. In a more recent approach, a group of multivalent glycodendrimers that bear different carbohydrates or glycomimetic ligands were synthesized and a very efficient binding to DC-SIGN was demonstrated, opening a new avenue to improve the efficacy of a wide spectrum prophylactic treatment to block virus uptake [37].

As abovementioned, apart from HS and DC-SIGN several other molecules were described for DENV binding, but no consistent antiviral approaches have been reported.

ENDOCYTOSIS AND FUSION FOR UNCOATING

After the interaction with attachment and receptor molecules, DENV penetrates into the cell by endocytosis and finally virion uncoating is triggered by the acid pH of the endocytic vesicle. DENV particles are internalized *via* clathrin-mediated endocytosis in most studied mammalian cells [7], but non classical clathrin-independent pathways may also be exploited depending on the host cell and virus serotype [38, 39].

These cellular processes can be interfered with several well-known biochemical inhibitors. However, these drugs are mainly used as valuable tools to elucidate the molecular mechanisms of virus entry but their level of cytotoxicity excludes a possible application in antiviral therapy. An exceptional approach of intending the use of this type of inhibitors to combat DENV infections is represented by chloroquine. Chloroquine is a weak base that raises the pH of acidic intracellular vesicles. Alkalinization of endosomes by chloroquine may prevent the low pH-induced fusion of viral and endosomal membranes and block DENV uncoating, whereas the pH increase within the TGN may also affect furin-dependent virion maturation and release from the cell. In fact, the infection of Vero and human monocytic U937 cells with DENV-2 was inhibited by chloroquine, and a reduction in the level of pro-inflammatory cytokines was observed [40, 41]. Since chloroquine has been clinically used as antimalarial drug and also as a secondary drug to treat chronic inflammatory diseases such as rheumatoid arthritis and lupus erythematosus [42, 43], two independent randomized, placebo-controlled small clinical trials were intended in Vietnam and in Brazil. In the first case, after 3 days of treatment no reduction on viremia, NS1 antigenemia, T cell activation or cytokine production were observed in treated patients in comparison to placebo [44], whereas in the second study the lack of effectiveness of chloroquine in patients was confirmed without significant differences in the duration and degree of the disease [45].

In this line of repurposing for new indications clinically approved drugs, a significant antiviral activity in human cell lines and in a mouse model was recently reported for prochlorperazine, a dopamine D2 receptor (D2R) antagonist approved to treat nausea, vomiting and headache in humans that are also common symptoms among dengue patients [46]. Additionally, this drug is a potent analog of chlorpromazine, a compound that interferes with the formation of the clathrin lattices in endosomes [47]. The blockade of DENV-2 infection by prochlorperazine was targeted to clathrin-associated mechanisms of viral entry, but also DENV-2 binding through D2R was affected. Further research with this compound is promising since prochlorperazine treatment in patients with dengue might have two beneficial effects: blocking DENV infection by antiviral activity and relieving clinical symptoms.

LIPID METABOLISM

Lipid metabolism is involved along the different steps of the flavivirus multiplication cycle, from entry and fusion, through intracellular macromolecular biosynthesis and ending with virion assembly and release. DENV infection alters the lipid profile of infected cells, by affecting biosynthetic and trafficking pathways of specific lipids, and hijacks cellular membranes derived from the endoplasmic reticulum (ER) to rearrange the optimal sites for virus replication and assembly. This subject is currently being explored with promising results to provide the identification of new suitable targets for antiviral research [reviewed in 48, 49]. Additionally, several studies undertaken on samples from DENV patients have shown that there are distinct changes in their lipidome [50, 51].

The strict dependence of flavivirus replication on fatty acid biosynthesis was one of the processes found associated to the drastic alteration in the lipid profile of intracellular membranes induced by DENV. Fatty acid synthase (FASN), a key enzyme in this lipidic pathway, was demonstrated to be relocalized to sites of viral RNA replication in DENV-infected human cells. Accordingly, DENV-2 and DENV-4 multiplication was significantly reduced in human and mosquito cells in the presence of FASN inhibitors like cerulenin, C75 and orlistat [52 - 55]. For C75, the most potent inhibitor, the requirement of fatty acid biosynthesis for DENV-2 multiplication was temporally located at a stage after virus entry and previous to virus assembly or release, confirming a probable effect on RNA replication [54].

In addition to fatty acid synthesis, the requisite of an active biogenesis of cholesterol has also been documented in DENV-infected cells. At early stages after DENV infection, an increase in cholesterol levels was found and it was related with an augment in the activity of hydroxyl methyl glutaryl-CoA (HMG-CoA) reductase, the enzyme that catalyzes the initial step in cholesterol biosynthesis [56]. Concomitantly, the treatment with statins, known cardiovascular drugs that inhibit HMG-CoA reductase, blocked the *in vitro* DENV-2 infection in diverse epithelial, endothelial and myeloid cells, affecting viral assembly [57, 58]. DENV-2 infection was also affected when the cholesterol intake in infected cells was disrupted using a cholesterol transport inhibitor, U18666A [59]. The antiviral activity resulted from a dual effect: viral trapping in the late endosome/lysosome compartments and suppression of *de novo* sterol biosynthesis. The authors also observed an additive antiviral activity of U18666A and C75, confirming that DENV relies on both cellular cholesterol and fatty acid biosynthesis for productive infection. Cholesterol is also an essential component of virion envelope to assess a productive infection, since incubation of a DENV suspension with cholesterol-reactive compounds such as methyl-β-cyclodextrin or nystatin inactivated viral particles [60]. The anti-DENV-2 activity of lovastatin was also evaluated *in vivo* and a survival increase was reported in the AG129 mouse model [61]. However, when a clinical trial with lovastatin was performed in 300 Vietnamese dengue patients no evidence of a beneficial effect on any of the clinical manifestations or on dengue viremia was demonstrated [62].

Other tested point of attack to combat DENV infections has been the interaction of the capsid C protein with lipid droplets (LD), lipid rich ER-derived organelles that regulate the storage and hydrolysis of neutral lipids, serving as reservoir of cholesterol and acyl-glycerols for membrane formation and maintenance [63]. These organelles increased in number in DENV-2 infected cells and accumulated C protein in the surface, providing a probable platform for genome encapsidation and nucleocapsid formation [52]. Nordihydroguaiaretic acid, a hypolipidemic agent with antioxidant and anti-inflammatory properties, impaired *in vitro* DENV-4 production apparently due to a reduction in the number of LD that led to inhibition of genome replication and virion morphogenesis [64]. A similar result was obtained using PF-429242, an active-site-directed inhibitor of human subtilisin kexin isozyme-1 (SKI-1)/site-1 protease (S1P). The loss of SKI-1/S1P enzymatic activity in human hepatoma cells by PF-429242 treatment resulted in a robust reduction of the LD number together with inhibition of infective particle production of the four DENV serotypes through blockade of virion assembly and release [65]. No *in vivo* assays of these LD inhibitors have been yet reported.

PROTEIN TRANSLATION

All viruses rely entirely upon the host cell machinery for viral protein synthesis. For DENV, as well as for other positive-stranded RNA viruses, translation is the first biosynthetic step after genome uncoating and represents a critical determinant of the productive cycle of multiplication [66]. The translation process consists of three steps: initiation, elongation and termination. In general, the known inhibitors of any of these steps have shown cytotoxic effects that have impeded their development as antiviral drugs. An exception has been reported for lactimidomycin, a product isolated from *Streptomyces amphibiosporus* that inhibits the first round of polypeptide elongation through binding to the ribosome E-site. A potent inhibition of DENV-2 infection in cell culture was detected at concentrations that did not affect cell viability [67]. Although the compound showed a broad inhibitory spectrum against several RNA viruses, further studies are required to validate the suitability of viral translation as a druggable host cell antiviral target.

UNFOLDED PROTEIN RESPONSE

It is known that DENV infection induces cellular ER stress leading to the activation of the unfolded protein response (UPR) signaling network, which in turn modulates various signaling pathways associated with cell survival [68]. UPR activation results in the degradation of misfolded proteins, upregulation of ER chaperones and phosphorylation of eukaryotic translation initiation factor 2α (eIF2α), which in turn inhibits RNA translation. However, *in vitro* studies have shown that phosphorylation of eIF2α occurred during initial stages of infection and later post-infection DENV-2 promoted eIF2α dephosphorylation allowing the synthesis of viral and cellular proteins [69].

Since NS5 viral protein traffics into and out of the nucleus during infection, a high-throughput screen was performed to identify small inhibitors of the interaction between NS5 and host nuclear transport protein. This study allowed the identification of the synthetic retinoid N-(4-hydroxyphenyl) retinamide (4-

HPR), a compound that exhibited antiviral activity against all serotypes of DENV in human PBMCs and also against ADE-mediated DENV-1 infection in cell culture and DENV-2 infection in a lethal mouse model [70]. Similar results were obtained independently by Carocci *et al.* [71] both *in vitro* and *in vivo* for DENV-2. The analysis of 4-HPR mechanism of action revealed that this compound acts promoting UPR response and inducing eIF2α phosphorylation [72]. It is still unclear whether the ability of 4-HPR to affect the interaction of NS5 with nuclear transport proteins drives, directly or indirectly, the activation of UPR. It is noteworthy that safety and bioavailability of 4-HPR has been well established in clinical trials performed to evaluate the efficacy of this compound for the treatment of other health disorders such as psoriasis and cancer [72].

UBIQUITIN PROTEASOME PATHWAY

The ubiquitin-proteasome pathway (UPP), the major proteolytic system in eukaryotes, is a key player in maintaining cellular protein homeostasis. A differential expression of several components of the UPP was detected in DENV-2 infected cells and treatment with the UPP inhibitors UBEI-41, MG132 and IU1 caused a significant reduction of viral infectivity in cell cultures [73 - 75]. These evidences, together with the fact that several UPP inhibitors have been licensed for therapeutic use, make this pathway an attractive target for antiviral intervention. Using an *in vitro* ADE model, THP-1 monocytic cells infected with DENV opsonized with enhancing levels of humanized 3H5 monoclonal antibody (h3H5), Choy *et al.* [76] demonstrated that treatment with the proteasome inhibitor β-lactone caused a significant dose-dependent reduction in DENV-2 infectious titers. However, no detectable decrease in RNA genome levels was observed indicating that β-lactone impaired DENV egress from infected cells. Similar results were obtained with bortezomib, a licensed reversible proteasome inhibitor used to treat multiple myeloma and mantle cell lymphoma. Moreover, bortezomib reduced DENV- 2 replication and the subsequent pro-inflammatory response in a mouse model [76].

NUCLEOTIDE METABOLISM

Nucleotide metabolism is one of the more exploited host metabolic pathways as potential antiviral targets for several human viruses, including DENV, with focus in the inhibition of cellular enzymes involved in nucleotide biosynthesis and the consequent blockade of viral RNA replication. One of the most widely investigated antiviral compounds was ribavirin (1-β-D-ribofuranosyl-1-2,4-triazole-3-carboxamide), a guanosine analog with broad spectrum of antiviral activity against several RNA and DNA viruses, including the four serotypes of DENV [77 - 79]. The inhibitory effect of ribavirin against DENV in monkey kidney and human hepatoma cells was weak and was completely reversed by the addition of exogenous guanosine, indicating that it was mainly exerted through competitive inhibition of inosine monophosphate dehydrogenase (IMPDH), a key cellular enzyme involved in guanosine biosynthesis [77, 79, 80]. Furthermore, ribavirin was not effective *in vivo* when tested in rhesus monkeys or in a dengue fever viremia model of AG129 mice deficient for the interferon (IFN) α/β and γ receptors [81, 82].

A recent interesting strategy to improve the effectiveness of ribavirin was reported by combination of this antiviral drug with an anti-inflammation agent. The combined treatment of infected cells with ribavirin and a plant derived anti-inflammatory compound showed greater reduction of infective virus production and cytokine/chemoquine expression, both factors contributing to control DENV infection [83]. In this line of combination therapy, a synergistic inhibition of DENV replication was also achieved by the simultaneous treatment with ribavirin as inhibitor of the guanosine biosynthesis pathway and a guanosine analog designated INX-08189 that incorporates into the nascent viral RNA leading to chain termination [84]. These investigations provide a new therapeutic approach for DENV infection that merits further studies since drug combination would allow get efficacy at lower compound doses with concomitant reduced toxicity.

The importance of IMPDH as a target for DENV therapy was corroborated through the evaluation of mycophenolic acid, an uncompetitive inhibitor of the enzyme, with very potent antiviral activity against DENV [77, 79]. However, a serious drawback to the perspective of therapeutic trials with mycophenolic acid or its derivatives is given by the immunosuppressive potential of the drug linked to the described immunopathogenesis of dengue severe syndrome. More recently, other compounds such as the nucleoside analog 1-β-D-ribofuranosyl-3-ethynyl-[1, 2, 4]triazole (ETAR) and heterocyclic derivatives of *N*-allyl acridones have shown antiviral activity against the four DENV serotypes mainly or partially mediated by IMPDH inhibition [85 - 87]. Both inhibitors exhibited substantially higher efficacy *in vitro* than ribavirin, but *in vivo* assays have not been still reported.

Several classes of compounds targeted to enzymes involved in pyrimidine biosynthesis have also been assayed as potential DENV inhibitors. Orotidine monophosphate (OMP) decarboxylase, an essential enzyme for the conversion of OMP to uridine monophosphate (UMP), was blocked with 6-azauridine, resulting in inhibition of DENV replication but also significant cytostatic activity was associated [78]. Dihydroorotate dehydrogenase (DHODH), the fourth enzyme in the *de novo* pyrimidine biosynthesis pathway, is another host factor considered as potential antiviral strategy. Brequinar and NITD-982 are DHODH inhibitors and both compounds have shown a very potent and selective anti-DENV-2 activity in cell culture through depletion of the intracellular pyrimidine pool whereas no efficacy was achieved in the AG129 mouse model [88, 89]. The authors ascribed these discordant results to high concentrations of plasma uridine in treated animals derived from exogenous uptake from the diet that could preclude the *in vivo* efficacy of this class of inhibitors.

KINASES

Mitogen-activated Protein Kinases

Mitogen-activated protein kinases (MAPKs) are families of serine/threonine kinases that regulate a widespread of cell activities including transcription, protein biosynthesis, cell cycle control, apoptosis, and differentiation. MAPKs preserved a distinct and evolutionarily conserved Thr-X-Tyr motif and the activation of each MAPK cascade can be controlled by phosphatases that dephosphorylate either the phospho-threonine and/or the phospho-tyrosine residue. MAPK signaling pathways are activated by a great number of membrane receptors and regulate very specific cellular responses. The best known MAPKs families are the extracellular signal-regulated kinases 1 and 2 (ERK 1/2), the c-Jun N-terminal kinase (JNK) and p38. ERK pathway is usually associated with growth or proliferation signals whereas JNK and p38 are associated with the response to environmental and inflammatory stress (Fig. **1**). Dysregulation of MAPK signaling pathways plays an important role in the development of several diseases such as diabetes, cancer, neurodegenerative diseases and inflammation related disorders [90 - 93].

DENV infection activates several cellular signaling pathways including MAPK cascades and these signaling routes represent potential targets for new antiviral strategies.

ERK Pathway

The principal components of this signal cascade are Raf, MEK 1/2 and ERK 1/2. Activation of ERK 1 and 2 allows their translocation to the nucleus where they phosphorylate transcription factors and other nuclear proteins that trigger changes in gene expression. In addition, ERK 1/2 mediate phosphorylation of several cytoplasmic substrates and also play an important role in innate immunity and inflammation acting as repressors of some cytokine genes [94].

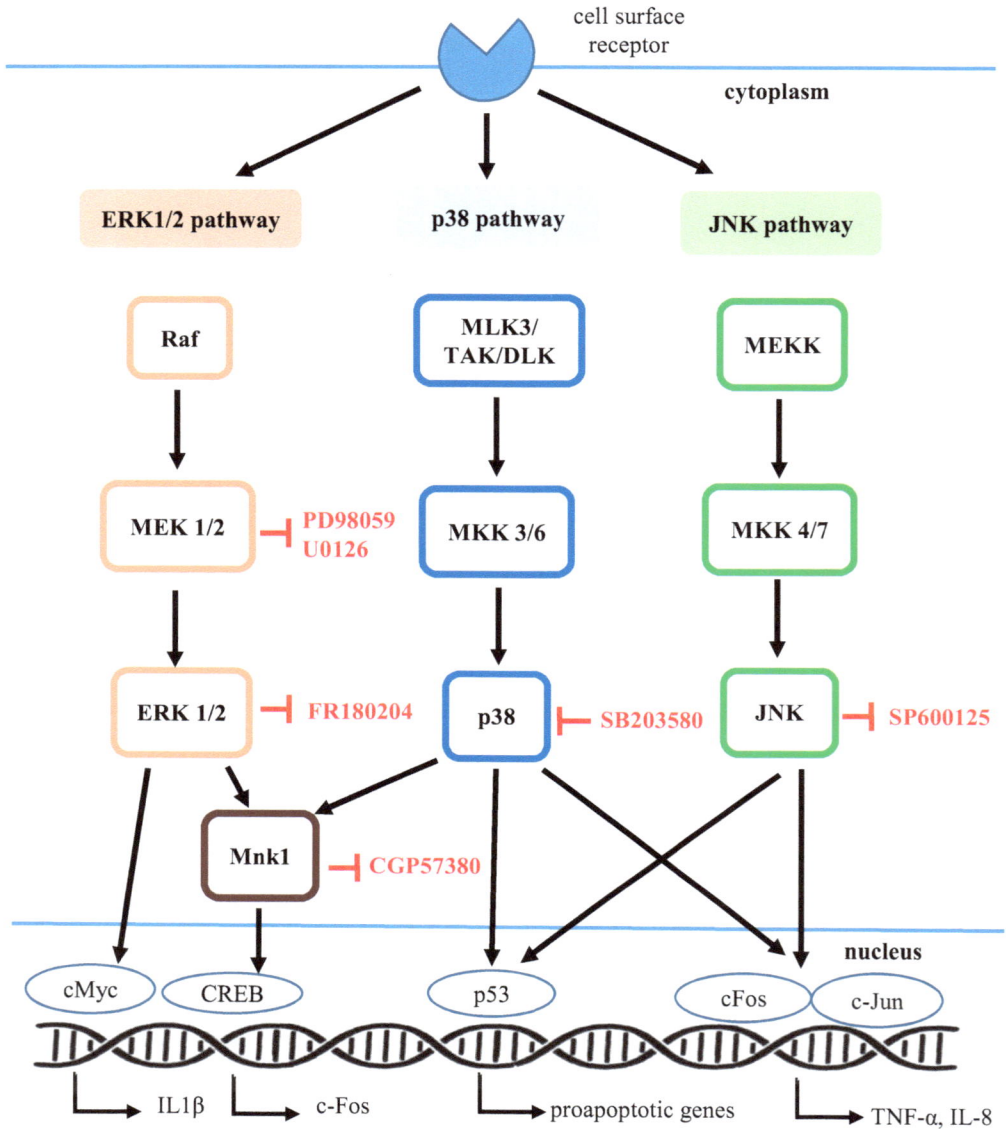

Fig. (1). Mitogen-activated protein kinase pathways involved in DENV pathogenesis. The main components of ERK 1/2, p38 and JNK pathways and the major nuclear transcription factors activated by each signaling cascade are represented. Chemical inhibitors acting at different levels of each pathway are also indicated. ERK: extracellular signal-regulated kinase; Raf: rapidly accelerated fibrosarcoma; MEK: mitogen activated protein kinase kinase, MLK3: mixed-lineage kinase 3; TAK: transforming growth factor β activated kinase; DLK: dual leucine bearing zipper kinase; MKK: mitogen activated protein kinase kinase; MEKK: mitogen activated protein kinase kinase kinase; JNK: c-Jun N-terminal kinase; Mnk1: MAPK-interacting kinase 1; CREB: cAMP response element-binding; IL1β: interleukin 1 beta; TNF-α: tumor necrosis factor alpha; IL-8: interleukin 8.

The requirement of the activation of ERK pathway for DENV replication seems to be dependent on the cell type. ERK phosphorylation was reported during the first minutes of DENV- 2 infection in human umbilical vein endothelial cells, liver epithelial cells and macrophages [95 - 97]. On the other hand, no activation of ERK was observed in hepatoma Huh7 cells and even a blockade of ERK signaling cascade was found in DENV-2 infected A549 cells [95, 98]. In the case of primary PBMCs infected with DENV-2 no activation of ERK was observed, however, infection with antibody-opsonized DENV-2 particles induced a strong phosphorylation of ERK 1/2 pathway after the first hour of infection, which indicates that entry of immune complexes would trigger ERK activation in this type of cells [99].

It has been demonstrated that there is a relationship between the level of the proinflammatory cytokine interleukin 8 (IL-8) and the severity of the symptoms in dengue patients. In endothelial cells infected with a DENV-2 hemorrhagic fever strain the compound PD98059, a non-competitive ATP inhibitor of the kinases MEK 1/2 that mediate the phosphorylation of ERK 1/2, caused a reduction in IL-8 production [95] and viral induced cell permeability [96]. In addition, inhibition of ERK signaling by PD98059 in PMBC cells infected with antibody-opsonized DENV-2 particles reduced the production of IL-1β, a cytokine also implied in severe dengue pathology. The same study showed that activation of ERK pathway is critical for cytokine induction but dispensable for viral production [99]. On the contrary, the inhibitor U0126, also affecting MEK 1/2, decreased DENV production in human HEK293 and hamster BHK-21 cells [100, 101].

In vivo studies demonstrated that DENV-2 infection in BALB/c mice induced ERK1/2 phosphorylation in liver tissue samples. Treatment with FR180204, a competitive ATP inhibitor of ERK pathway with high selectivity, did not reduce viral production but decreased caspase-3 cleavage and apoptosis in liver cells. In DENV-2 infected mice, the raise of liver aminotransferases and tumor necrosis factor alpha (TNF-α) expression were also reduced by FR180204 treatment [102]. The fact that ERK inhibition attenuates DENV-2 pathogenesis together with recent advances in the evaluation of ERK inhibitors in cancer clinical trials make this signaling pathway an interesting therapeutic target to reduce severe symptoms of DENV infection.

JNK Pathway

JNK1, JNK2 and JNK3 shared more than 85% amino acid identity. JNK1 and JNK2 are ubiquitously expressed and JNK3 is expressed principally in neuronal tissues. JNK pathway is activated in response to cellular stresses such as heat shock, ionizing radiation, oxidative stress, DNA damage, DNA and protein synthesis inhibition, and in minor extent by growth factors. The JNK signaling pathway plays an important role in cytokine production, inflammatory response, cell proliferation, differentiation or apoptosis. Activation of JNK induces its translocation to the nucleus, where JNK phosphorylate a series of transcription factors [103].

Regarding virus infection, it has been reported that JNK pathway is involved in the replication of several viruses including JEV [104] and, like ERK cascade, JNK signaling pathway has also been reported to be involved in DENV pathogenesis. In human macrophages infected with infectious DENV-2 or UV-inactivated DENV-2 particles JNK phosphorylation was only observed within the first minutes after infection suggesting that the interaction of viral particles with the cell surface may trigger JNK activation. Interestingly, treatment with SP60025, a reversible ATP competitive inhibitor of JNK and several other kinases [105], reduced extracellular NS1 levels and virus yield indicating that activation of JNK would be essential for multiplication of DENV-2 in macrophages [97]. On the other hand, whereas DENV-2 infection in PBMCs caused a poor activation of JNK during the first 2 hours of infection, in a model of ADE infection of PBMCs JNK phosphorylation was not detected; however, inhibition of JNK by the compound SP600125 reduced IL1-β secretion induced by DENV-2 immunocomplex infection [99].

In vivo studies corroborated JNK phosphorylation in liver tissue samples obtained from DENV-2 infected mice and, using this animal model, treatment with SP600125 caused JNK dephosphorylation without affecting DENV replication. However, the inhibitor was able to reduce liver transaminases levels and prevented the rise in red blood cell count induced by the infection [106]. SP600125 also blocked the production of factors associated with disease severity and apoptosis induction such as TNF-α and TNF-related apoptosis –inducing ligand (TRAIL) [106, 107]. The inhibition of cellular apoptosis triggered by extrinsic and intrinsic pathways in DENV-2 infected mice treated with SP600125 was also demonstrated however, as it was mentioned above, the inhibitor also affected p38 cascade activation [106]. Therefore, development of more specific inhibitors of JNK is further required to assess the importance of this cascade for DENV replication and evaluate the potential of this pathway as a therapeutic target.

p38 Pathway

There are four p38 family members (α, β, γ and δ) that share only 60% amino acid identity, suggesting highly diverse functions. p38α and p38β are ubiquitously expressed whereas p38γ and p38δ have more restricted expression pattern. p38 pathway is activated principally by cellular stressors such as UV radiation, oxidative stress, hypoxia, pro-inflammatory cytokines and less often growth factors, and plays an important role in inflammatory responses, apoptosis, cellular senescence and cell cycle checkpoints. p38 isoforms are present in the nucleus and cytoplasm in resting cells and upon activation, p38 isoforms phosphorylate a large number of substrates in many cellular compartments, including the cytoplasm and the nucleus [108].

An important role for the p38 pathway on DENV pathogenesis has been proposed. Phosphorylation of p38 at early times of DENV-2 infection in HUVEC and human macrophages was reported [95, 97] while p38 remained activated along the infection in HepG2 and Huh7 cells [98, 109]. The compound SB203580, a competitive inhibitor of p38α and p38β, caused a minor reduction in DENV-2 production in human macrophages and Huh7 cells [97, 98] and had no significant effect on virus yields in PBMCs, monocytic THP-1 cells and pre-basophilic KU812 cells infected with DENV-2 immune complexes [110, 111]. On the contrary, DENV-2 production was strongly inhibited by CGP57380 (Fig. **1**), a specific inhibitor of MAPK-interacting kinase 1 (Mnk1), a p38 downstream kinase shared with ERK 1/2 pathway [98].

Activation of p38 would be related with the induction of important cytokines involved in DENV pathogenesis. At the endothelial level, this activation was correlated with the up-regulation of tissue factors and protease-activated receptors, which suggests that it is implied in the coagulation-inflammation processes in dengue hemorrhagic cases [95]. Treatment with p38 inhibitors produced a reduction in the expression of TNF-α, an upregulated cytokine during DENV-2 infection, in DENV infected Hep-G2 cells and in DENV immune complex infected PBMCs, THP-1 and KU812 cells [110, 111]. Furthermore, treatment with the inhibitor SB203580 reduced apoptosis in HepG2 cells, IL-1β secretion and IL-8 levels in PMBCs, and CCL5 expression in THP-1 and KU182 cells. Therefore, p38 would be a good target to reduce overproduction of TNF-α and proinflammatory cytokines that are responsible of most of the severe symptoms in DHF/DSS patients [112, 117].

In vivo studies in different animal models have shown that treatment with SB203580 blocked DENV-2 induced upregulation of cytokines TNF-α and IL-6 in blood and liver samples [111, 113]. The inhibitor also reduced the expression of cytokine IL-10 and chemokines CCL-5 and CXCL-10 in liver samples from DENV-2 infected Balb/c mice and caused a decrease in proinflammatory metalloproteinase-9 levels in blood samples from infected AG129 mice. In addition, SB203580 improved the hematological profile by preventing the reduction of white blood cells and platelets in infected Balb/c mice and the increase of red blood cells and hematocrits in infected AG129 mice. In both models, no effect on viral production was observed after treatment with the inhibitor [111, 113].

Other Kinases

The activity of diverse kinases is crucial for the biochemical signal transduction in many pathways involved in the regulation of cell survival and immune response affecting DENV replication.

Src, Abl and Fyn Kinases

The screening of a collection of well-annotated kinase inhibitors, including compounds that have been approved or that are in late stages of clinical development, allowed the identification of several inhibitors of Src and Abl family kinases (SFK and AFK) that were active against DENV in different types of cell cultures. Former studies about the mode of action of two SFK and AFK inhibitors, dasatinib, which is a relatively nonselective ATP-competitive inhibitor, and AZD0530, which is a considerable more selective SFK and AFK inhibitor, revealed that these compounds would impair virion assembly in the four DENV serotypes [114]. A more detailed analysis of the mechanism of action of these compounds indicated that AZD0530 and dasatinib efficiently prevented DENV-2 RNA replication and this study suggests that even though Src and Abl kinases seem to be relevant for viral replication, the main target of the inhibitors would be Fyn kinase. Small interfering RNA (siRNA) silencing of Fyn kinase expression also abrogated DENV-2 replication and interestingly, a single mutation in NS4B protein is sufficient to overcome the inhibitory effects of AZD0530, dasatinib or Fyn kinase knockdown. The above results indicate that Fyn kinase, and possible members of AFK and SFK, would be involved in the phosphorylation of viral or host factors required for viral RNA replication [115]. Based on these previously reported results, Vincetti *et al.* [116] performed a structural virtual screening to find Src inhibitors that would interact with an allosteric pocket on NS5 polymerase that could be exploited for the development of non-nucleoside inhibitors. An allosteric inhibitor that was able to target both NS5-NS3 interaction and the host Src and Fyn kinases was identified being a promising multi-target compound for further antiviral studies [116].

Another compound named GNF-2, which is an allosteric Abl kinase inhibitor that exhibited anti DENV-2 *in vitro* activity, has a dual mechanism of antiviral action via both host and viral targets [117]. Besides its inhibitory effect on Abl kinase activity that prevented viral replication, GNF-2 would also interact with DENV-2 glycoprotein E, in the pre-fusion conformation, inhibiting conformational changes required for membrane fusion during viral entry [117].

AP2-associated Protein Kinase 1 and Cyclin G-associated Kinase

Intracellular membrane trafficking is highly relevant for DENV multiplication and this process relies on the interactions between adaptor proteins (AP1 to AP5) and the transmembrane cargo during endocytosis and transport through the secretory pathway. The host AP2-associated protein kinase 1 (AAK1) and cyclin G–associated kinase (GAK) regulate receptor-mediated endocytosis and trans-Golgi network (TGN) transport by recruiting AP proteins and enhancing their binding affinity for sorting motifs within the cargo. Imidazo[1,2-b] pyridazine-based inhibitors of AAK1 and two isothiazolo[5,4-b] pyridines inhibitors of GAK, displayed *in vitro* antiviral activity against DENV-2 with minimal or no cytotoxicity. Moreover, sunitinib and erlotinib, approved anticancer drugs with potent binding to AAK1 and GAK, also exhibited anti-DENV-2 activity and treatment with combinations of these drugs achieved synergistic inhibition of DENV-2 infection *in vitro* as well as a significant reduction of viral load in serum, spleen and liver from mice treated with both compounds. In addition, the inhibition of AP2 phosphorylation was detected in treated mice, reinforcing the involvement of AAK1 and GAK in the antiviral activity of these compounds [118].

Phosphatidylinositol 3 Kinase/Akt Pathway

It has been established that DENV-2 infection activates the phosphatidylinositol 3 kinase (PI3K)/Akt pathway and this activation would maintain cell survival and promote IL-10 production [119]. AR-12, a potent inhibitor of PI3K/Akt signaling, exhibited antiviral activity against the four DENV serotypes. Treatment of cell cultures both before and after infection inhibited DENV-2 replication without inducing apoptosis. In addition to PI3K/Akt signaling, DENV-2 stimulates the expression of cellular chaperone proteins, such as glucose-regulated protein 78 (GRP78) that would be important for DENV replication. AR-12 treatment suppressed not only PI3K/Akt activation but also diminished GRP78 expression. A recently developed DENV-2 infected suckling mouse model was used to assess the *in vivo* antiviral activity of AR-12 revealing that in accordance with *in vitro* studies, treatment of mice with AR-12, either before or after viral infection, suppressed viral replication and reduced mortality in infected mice, providing evidence that AR-12 has potential as an anti-DENV compound [120].

PROTEIN PROCESSING

Endoplasmic Reticulum α-glucosidases

During DENV protein synthesis in ribosomes at ER membranes, prM, the intracellular glycosylated precursor of M protein, rapidly associates with the E glycoprotein forming heterodimers. Newly synthesized viral genomes associate with C protein to form nucleocapsids, which bud into the lumen of the ER at microdomains enriched with prM-E heterodimers leading to the assembly of immature viral particles. These non-infectious viral particles are transported to the TGN where the host protease furin cleaves prM into M protein, giving rise to the mature infectious viral particles that are released to the extracellular milieu via the secretory pathway [121].

Experimental evidences indicate that N-linked oligosaccharide processing events in the ER are important for the secretion of infectious virus. ER α-glucosidases I and II are involved in the trimming of the glucose residues on the oligosaccharide precursor Glc3Man9GlcNAc2. An early study demonstrated that the indolizidine alkaloid castanospermine (CST) and the iminosugar deoxynojirimycin (DNJ), which are ER α-glucosidase inhibitors, affected DENV-1 production in mouse neuroblastoma cells [122]. Inhibition of α-glucosidase activity would impair the correct folding of DENV glycoproteins prM and E, and even though treatment with CST or DNJ did not prevent the heterodimeric association between prM and E, the prM-E complexes carrying unprocessed N-linked oligosaccharides appeared to be unstable disturbing early stages on virus morphogenesis [122]. Other two known sulfonium-ion α-glucosidase inhibitors, kotalanol and its de-sulfonated derivative, also displayed anti-DENV-2 activity in cell cultures [123].

Chang *et al.* [124, 125] reported the *in vitro* anti-DENV-2 activity of DNJ derivatives and one of these compounds, named CM-10-18, reduced the peak viremia of DENV in AG129 mice and significantly protected mice from death and/or disease progress [126]. Interestingly, combination therapy of ribavirin with CM-10-18 rendered a significantly enhanced *in vivo* antiviral activity [125]. Besides their inhibitory effect on ER α-glucosidases, some iminosugars are able to disturb glycolipid processing, however the latter activity would not be responsible for the antiviral effect against DENV-2 [127].

On the other hand, CST proved to be effective against the four DENV serotypes in cell cultures and prevented mortality in DENV-2 infected mice [128]. A water soluble oral pro-drug of the natural alkaloid CST, named celgosivir, was about 100 times more effective against DENV-2 than CST in cell cultures. In addition to the effect on prM and E glycoprotein processing, celgosivir strongly affected viral replication by causing the misfolding and accumulation of NS1 in the ER [129].

AG129 mice infected with non-mouse-adapted DENV-2 strains exhibit severe disease, including high viremia and death. Moreover, immunization of AG129 mice with a mouse monoclonal antibody against DENV E protein (4G2) prior to DENV-2 infection leads to an increased plasma leakage and mortality, constituting a murine model that recapitulates ADE. Rathore *et al.* [129] reported that celgosivir reduced viremia and increased survival in both primary and ADE mouse models of DENV infection.

While twice daily treatment with celgosivir conferred protection in AG129 mice [130], no reduction in serum viral loads was detected when celgosivir was administered twice daily to dengue infected patients in a clinical trial. This discrepancy between pre-clinical and clinical studies could be ascribed to the fact that in the clinical trial celgosivir treatment was initiated when patients were already viremic [131, 132]. In accordance with this assumption, the lack of efficacy of the twice-daily regimen of celgosivir administration after the onset of viremia was also evident in a new mouse model using DENV-1 or DENV-2 isolated from patients [133]. However, using the same mouse models, Watanabe *et al.* [133], reported that a schedule of four times daily treatment with celgosivir significantly reduced viremia even when treatment was initiated during the peak of viremia, suggesting that changes in dosing schedule might also increase viral clearance in acute dengue patients. Based on these experimental evidences a clinical trial to assess the effectiveness of the four times daily schedule of celgosivir administration is currently being conducted [133]. In addition, an iminosugar called UV-4, which also displayed anti-DENV activity in several mouse models, including the ADE mouse model of severe DENV-2 infection in AG129 mice, is actually being evaluated in a clinical trial against dengue fever [134, 135].

Furin

Furin is a type I transmembrane protein mainly located in the Golgi and TGN that belongs to the family of secretory proprotein convertases and contains a subtilisin-like protease domain. As it was above mentioned, furin catalyzes the essential removal of the pr segment from the prM precursor of the membrane glycoprotein M in the TGN compartment. The cleaved pr peptide remains associated as long as progeny virions are being transported along the secretory pathway and the exposition to neutral pH in the extracellular space promotes pr dissociation providing fusion-competent infectious virus particles. In recent studies, it was shown that several peptidomimetic furin inhibitors, which act as competitive substrate analogs, hindered viral protein maturation [136] and DENV-2 replication in Huh-7 cells [137]. The relevance of these novel inhibitors as potential candidates for DENV chemotherapy relies on further studies about their inhibitory action against the other DENV serotypes and their ability to prevent *in vivo* viral replication. Interestingly, another study reported that the flavonoid luteolin, a natural compound isolated from plants used in traditional Chinese medicine, inhibited *in vitro* infection of the four DENV serotypes and *in vivo* DENV-1 replication, and mechanistic studies suggest that luteolin would exert its antiviral action through the inhibition of furin activity [138].

Endoplasmic Reticulum Associated Signal Peptidase

A genome-wide CRISPR/cas9-based study allowed the identification of ER associated signal peptidase as an important cell factor involved in the proper cleavage of flavivirus prM and E proteins from viral polyprotein precursor [139]. Recently, the antiviral activity against all DENV serotypes and ZIKV of cavinafungin, a linear lipopeptide isolated from the fungus *Colispora cavincola*, has been demonstrated. Remarkably, using a genome-wide CRISPR/Cas9 chemogenomic profiling approach, Estoppey *et al.* [140] identified signal peptidase as cavinafungin antiviral target and they also demonstrated that mutations in the catalytic subunit of the enzyme caused cavinafungin resistance. Therefore, the ER signal peptidase can be considered as a novel therapeutic target to prevent the formation of infectious DENV particles.

INNATE ANTIVIRAL RESPONSE

The identification and characterization of antiviral genes with the ability to interfere with virus replication has established innate immunity as the first line of antiviral defense. Innate immunity includes the IFN activity, with the induction of cytokines, interferon-stimulated genes (ISG) and inflammatory responses that result in virus-specific acquired immune responses, and host molecules that directly bind viral molecules, such as the cell-intrinsic restriction factors (Fig. **2**).

Interferon Activity

Innate immunity to DENV is triggered by activation of cellular sensors. The two key cellular sensors are Toll-like receptor 3 (TLR3), which senses double-stranded RNA (dsRNA) within endosomes, and the RNA helicase retinoic acid-inducible gene I (RIG-I), which senses intracellular dsRNA or single-stranded viral RNA. Signaling initiated by TLR3 and RIG-I is transmitted through the adaptor proteins Toll/IL-1 receptor domain-containing adaptor inducing IFN- β (TRIF) and mitochondrial antiviral-signaling protein (MAVS) respectively, to interact with TNF receptor-associated factor 3 (TRAF3) and converge on the transcription factors, IFN regulatory factor 3 (IRF3) and NF-κB. IRF3 is phosphorylated by IKK-ε and TANK-binding kinase 1 (TBK1), resulting in its dimerization and nuclear translocation.

Activated IRF3 and NF-κB translocate to the nucleus, where they activate IFN-β gene transcription. The secreted type I IFN cytokine stimulates the IFN-α/β receptor (IFNAR-1 and -2) through autocrine or paracrine interaction and then activates the Janus kinase-signal transducer and activator of transcription (JAK-STAT) signaling pathway [141]. Phosphorylated STAT-1 and STAT-2 recruit IRF9 to form a complex known as IFN-stimulated gene factor 3 (ISGF3), which translocates into the nucleus, binds to IFN-stimulated response elements (ISRE) and induces the transcription of ISGs, many of which confer antiviral effects against flaviviruses [142] (Fig. **2**).

It has been observed that IFNα/β inhibits DENV replication if it is added prior to infection [143]. Depending on the cell type, IFN dose, and time of treatment, microarray studies have identified 50–1000 potential ISGs implicated in flaviviruses suppression [144 - 146]. However, DENV can replicate in cells if IFN treatment occurs post infection. DENV is very efficient at modulating innate immunity and this property allows the virus to successfully establish infection in humans. Though strain and cell-type dependent differences do appear to exist, there are three common observations seen when DENV infects human and non-human primate cells: type I IFN signaling is impaired, type I IFN-mediated STAT1 phosphorylation is inhibited, and total STAT2 protein levels decrease.

DENV inhibits type I IFN signaling through the use of the NS proteins [147] (Fig. **2**). It was observed that the combined action of DENV-2 NS2A along with NS4A and NS4B is sufficient to block IFN signaling completely through a reduction in STAT1 phosphorylation, diminishing its nuclear localization and preventing IFN-β promoter driven transcription [148]. Furthermore, studies have shown that the DENV-2 NS2B-NS3 protease interferes with type I IFN induction via cleavage of stimulator of the interferon gene (STING) [149]. Also, through the direct interaction and modulation of IκB kinase ε, DENV-2 NS2B-NS3 disrupts RIG-I signaling, blocks serine 386 phosphorylation and nuclear transport of IRF3 thereby decreasing IFN production [150]. Finally, it was reported that NS5 inhibition of STAT1/2 activation or translocation prevents the upregulation of ISGs and the establishment of an antiviral state. DENV NS5 binds and degrades STAT2 by targeting it for UPP degradation [151, 152].

Interestingly, it has been also shown that during DENV infection the abundantly produced subgenomic flaviviral RNA (sfRNA) colocalizes, interacts and antagonizes a group of proteins implicated in modulating viral infection through the regulation of the expression and translation of several ISGs [153, 154]. In addition, TRIM25, another modulator of the type I IFN response, has also been identified as a target of DENV-2 sfRNA [155]. TRIM25 functions as an E3 ligase, which adds poly-ubiquitin chains to the amino-terminal of the caspase activation and recruitment domains (CARDs) of RIG-I [156]. This is thought to facilitate the interaction between RIG-I and MAVS, thus modulating downstream signaling of the type I IFN response [155].

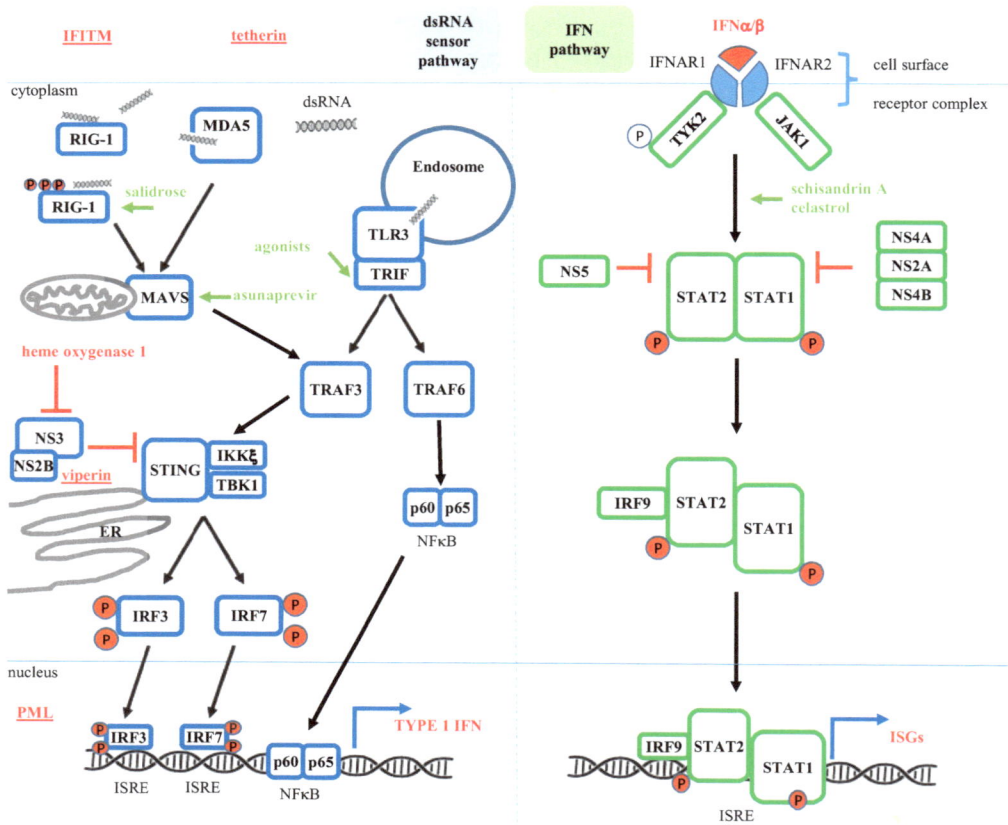

Fig. (2). Sensing of DENV dsRNA, activation of the IFN pathway and induction of ISGs. Schematic representation of the DENV type I IFN signaling inhibition are depicted in red. Pharmacological stimulation of the IFN pathway suggested against dengue infection are indicated in green. Cell-intrinsic restriction factors suppressing DENV replication are underlined and indicated in red. dsRNA: double stranded RNA; IFNAR: interferon-α/β receptor; IKK-ε: IκB kinase ε; IRF: interferon regulatory transcription factor; ISRE: interferon-stimulated response element; JAK: Janus kinase; MAVS: mitochondrial antiviral-signaling protein; MDA5: melanoma Differentiation-Associated protein 5; RIG-1: retinoic acid-inducible gene I; STAT: signal transducer and activator of transcription factor; TBK1: TANK-binding kinase 1; TLR: toll-like receptor. TRAF: TNF receptor associated factors; TRIF: TIR-domain-containing adapter-inducing interferon-β; TYK: non-receptor tyrosine-protein kinase.

Clinical utilization of IFN itself is associated with significant undesirable attributes, including high cost, dosing feasibility, and adverse side effects [157 - 159]. Clinical-grade IFN is costly to produce and requires repeated delivery due to a short *in vivo* half-life, and these factors contribute to a high overall expense.

Alternatively, the pharmacological targeting of the abovementioned enzymatic activity of flaviviral proteins, or their enzymatic-independent interactions with host immune molecules is an interesting approach for the development of antiviral therapies. Recently, it has been observed that human heme oxygenase 1 (HO-1) exerts *in vitro* antiviral activity against the four DENV serotypes. Infected Huh-7 cells treated with HO-1 showed a reduction of DENV protein synthesis and RNA replication. The anti-DENV effect exerted by HO-1 was mediated by biliverdin, which trigged the host antiviral IFN response by noncompetitively inhibiting the DENV NS2B/NS3 protease. In addition, it was reported that HO-1 induction in suckling mice infected with DENV delayed the mortality induced by DENV infection. Furthermore, similar antiviral effects were obtained when treating animals with andrographolide, which inhibited DENV both *in vitro* and *in vivo* by inducing HO-1 expression [160, 161].

Also, pharmacologic IFN stimulation has been suggested as a broad spectrum antiviral strategy (Fig. **2**). Molecules capable of yielding therapeutic effects via activation of IFN-mediated responses have been identified and biologically validated [162 - 166]. Yu *et al.* [167] have identified and characterized the mechanism by which schisandrin A increased IFN expression and activated JAK-STAT pathway to trigger antiviral innate responses against DENV replication. Importantly, it was observed that schisandrin A showed a potential antiviral activity against the four DENV serotypes *in vitro* and *in vivo*. Moreover, celastrol represents a potential anti- DENV agent that induces IFN-α expression and stimulates a downstream antiviral response against the four serotypes, making the therapy a promising drug for the treatment of DENV-infected patients [168]. In addition, several groups have pursued studies using novel agonists of IRF3-terminal pathways as treatments against RNA viruses, including DENV [169]. It has been reported that salidroside (p-hydroxyphenethyl-b-D-glucoside, $C_{14}H_{20}O_7$), a main bioactive compound of *Rhodiola rosea L.* (*Crassulaceae*), inhibited DENV-2 infection in THP-1 cells by enhancing host innate immune factors such as RIG-I, IRF-3, IRF-7, IFN- α, PKR and P-eIF2 α [170]. More recently, Tsai *et al.* [171] revealed that the anti-DENV-2 activity of asunaprevir is exerted through the activation of MAVS. Also, Chiang *et al.* [172] have described a novel sequence-specific RIG-I agonist that was effective against a broad range of RNA viruses. While molecules described thus far as efficacious immunostimulators are agonists of the MAVS or STING pathways, also a novel synthetic compound (1-(2-fluorophenyl)-2-(5-isopropyl-1,3,4-thiadiazol-2-yl)-1,2-dihydrochromeno[2,3-c]pyrrole-3,9-dione) that induces TRIF-dependent responses has been recently reported [173]. This small molecule, capable of rendering human cells resistant to DENV-2 multiplication via the targeting of TRIF pathway and of eliciting proinflammatory responses from human immune cells, represents a promising perspective for chemotherapy. Furthermore, Fusco *et al.* [174] identified 56 IFN antiviral effector genes against fully infectious DENV-2. Among them, the helicase with zinc finger 2 (HELZ2) was a potent IFN effector mediating suppression of DENV-2 infection, making this gene a possible candidate to be stimulated. Another pathway involving purinergic signaling in the context of DENV-2 infection has been recently reported as a potential target for modulation [175].

Lastly, there are reports showing antiviral and immunomodulatory effects of different plant extracts against DENV-2 infection [176 - 178]. It is worth to mention that some studies have included *in vivo* antiviral activity against all DENV serotypes [179].

From all these investigations, it is clear that pharmacological IFN activation may represent a cost-effective and impactful antiviral strategy applicable for populations prone to virus emergence events.

Cell-intrinsic Restriction Factors

Cell-intrinsic restriction factors are proteins that are able to limit viral replication by targeting specific steps of the viral life cycle rendering cells less permissive or non-permissive to infection [180]. These proteins are expressed at low constitutive levels allowing an immediate response upon viral infection, and are often upregulated following IFN stimulation after viral infection. In particular, DENV infected cells attempt to restrain virus replication through the activation of different defense mechanisms involving cell-intrinsic restriction factors along the virus cycle [181]. Well-established restriction factors have been shown to interfere specifically with viral entry, early post-entry steps, viral budding and even to reduce the infectious quality of extracellular released particles [182]. On the other hand, DENV counteracts these cell antiviral responses through host-viral interactions and mechanisms involving cellular components to evade intrinsic innate immune pathways [183, 184].

Mechanistically, IFN induced transmembrane proteins (IFITM1, IFITM2 and IFITM3) are the only known ISG products that act by blocking entry and/or viral particle trafficking [185, 186]. In particular, Brass *et al.* [187] have demonstrated that the action of a single intrinsic immune effector, IFITM3, served as an essential barrier to infection *in vitro*. Interestingly, another study revealed that IFITM proteins could interfere with the ADE effect during secondary DENV infection, which bypassed the IFN-mediated restriction [188]. More importantly, genetic studies emphasize the pivotal role that IFITM3 plays in governing viral disease in humans. A number of polymorphisms within human IFITM3 have been identified that may potentially influence its function [189]. These studies must be considered in order to associate IFITM polymorphisms with the different manifestations of DENV infection outcome. Zhu *et al.* [190] have suggested future development of exosome-mediated antiviral strategies using IFITM3 as a therapeutic agent. It is worth noting that secreted or membrane-bound proteins are of particular interest in drug development, because their extracellular nature renders them more accessible for therapeutic intervention.

Moreover, post-entry viral steps have been also observed to be restricted by cellular antiviral factors. It has been shown that overexpression of viperin, a radical S-adenosyl-L-methionine domain-containing enzyme associated with the ER that is highly expressed during DENV infection, inhibits DENV RNA replication, consistent with several reported effects of viperin against the replication of other *Flaviviridae* members, like hepatitis C virus [191] and WNV [192]. Furthermore, Jiang *et al.* [193] have identified ISG20, a 3′-to-5′ exonuclease, as an inhibitor of DENV-1 and DENV-2 replication. Most recently, ISG15 was found to play an anti-DENV-2 function via protein ISGylation. In addition, ISG12b2 was recognized as a novel inner mitochondrial membrane ISG that regulates mitochondria-mediated apoptosis during DENV-2 infection [194, 195].

Three DENV proteins (C, NS3 and NS5) interact with the host nucleus and/or its components impairing the host cell response and ensuring a successful outcome of viral infection. Different studies now indicate that the viral protein nuclear targeting might have a critical role in subversion of host immunity. Interestingly, extracellular DENV production can be reduced by inhibiting cytoplasmic-nuclear traffic [196]. In line with this, Giovannoni *et al.* [197] have demonstrated that one nuclear mediator of the intrinsic antiviral defense against DENV-2 is the promyelocytic leukemia protein (PML). PML is a regulatory protein that is constitutively expressed, but in addition, the PML promoter contains elements that trigger its upregulation in response to the activation of the antiviral IFN pathway. Initial evidence that PML might be involved in counteracting the infection is based on the observation of PML bodies disassembly during DENV-2 infection [197].

Finally, tetherin (BST-2/CD317/HM1.24) is an IFN induced transmembrane protein that restricts the release of a broad range of enveloped viruses. Pan *et al.* [198] have reported tetherin as a functional mediator of the IFN response against DENV-2 infection. It was observed that tetherin inhibits the release of DENV-2 virions from Huh7 cells and limits viral cell-to-cell transmission.

Altogether, these studies should provide a better understanding of the cellular antiviral activity against DENV infection. It is very important to understand the functions of factors mediating intrinsic immunity, which may lead to the development of new pharmacological agents that can increase its activity and hence lead to treatments for this viral disease.

CONCLUDING REMARKS

The host-directed antiviral approach has extensively expanded in the last years for DENV infections in an attempt to get an effective wide spectrum agent able to be used against other pathogenic flaviviruses and to avoid the appearance of resistant variants. The studies described here included new compounds targeted to cellular molecules and pathways as well as the repurposing for DENV of drugs previously approved for other therapeutic medications. The latter strategy allows a less expensive process of antiviral development given the well-known information about safety, bioavailability and validation for compounds in human clinical use, in contrast with the challenge of totally new drugs that are costly and may limit the therapy uptake in low-income American and Asiatic countries where dengue is endemic. Concomitantly, the present cocirculation of different flaviviruses, like DENV and ZIKV, in some tropical regions increase the difficulties of a precise and rapid diagnosis, reinforcing the advantage of an antiviral agent directed to a cellular target shared by both viruses.

Recent advances in the knowledge of DENV interactions with the host cell have greatly contributed to the discovery of new molecules with antiviral activity against all DENV serotypes. Structure-based approaches to obtain potent inhibitors of cellular enzymes involved in different stages of DENV replicative cycle will be highly relevant for the development of novel host-directed antiviral compounds. Moreover, progress in the identification of cell factors restricting viral replication offers new insights for the design of compounds that stimulate the expression of molecules responsible for intrinsic immunity as an alternative therapeutic approach. Taking into account the ability of IFN system to induce cell refractory state to viral replication, as well as its role in the coordination of adaptive immune responses, the identification of new molecules capable of stimulating innate immune signaling, through the design of improved high-throughput screenings, would render a potentially high-impact broad spectrum antiviral strategy. Even though most experimental evidences showed that targeting MAPK signaling pathways does not impair DENV replication, MAPK inhibitors might be a promising alternative to attenuate dengue severe symptoms in a combined therapy with other molecules that hinder DENV multiplication. On the other hand, improved animal models for primary and ADE DENV infections are currently available being an extremely useful tool for an accurate assessment of the potential of new antiviral agents before evaluating their efficacy in clinical trials.

Unfortunately, up to now the clinical trials performed with host-targeted drugs, such as chloroquine, lovastatin and celgosivir have shown disappointing results. Interestingly, it was hypothesized that the failure may be due to an inadequate therapeutic schedule because the compound was given to patients with an ongoing infection at the time near of the peak viremia as well as with a low frequency of administration. The timing for the initiation of the therapy is not easy to manage because dengue is an acute infection allowing a very limited time window for medication, but an optimized dosing schedule is intended for the α-glucosidase inhibitor celgosivir in a therapeutic assay in progress in order to improve the effectiveness of the drug. In addition, no beneficial clinical effect was observed with the only virus-targeted drug tested in humans, the viral polymerase inhibitor balapiravir. Finally, although the occurrence of undesirable toxicity may be a disadvantage associated to compounds directed towards cellular components, the short-term treatments required for acute infectious diseases such as dengue might minimize the potential unwanted side effects.

CONSENT FOR PUBLICATION

Not applicable.

CONFLICT OF INTEREST

The authors declare no conflict of interest, financial or otherwise.

ACKNOWLEDGEMENTS

Research in the authors' laboratory was supported by Agencia Nacional de Promoción Científica y Tecnológica, Consejo Nacional de Investigaciones Científicas y Técnicas (CONICET) and Universidad de Buenos Aires (UBA), Argentina. V.M.Q is a PhD fellow of CONICET. C.C.G. and E.B.D. are members of the same Institution.

REFERENCES

[1]   Guzman MG, Harris E. Dengue. Lancet 2015; 385(9966): 453-65.
       [http://dx.doi.org/10.1016/S0140-6736(14)60572-9] [PMID: 25230594]

[2]   Bhatt S, Gething PW, Brady OJ, *et al.* The global distribution and burden of dengue. Nature 2013; 496(7446): 504-7.
       [http://dx.doi.org/10.1038/nature12060] [PMID: 23563266]

[3]   Halstead SB. Dengue. Lancet 2007; 370(9599): 1644-52.
       [http://dx.doi.org/10.1016/S0140-6736(07)61687-0] [PMID: 17993365]

[4]   Halstead SB, Russell PK. Protective and immunological behavior of chimeric yellow fever dengue vaccine. Vaccine 2016; 34(14): 1643-7.
       [http://dx.doi.org/10.1016/j.vaccine.2016.02.004] [PMID: 26873054]

[5]   Hidari KI, Suzuki T. Dengue virus receptor. Trop Med Health 2011; 39(4) (Suppl.): 37-43.

[http://dx.doi.org/10.2149/tmh.2011-S03] [PMID: 22500135]

[6]   Perera-Lecoin M, Meertens L, Carnec X, Amara A. Flavivirus entry receptors: an update. Viruses 2013; 6(1): 69-88.
[http://dx.doi.org/10.3390/v6010069] [PMID: 24381034]

[7]   Cruz-Oliveira C, Freire JM, Conceição TM, Higa LM, Castanho MA, Da Poian AT. Receptors and routes of dengue virus entry into the host cells. FEMS Microbiol Rev 2015; 39(2): 155-70.
[http://dx.doi.org/10.1093/femsre/fuu004] [PMID: 25725010]

[8]   Chen Y, Maguire T, Hileman RE, *et al.* Dengue virus infectivity depends on envelope protein binding to target cell heparan sulfate. Nat Med 1997; 3(8): 866-71.
[http://dx.doi.org/10.1038/nm0897-866] [PMID: 9256277]

[9]   Hilgard P, Stockert R. Heparan sulfate proteoglycans initiate dengue virus infection of hepatocytes. Hepatology 2000; 32(5): 1069-77.
[http://dx.doi.org/10.1053/jhep.2000.18713] [PMID: 11050058]

[10]   Germi R, Crance JM, Garin D, *et al.* Heparan sulfate-mediated binding of infectious dengue virus type 2 and yellow fever virus. Virology 2002; 292(1): 162-8.
[http://dx.doi.org/10.1006/viro.2001.1232] [PMID: 11878919]

[11]   Dalrymple N, Mackow ER. Productive dengue virus infection of human endothelial cells is directed by heparan sulfate-containing proteoglycan receptors. J Virol 2011; 85(18): 9478-85.
[http://dx.doi.org/10.1128/JVI.05008-11] [PMID: 21734047]

[12]   Lin YL, Lei HY, Lin YS, Yeh TM, Chen SH, Liu HS. Heparin inhibits dengue-2 virus infection of five human liver cell lines. Antiviral Res 2002; 56(1): 93-6.
[http://dx.doi.org/10.1016/S0166-3542(02)00095-5] [PMID: 12323403]

[13]   Lee E, Pavy M, Young N, Freeman C, Lobigs M. Antiviral effect of the heparan sulfate mimetic, PI-88, against dengue and encephalitic flaviviruses. Antiviral Res 2006; 69(1): 31-8.
[http://dx.doi.org/10.1016/j.antiviral.2005.08.006] [PMID: 16309754]

[14]   Kato D, Era S, Watanabe I, *et al.* Antiviral activity of chondroitin sulphate E targeting dengue virus envelope protein. Antiviral Res 2010; 88(2): 236-43.
[http://dx.doi.org/10.1016/j.antiviral.2010.09.002] [PMID: 20851716]

[15]   Ichiyama K, Gopala Reddy SB, Zhang LF, *et al.* Sulfated polysaccharide, curdlan sulfate, efficiently prevents entry/fusion and restricts antibody-dependent enhancement of dengue virus infection *in vitro*: a possible candidate for clinical application. PLoS Negl Trop Dis 2013; 7(4): e2188.
[http://dx.doi.org/10.1371/journal.pntd.0002188] [PMID: 23658845]

[16]   Vervaeke P, Alen M, Noppen S, Schols D, Oreste P, Liekens S. Sulfated Escherichia coli K5 polysaccharide derivatives inhibit dengue virus infection of human microvascular endothelial cells by interacting with the viral envelope protein E domain III. PLoS One 2013; 8(8): e74035.
[http://dx.doi.org/10.1371/journal.pone.0074035] [PMID: 24015314]

[17]   Pujol CA, Estévez JM, Carlucci MJ, Ciancia M, Cerezo AS, Damonte EB. Novel DL-galactan hybrids from the red seaweed *Gymnogongrus torulosus* are potent inhibitors of herpes simplex virus and dengue virus. Antivir Chem Chemother 2002; 13(2): 83-9.
[http://dx.doi.org/10.1177/095632020201300202] [PMID: 12238532]

[18]   Rodríguez MC, Merino ER, Pujol CA, Damonte EB, Cerezo AS, Matulewicz MC. Galactans from cystocarpic plants of the red seaweed Callophyllis variegata (Kallymeniaceae, Gigartinales). Carbohydr Res 2005; 340(18): 2742-51.
[http://dx.doi.org/10.1016/j.carres.2005.10.001] [PMID: 16289051]

[19]   Talarico LB, Pujol CA, Zibetti RG, *et al.* The antiviral activity of sulfated polysaccharides against dengue virus is dependent on virus serotype and host cell. Antiviral Res 2005; 66(2-3): 103-10.
[http://dx.doi.org/10.1016/j.antiviral.2005.02.001] [PMID: 15911027]

[20]   Hidari KI, Takahashi N, Arihara M, Nagaoka M, Morita K, Suzuki T. Structure and anti-dengue virus

activity of sulfated polysaccharide from a marine alga. Biochem Biophys Res Commun 2008; 376(1): 91-5.
[http://dx.doi.org/10.1016/j.bbrc.2008.08.100] [PMID: 18762172]

[21]   Pujol CA, Ray S, Ray B, Damonte EB. Antiviral activity against dengue virus of diverse classes of algal sulfated polysaccharides. Int J Biol Macromol 2012; 51(4): 412-6.
[http://dx.doi.org/10.1016/j.ijbiomac.2012.05.028] [PMID: 22652218]

[22]   Ono L, Wollinger W, Rocco IM, Coimbra TL, Gorin PA, Sierakowski MR. *In vitro* and *in vivo* antiviral properties of sulfated galactomannans against yellow fever virus (BeH111 strain) and dengue 1 virus (Hawaii strain). Antiviral Res 2003; 60(3): 201-8.
[http://dx.doi.org/10.1016/S0166-3542(03)00175-X] [PMID: 14638396]

[23]   Qiu H, Tang W, Tong X, Ding K, Zuo J. Structure elucidation and sulfated derivatives preparation of two α-D-glucans from Gastrodia elata Bl. and their anti-dengue virus bioactivities. Carbohydr Res 2007; 342(15): 2230-6.
[http://dx.doi.org/10.1016/j.carres.2007.06.021] [PMID: 17637459]

[24]   Talarico LB, Damonte EB. Interference in dengue virus adsorption and uncoating by carrageenans. Virology 2007; 363(2): 473-85.
[http://dx.doi.org/10.1016/j.virol.2007.01.043] [PMID: 17337028]

[25]   Talarico LB, Noseda MD, Ducatti DR, Duarte ME, Damonte EB. Differential inhibition of dengue virus infection in mammalian and mosquito cells by iota-carrageenan. J Gen Virol 2011; 92(Pt 6): 1332-42.
[http://dx.doi.org/10.1099/vir.0.028522-0] [PMID: 21325483]

[26]   Marks RM, Lu H, Sundaresan R, *et al.* Probing the interaction of dengue virus envelope protein with heparin: assessment of glycosaminoglycan-derived inhibitors. J Med Chem 2001; 44(13): 2178-87.
[http://dx.doi.org/10.1021/jm000412i] [PMID: 11405655]

[27]   Damonte EB, Matulewicz MC, Cerezo AS. Sulfated seaweed polysaccharides as antiviral agents. Curr Med Chem 2004; 11(18): 2399-419.
[http://dx.doi.org/10.2174/0929867043364504] [PMID: 15379705]

[28]   Acosta EG, Piccini LE, Talarico LB, Castilla V, Damonte EB. Changes in antiviral susceptibility to entry inhibitors and endocytic uptake of dengue-2 virus serially passaged in Vero or C6/36 cells. Virus Res 2014; 184: 39-43.
[http://dx.doi.org/10.1016/j.virusres.2014.02.011] [PMID: 24583230]

[29]   Talarico LB, Duarte ME, Zibetti RG, Noseda MD, Damonte EB. An algal-derived DL-galactan hybrid is an efficient preventing agent for *in vitro* dengue virus infection. Planta Med 2007; 73(14): 1464-8.
[http://dx.doi.org/10.1055/s-2007-990241] [PMID: 17948168]

[30]   Talarico LB, Damonte EB. Characterization of *in vitro* dengue virus resistance to carrageenan. J Med Virol 2016; 88(7): 1120-9.
[http://dx.doi.org/10.1002/jmv.24457] [PMID: 26694200]

[31]   Guzman MG, Alvarez M, Halstead SB. Secondary infection as a risk factor for dengue hemorrhagic fever/dengue shock syndrome: an historical perspective and role of antibody-dependent enhancement of infection. Arch Virol 2013; 158(7): 1445-59.
[http://dx.doi.org/10.1007/s00705-013-1645-3] [PMID: 23471635]

[32]   Navarro-Sanchez E, Altmeyer R, Amara A, *et al.* Dendritic-cell-specific ICAM3-grabbing non-integrin is essential for the productive infection of human dendritic cells by mosquito-cell-derived dengue viruses. EMBO Rep 2003; 4(7): 723-8.
[http://dx.doi.org/10.1038/sj.embor.embor866] [PMID: 12783086]

[33]   Lozach PY, Burleigh L, Staropoli I, *et al.* Dendritic cell-specific intercellular adhesion molecule 3-grabbing non-integrin (DC-SIGN)-mediated enhancement of dengue virus infection is independent of DC-SIGN internalization signals. J Biol Chem 2005; 280(25): 23698-708.
[http://dx.doi.org/10.1074/jbc.M504337200] [PMID: 15855154]

[34] Pokidysheva E, Zhang Y, Battisti AJ, *et al.* Cryo-EM reconstruction of dengue virus in complex with the carbohydrate recognition domain of DC-SIGN. Cell 2006; 124(3): 485-93.
[http://dx.doi.org/10.1016/j.cell.2005.11.042] [PMID: 16469696]

[35] Alen MM, Kaptein SJ, De Burghgraeve T, Balzarini J, Neyts J, Schols D. Antiviral activity of carbohydrate-binding agents and the role of DC-SIGN in dengue virus infection. Virology 2009; 387(1): 67-75.
[http://dx.doi.org/10.1016/j.virol.2009.01.043] [PMID: 19264337]

[36] Alen MM, De Burghgraeve T, Kaptein SJ, Balzarini J, Neyts J, Schols D. Broad antiviral activity of carbohydrate-binding agents against the four serotypes of dengue virus in monocyte-derived dendritic cells. PLoS One 2011; 6(6): e21658.
[http://dx.doi.org/10.1371/journal.pone.0021658] [PMID: 21738755]

[37] Varga N, Sutkeviciute I, Ribeiro-Viana R, *et al.* A multivalent inhibitor of the DC-SIGN dependent uptake of HIV-1 and Dengue virus. Biomaterials 2014; 35(13): 4175-84.
[http://dx.doi.org/10.1016/j.biomaterials.2014.01.014] [PMID: 24508075]

[38] Acosta EG, Castilla V, Damonte EB. Alternative infectious entry pathways for dengue virus serotypes into mammalian cells. Cell Microbiol 2009; 11(10): 1533-49.
[http://dx.doi.org/10.1111/j.1462-5822.2009.01345.x] [PMID: 19523154]

[39] Piccini LE, Castilla V, Damonte EB. Dengue-3 virus entry into Vero cells: role of clathrin-mediated endocytosis in the outcome of infection. PLoS One 2015; 10(10): e0140824.
[http://dx.doi.org/10.1371/journal.pone.0140824] [PMID: 26469784]

[40] Farias KJ, Machado PR, da Fonseca BA. Chloroquine inhibits dengue virus type 2 replication in Vero cells but not in C6/36 cells. Scientific World Journal 2013; 2013: 282734.

[41] Farias KJ, Machado PR, de Almeida Junior RF, de Aquino AA, da Fonseca BA. Chloroquine interferes with dengue-2 virus replication in U937 cells. Microbiol Immunol 2014; 58(6): 318-26.
[http://dx.doi.org/10.1111/1348-0421.12154] [PMID: 24773578]

[42] Thomé R, Lopes SC, Costa FT, Verinaud L. Chloroquine: modes of action of an undervalued drug. Immunol Lett 2013; 153(1-2): 50-7.
[http://dx.doi.org/10.1016/j.imlet.2013.07.004] [PMID: 23891850]

[43] Wozniacka A, McCauliffe DP. Optimal use of antimalarials in treating cutaneous lupus erythematosus. Am J Clin Dermatol 2005; 6(1): 1-11.
[http://dx.doi.org/10.2165/00128071-200506010-00001] [PMID: 15675885]

[44] Tricou V, Minh NN, Van TP, *et al.* A randomized controlled trial of chloroquine for the treatment of dengue in Vietnamese adults. PLoS Negl Trop Dis 2010; 4(8): e785.
[http://dx.doi.org/10.1371/journal.pntd.0000785] [PMID: 20706626]

[45] Borges MC, Castro LA, Fonseca BA. Chloroquine use improves dengue-related symptoms. Mem Inst Oswaldo Cruz 2013; 108(5): 596-9.
[http://dx.doi.org/10.1590/S0074-02762013000500010] [PMID: 23903975]

[46] Simanjuntak Y, Liang J-J, Lee Y-L, Lin Y-L. Repurposing of prochlorperazine for use against dengue virus infection. J Infect Dis 2015; 211(3): 394-404.
[http://dx.doi.org/10.1093/infdis/jiu377] [PMID: 25028694]

[47] Wang LH, Rothberg KG, Anderson RG. Mis-assembly of clathrin lattices on endosomes reveals a regulatory switch for coated pit formation. J Cell Biol 1993; 123(5): 1107-17.
[http://dx.doi.org/10.1083/jcb.123.5.1107] [PMID: 8245121]

[48] Villareal VA, Rodgers MA, Costello DA, Yang PL. Targeting host lipid synthesis and metabolism to inhibit dengue and hepatitis C viruses. Antiviral Res 2015; 124: 110-21.
[http://dx.doi.org/10.1016/j.antiviral.2015.10.013] [PMID: 26526588]

[49] Martín-Acebes MA, Vázquez-Calvo Á, Saiz JC. Lipids and flaviviruses, present and future

perspectives for the control of dengue, Zika, and West Nile viruses. Prog Lipid Res 2016; 64: 123-37.
[http://dx.doi.org/10.1016/j.plipres.2016.09.005] [PMID: 27702593]

[50]   Cui L, Lee YH, Kumar Y, *et al.* Serum metabolome and lipidome changes in adult patients with primary dengue infection. PLoS Negl Trop Dis 2013; 7(8): e2373.
[http://dx.doi.org/10.1371/journal.pntd.0002373] [PMID: 23967362]

[51]   Durán A, Carrero R, Parra B, *et al.* Association of lipid profile alterations with severe forms of dengue in humans. Arch Virol 2015; 160(7): 1687-92.
[http://dx.doi.org/10.1007/s00705-015-2433-z] [PMID: 25936955]

[52]   Samsa MM, Mondotte JA, Iglesias NG, *et al.* Dengue virus capsid protein usurps lipid droplets for viral particle formation. PLoS Pathog 2009; 5(10): e1000632.
[http://dx.doi.org/10.1371/journal.ppat.1000632] [PMID: 19851456]

[53]   Heaton NS, Perera R, Berger KL, *et al.* Dengue virus nonstructural protein 3 redistributes fatty acid synthase to sites of viral replication and increases cellular fatty acid synthesis. Proc Natl Acad Sci USA 2010; 107(40): 17345-50.
[http://dx.doi.org/10.1073/pnas.1010811107] [PMID: 20855599]

[54]   Perera R, Riley C, Isaac G, *et al.* Dengue virus infection perturbs lipid homeostasis in infected mosquito cells. PLoS Pathog 2012; 8(3): e1002584.
[http://dx.doi.org/10.1371/journal.ppat.1002584] [PMID: 22457619]

[55]   Tongluan N, Ramphan S, Wintachai P, *et al.* Involvement of fatty acid synthase in dengue virus infection. Virol J 2017; 14(1): 28.
[http://dx.doi.org/10.1186/s12985-017-0685-9] [PMID: 28193229]

[56]   Soto-Acosta R, Mosso C, Cervantes-Salazar M, *et al.* The increase in cholesterol levels at early stages after dengue virus infection correlates with an augment in LDL particle uptake and HMG-CoA reductase activity. Virology 2013; 442(2): 132-47.
[http://dx.doi.org/10.1016/j.virol.2013.04.003] [PMID: 23642566]

[57]   Rothwell C, Lebreton A, Young Ng C, *et al.* Cholesterol biosynthesis modulation regulates dengue viral replication. Virology 2009; 389(1-2): 8-19.
[http://dx.doi.org/10.1016/j.virol.2009.03.025] [PMID: 19419745]

[58]   Martínez-Gutierrez M, Castellanos JE, Gallego-Gómez JC. Statins reduce dengue virus production via decreased virion assembly. Intervirology 2011; 54(4): 202-16.
[http://dx.doi.org/10.1159/000321892] [PMID: 21293097]

[59]   Poh MK, Shui G, Xie X, Shi PY, Wenk MR, Gu F. U18666A, an intra-cellular cholesterol transport inhibitor, inhibits dengue virus entry and replication. Antiviral Res 2012; 93(1): 191-8.
[http://dx.doi.org/10.1016/j.antiviral.2011.11.014] [PMID: 22146564]

[60]   Carro AC, Damonte EB. Requirement of cholesterol in the viral envelope for dengue virus infection. Virus Res 2013; 174(1-2): 78-87.
[http://dx.doi.org/10.1016/j.virusres.2013.03.005] [PMID: 23517753]

[61]   Martinez-Gutierrez M, Correa-Londoño LA, Castellanos JE, Gallego-Gómez JC, Osorio JE. Lovastatin delays infection and increases survival rates in AG129 mice infected with dengue virus serotype 2. PLoS One 2014; 9(2): e87412.
[http://dx.doi.org/10.1371/journal.pone.0087412] [PMID: 24586275]

[62]   Whitehorn J, Nguyen CV, Khanh LP, *et al.* Lovastatin for the treatment of adult patients with dengue: a randomized, double-blind, placebo-controlled trial. Clin Infect Dis 2016; 62(4): 468-76.
[PMID: 26565005]

[63]   Walther TC, Farese RV Jr. Lipid droplets and cellular lipid metabolism. Annu Rev Biochem 2012; 81: 687-714.
[http://dx.doi.org/10.1146/annurev-biochem-061009-102430] [PMID: 22524315]

[64]   Soto-Acosta R, Bautista-Carbajal P, Syed GH, Siddiqui A, Del Angel RM. Nordihydroguaiaretic acid

(NDGA) inhibits replication and viral morphogenesis of dengue virus. Antiviral Res 2014; 109: 132-40.
[http://dx.doi.org/10.1016/j.antiviral.2014.07.002] [PMID: 25017471]

[65] Hyrina A, Meng F, McArthur SJ, Eivemark S, Nabi IR, Jean F. Human Subtilisin Kexin Isozyme-1 (SKI-1)/Site-1 Protease (S1P) regulates cytoplasmic lipid droplet abundance: A potential target for indirect-acting anti-dengue virus agents. PLoS One 2017; 12(3): e0174483.
[http://dx.doi.org/10.1371/journal.pone.0174483] [PMID: 28339489]

[66] Edgil D, Diamond MS, Holden KL, Paranjape SM, Harris E. Translation efficiency determines differences in cellular infection among dengue virus type 2 strains. Virology 2003; 317(2): 275-90.
[http://dx.doi.org/10.1016/j.virol.2003.08.012] [PMID: 14698666]

[67] Carocci M, Yang PL. Lactimidomycin is a broad-spectrum inhibitor of dengue and other RNA viruses. Antiviral Res 2016; 128: 57-62.
[http://dx.doi.org/10.1016/j.antiviral.2016.02.005] [PMID: 26872864]

[68] Paradkar PN, Ooi EE, Hanson BJ, Gubler DJ, Vasudevan SG. Unfolded protein response (UPR) gene expression during antibody-dependent enhanced infection of cultured monocytes correlates with dengue disease severity. Biosci Rep 2011; 31(3): 221-30.
[http://dx.doi.org/10.1042/BSR20100078] [PMID: 20858223]

[69] Peña J, Harris E. Early dengue virus protein synthesis induces extensive rearrangement of the endoplasmic reticulum independent of the UPR and SREBP-2 pathway. PLoS One 2012; 7(6): e38202.
[http://dx.doi.org/10.1371/journal.pone.0038202] [PMID: 22675522]

[70] Fraser JE, Watanabe S, Wang C, *et al.* A nuclear transport inhibitor that modulates the unfolded protein response and provides in vivo protection against lethal dengue virus infection. J Infect Dis 2014; 210(11): 1780-91.
[http://dx.doi.org/10.1093/infdis/jiu319] [PMID: 24903662]

[71] Carocci M, Hinshaw SM, Rodgers MA, *et al.* The bioactive lipid 4-hydroxyphenyl retinamide inhibits flavivirus replication. Antimicrob Agents Chemother 2015; 59(1): 85-95.
[http://dx.doi.org/10.1128/AAC.04177-14] [PMID: 25313218]

[72] Fraser JE, Wang C, Chan KW, Vasudevan SG, Jans DA. Novel dengue virus inhibitor 4-HPR activates ATF4 independent of protein kinase R-like Endoplasmic Reticulum Kinase and elevates levels of eIF2α phosphorylation in virus infected cells. Antiviral Res 2016; 130: 1-6.
[http://dx.doi.org/10.1016/j.antiviral.2016.03.006] [PMID: 26965420]

[73] Kanlaya R, Pattanakitsakul SN, Sinchaikul S, Chen ST, Thongboonkerd V. The ubiquitin-proteasome pathway is important for dengue virus infection in primary human endothelial cells. J Proteome Res 2010; 9(10): 4960-71.
[http://dx.doi.org/10.1021/pr100219y] [PMID: 20718508]

[74] Fernandez-Garcia MD, Meertens L, Bonazzi M, Cossart P, Arenzana-Seisdedos F, Amara A. Appraising the roles of CBLL1 and the ubiquitin/proteasome system for flavivirus entry and replication. J Virol 2011; 85(6): 2980-9.
[http://dx.doi.org/10.1128/JVI.02483-10] [PMID: 21191016]

[75] Nag DK, Finley D. A small-molecule inhibitor of deubiquitinating enzyme USP14 inhibits Dengue virus replication. Virus Res 2012; 165(1): 103-6.
[http://dx.doi.org/10.1016/j.virusres.2012.01.009] [PMID: 22306365]

[76] Choy MM, Zhang SL, Costa VV, Tan HC, Horrevorts S, Ooi EE. Proteasome Inhibition Suppresses Dengue Virus Egress in Antibody Dependent Infection. PLoS Negl Trop Dis 2015; 9(11): e0004058.
[http://dx.doi.org/10.1371/journal.pntd.0004058] [PMID: 26565697]

[77] Diamond MS, Zachariah M, Harris E. Mycophenolic acid inhibits dengue virus infection by preventing replication of viral RNA. Virology 2002; 304(2): 211-21.
[http://dx.doi.org/10.1006/viro.2002.1685] [PMID: 12504563]

[78]   Crance JM, Scaramozzino N, Jouan A, Garin D. Interferon, ribavirin, 6-azauridine and glycyrrhizin: antiviral compounds active against pathogenic flaviviruses. Antiviral Res 2003; 58(1): 73-9.
[http://dx.doi.org/10.1016/S0166-3542(02)00185-7] [PMID: 12719009]

[79]   Takhampunya R, Ubol S, Houng HS, Cameron CE, Padmanabhan R. Inhibition of dengue virus replication by mycophenolic acid and ribavirin. J Gen Virol 2006; 87(Pt 7): 1947-52.
[http://dx.doi.org/10.1099/vir.0.81655-0] [PMID: 16760396]

[80]   Leyssen P, Balzarini J, De Clercq E, Neyts J. The predominant mechanism by which ribavirin exerts its antiviral activity in vitro against flaviviruses and paramyxoviruses is mediated by inhibition of IMP dehydrogenase. J Virol 2005; 79(3): 1943-7.
[http://dx.doi.org/10.1128/JVI.79.3.1943-1947.2005] [PMID: 15650220]

[81]   Malinoski FJ, Hasty SE, Ussery MA, Dalrymple JM. Prophylactic ribavirin treatment of dengue type 1 infection in rhesus monkeys. Antiviral Res 1990; 13(3): 139-49.
[http://dx.doi.org/10.1016/0166-3542(90)90029-7] [PMID: 2353804]

[82]   Schul W, Liu W, Xu HY, Flamand M, Vasudevan SG. A dengue fever viremia model in mice shows reduction in viral replication and suppression of the inflammatory response after treatment with antiviral drugs. J Infect Dis 2007; 195(5): 665-74.
[http://dx.doi.org/10.1086/511310] [PMID: 17262707]

[83]   Rattanaburee T, Junking M, Panya A, et al. Inhibition of dengue virus production and cytokine/chemokine expression by ribavirin and compound A. Antiviral Res 2015; 124: 83-92.
[http://dx.doi.org/10.1016/j.antiviral.2015.10.005] [PMID: 26542647]

[84]   Yeo KL, Chen YL, Xu HY, et al. Synergistic suppression of dengue virus replication using a combination of nucleoside analogs and nucleoside synthesis inhibitors. Antimicrob Agents Chemother 2015; 59(4): 2086-93.
[http://dx.doi.org/10.1128/AAC.04779-14] [PMID: 25624323]

[85]   McDowell M, Gonzales SR, Kumarapperuma SC, Jeselnik M, Arterburn JB, Hanley KA. A novel nucleoside analog, 1-β-d-ribofuranosyl-3-ethynyl-[1,2,4]triazole (ETAR), exhibits efficacy against a broad range of flaviviruses in vitro. Antiviral Res 2010; 87(1): 78-80.
[http://dx.doi.org/10.1016/j.antiviral.2010.04.007] [PMID: 20416341]

[86]   Sepúlveda CS, Fascio ML, Mazzucco MB, et al. Synthesis and evaluation of N-substituted acridones as antiviral agents against haemorrhagic fever viruses. Antivir Chem Chemother 2008; 19(1): 41-7.
[http://dx.doi.org/10.1177/095632020801900106] [PMID: 18610557]

[87]   Mazzucco MB, Talarico LB, Vatansever S, et al. Antiviral activity of an N-allyl acridone against dengue virus. J Biomed Sci 2015; 22: 29.
[http://dx.doi.org/10.1186/s12929-015-0134-2] [PMID: 25908170]

[88]   Qing M, Zou G, Wang QY, et al. Characterization of dengue virus resistance to brequinar in cell culture. Antimicrob Agents Chemother 2010; 54(9): 3686-95.
[http://dx.doi.org/10.1128/AAC.00561-10] [PMID: 20606073]

[89]   Wang QY, Bushell S, Qing M, et al. Inhibition of dengue virus through suppression of host pyrimidine biosynthesis. J Virol 2011; 85(13): 6548-56.
[http://dx.doi.org/10.1128/JVI.02510-10] [PMID: 21507975]

[90]   Cuenda A, Rousseau S. p38 MAP-kinases pathway regulation, function and role in human diseases. Biochim Biophys Acta 2007; 1773: 1358-75.

[91]   Wagner EF, Nebreda AR. Signal integration by JNK and p38 MAPK pathways in cancer development. Nat Rev Cancer 2009; 9(8): 537-49.
[http://dx.doi.org/10.1038/nrc2694] [PMID: 19629069]

[92]   Keshet Y, Seger R. The MAP kinase signaling cascades: a system of hundreds of components regulates a diverse array of physiological functions. Methods Mol Biol 2010; 661: 3-38.
[http://dx.doi.org/10.1007/978-1-60761-795-2_1] [PMID: 20811974]

[93]   Rauch N, Rukhlenko OS, Kolch W, Kholodenko BN. MAPK kinase signalling dynamics regulate cell fate decisions and drug resistance. Curr Opin Struct Biol 2016; 41: 151-8.
[http://dx.doi.org/10.1016/j.sbi.2016.07.019] [PMID: 27521656]

[94]   Zehorai E, Yao Z, Plotnikov A, Seger R. The subcellular localization of MEK and ERK--a novel nuclear translocation signal (NTS) paves a way to the nucleus. Mol Cell Endocrinol 2010; 314(2): 213-20.
[http://dx.doi.org/10.1016/j.mce.2009.04.008] [PMID: 19406201]

[95]   Huerta-Zepeda A, Cabello-Gutiérrez C, Cime-Castillo J, *et al.* Crosstalk between coagulation and inflammation during Dengue virus infection. Thromb Haemost 2008; 99(5): 936-43.
[PMID: 18449425]

[96]   Cabello-Gutiérrez C, Manjarrez-Zavala ME, Huerta-Zepeda A, *et al.* Modification of the cytoprotective protein C pathway during Dengue virus infection of human endothelial vascular cells. Thromb Haemost 2009; 101(5): 916-28.
[PMID: 19404546]

[97]   Ceballos-Olvera I, Chávez-Salinas S, Medina F, Ludert JE, del Angel RM. JNK phosphorylation, induced during dengue virus infection, is important for viral infection and requires the presence of cholesterol. Virology 2010; 396(1): 30-6.
[http://dx.doi.org/10.1016/j.virol.2009.10.019] [PMID: 19897220]

[98]   Roth H, Magg V, Uch F, *et al.* Flavivirus infection uncouples translation suppression from cellular stress responses. MBio 2017; 8(1): e02150-16.
[http://dx.doi.org/10.1128/mBio.02150-16] [PMID: 28074025]

[99]   Callaway JB, Smith SA, McKinnon KP, de Silva AM, Crowe JE Jr, Ting JP. Spleen tyrosine kinase (Syk) mediates IL-1β induction by primary human monocytes during antibody-enhanced dengue virus infection. J Biol Chem 2015; 290(28): 17306-20.
[http://dx.doi.org/10.1074/jbc.M115.664136] [PMID: 26032420]

[100]   Albarnaz JD, De Oliveira LC, Torres AA, *et al.* MEK/ERK activation plays a decisive role in yellow fever virus replication: implication as an antiviral therapeutic target. Antiviral Res 2014; 111: 82-92.
[http://dx.doi.org/10.1016/j.antiviral.2014.09.004] [PMID: 25241249]

[101]   Smith JL, Stein DA, Shum D, *et al.* Inhibition of dengue virus replication by a class of small-molecule compounds that antagonize dopamine receptor d4 and downstream mitogen-activated protein kinase signaling. J Virol 2014; 88(10): 5533-42.
[http://dx.doi.org/10.1128/JVI.00365-14] [PMID: 24599995]

[102]   Sreekanth GP, Chuncharunee A, Sirimontaporn A, *et al.* Role of ERK1/2 signaling in dengue virus-induced liver injury. Virus Res 2014; 188: 15-26.
[http://dx.doi.org/10.1016/j.virusres.2014.03.025] [PMID: 24704674]

[103]   Bode AM, Dong Z. The functional contrariety of JNK. Mol Carcinog 2007; 46(8): 591-8.
[http://dx.doi.org/10.1002/mc.20348] [PMID: 17538955]

[104]   Huang M, Xu A, Wu X, *et al.* Japanese encephalitis virus induces apoptosis by the IRE1/JNK pathway of ER stress response in BHK-21 cells. Arch Virol 2016; 161(3): 699-703.
[http://dx.doi.org/10.1007/s00705-015-2715-5] [PMID: 26660165]

[105]   Bain J, Plater L, Elliott M, *et al.* The selectivity of protein kinase inhibitors: a further update. Biochem J 2007; 408(3): 297-315.
[http://dx.doi.org/10.1042/BJ20070797] [PMID: 17850214]

[106]   Sreekanth GP, Chuncharunee A, Cheunsuchon B, Noisakran S, Yenchitsomanus PT, Limjindaporn T. JNK1/2 inhibitor reduces dengue virus-induced liver injury. Antiviral Res 2017; 141: 7-18.
[http://dx.doi.org/10.1016/j.antiviral.2017.02.003] [PMID: 28188818]

[107]   Arias J, Valero N, Mosquera J, *et al.* Increased expression of cytokines, soluble cytokine receptors, soluble apoptosis ligand and apoptosis in dengue. Virology 2014; 452-453: 42-51.

[http://dx.doi.org/10.1016/j.virol.2013.12.027] [PMID: 24606681]

[108] Cuadrado A, Nebreda AR. Mechanisms and functions of p38 MAPK signalling. Biochem J 2010; 429(3): 403-17.
[http://dx.doi.org/10.1042/BJ20100323] [PMID: 20626350]

[109] Nagila A, Netsawang J, Suttitheptumrong A, *et al.* Inhibition of p38MAPK and CD137 signaling reduce dengue virus-induced TNF-α secretion and apoptosis. Virol J 2013; 10: 105.
[http://dx.doi.org/10.1186/1743-422X-10-105] [PMID: 23557259]

[110] Morchang A, Yasamut U, Netsawang J, *et al.* Cell death gene expression profile: role of RIPK2 in dengue virus-mediated apoptosis. Virus Res 2011; 156(1-2): 25-34.
[http://dx.doi.org/10.1016/j.virusres.2010.12.012] [PMID: 21195733]

[111] Fu Y, Yip A, Seah PG, Blasco F, Shi PY, Hervé M. Modulation of inflammation and pathology during dengue virus infection by p38 MAPK inhibitor SB203580. Antiviral Res 2014; 110: 151-7.
[http://dx.doi.org/10.1016/j.antiviral.2014.08.004] [PMID: 25131378]

[112] Yeh CJ, Lin PY, Liao MH, *et al.* TNF-alpha mediates pseudorabies virus-induced apoptosis via the activation of p38 MAPK and JNK/SAPK signaling. Virology 2008; 381(1): 55-66.
[http://dx.doi.org/10.1016/j.virol.2008.08.023] [PMID: 18799179]

[113] Sreekanth GP, Chuncharunee A, Sirimontaporn A, *et al.* SB203580 Modulates p38 MAPK Signaling and Dengue Virus-Induced Liver Injury by Reducing MAPKAPK2, HSP27, and ATF2 Phosphorylation. PLoS One 2016; 11(2): e0149486.
[http://dx.doi.org/10.1371/journal.pone.0149486] [PMID: 26901653]

[114] Chu JJ, Yang PL. c-Src protein kinase inhibitors block assembly and maturation of dengue virus. Proc Natl Acad Sci USA 2007; 104(9): 3520-5.
[http://dx.doi.org/10.1073/pnas.0611681104] [PMID: 17360676]

[115] de Wispelaere M, LaCroix AJ, Yang PL. The small molecules AZD0530 and dasatinib inhibit dengue virus RNA replication via Fyn kinase. J Virol 2013; 87(13): 7367-81.
[http://dx.doi.org/10.1128/JVI.00632-13] [PMID: 23616652]

[116] Vincetti P, Caporuscio F, Kaptein S, *et al.* Discovery of multitarget antivirals acting on both the dengue virus NS5-NS3 interaction and the host Src/Fyn kinases. J Med Chem 2015; 58(12): 4964-75.
[http://dx.doi.org/10.1021/acs.jmedchem.5b00108] [PMID: 26039671]

[117] Clark MJ, Miduturu C, Schmidt AG, *et al.* GNF-2 inhibits dengue virus by targeting Abl kinases and the viral E protein. Cell Chem Biol 2016; 23(4): 443-52.
[http://dx.doi.org/10.1016/j.chembiol.2016.03.010] [PMID: 27105280]

[118] Bekerman E, Neveu G, Shulla A, *et al.* Anticancer kinase inhibitors impair intracellular viral trafficking and exert broad-spectrum antiviral effects. J Clin Invest 2017; 127(4): 1338-52.
[http://dx.doi.org/10.1172/JCI89857] [PMID: 28240606]

[119] Chang TH, Liao CL, Lin YL. Flavivirus induces interferon-beta gene expression through a pathway involving RIG-I-dependent IRF-3 and PI3K-dependent NF-kappaB activation. Microbes Infect 2006; 8(1): 157-71.
[http://dx.doi.org/10.1016/j.micinf.2005.06.014] [PMID: 16182584]

[120] Chen HH, Chen CC, Lin YS, *et al.* AR-12 suppresses dengue virus replication by down-regulation of PI3K/AKT and GRP78. Antiviral Res 2017; 142: 158-68.
[http://dx.doi.org/10.1016/j.antiviral.2017.02.015] [PMID: 28238876]

[121] Acosta EG, Kumar A, Bartenschlager R. Revisiting dengue virus-host cell interaction: new insights into molecular and cellular virology. Adv Virus Res 2014; 88: 1-109.
[http://dx.doi.org/10.1016/B978-0-12-800098-4.00001-5] [PMID: 24373310]

[122] Courageot MP, Frenkiel MP, Dos Santos CD, Deubel V, Desprès P. Alpha-glucosidase inhibitors reduce dengue virus production by affecting the initial steps of virion morphogenesis in the endoplasmic reticulum. J Virol 2000; 74(1): 564-72.

[http://dx.doi.org/10.1128/JVI.74.1.564-572.2000] [PMID: 10590151]

[123]   Mohan S, McAtamney S, Jayakanthan K, Eskandari R, von Itzstein M, Pinto BM. Antiviral activities of sulfonium-ion glucosidase inhibitors and 5-thiomannosylamine disaccharide derivatives against dengue virus. Int J Antimicrob Agents 2012; 40(3): 273-6.
[http://dx.doi.org/10.1016/j.ijantimicag.2012.05.002] [PMID: 22784856]

[124]   Chang J, Wang L, Ma D, *et al*. Novel imino sugar derivatives demonstrate potent antiviral activity against flaviviruses. Antimicrob Agents Chemother 2009; 53(4): 1501-8.
[http://dx.doi.org/10.1128/AAC.01457-08] [PMID: 19223639]

[125]   Chang J, Schul W, Butters TD, *et al*. Combination of α-glucosidase inhibitor and ribavirin for the treatment of dengue virus infection *in vitro* and *in vivo*. Antiviral Res 2011; 89(1): 26-34.
[http://dx.doi.org/10.1016/j.antiviral.2010.11.002] [PMID: 21073903]

[126]   Chang J, Schul W, Yip A, Xu X, Guo JT, Block TM. Competitive inhibitor of cellular α-glucosidases protects mice from lethal dengue virus infection. Antiviral Res 2011; 92(2): 369-71.
[http://dx.doi.org/10.1016/j.antiviral.2011.08.003] [PMID: 21854808]

[127]   Sayce AC, Alonzi DS, Killingbeck SS, *et al*. Iminosugars inhibit dengue virus production via inhibition of ER alpha-glucosidases-not glycolipid processing enzymes. PLoS Negl Trop Dis 2016; 10(3): e0004524.
[http://dx.doi.org/10.1371/journal.pntd.0004524] [PMID: 26974655]

[128]   Whitby K, Pierson TC, Geiss B, *et al*. Castanospermine, a potent inhibitor of dengue virus infection *in vitro* and *in vivo*. J Virol 2005; 79(14): 8698-706.
[http://dx.doi.org/10.1128/JVI.79.14.8698-8706.2005] [PMID: 15994763]

[129]   Rathore AP, Paradkar PN, Watanabe S, *et al*. Celgosivir treatment misfolds dengue virus NS1 protein, induces cellular pro-survival genes and protects against lethal challenge mouse model. Antiviral Res 2011; 92(3): 453-60.
[http://dx.doi.org/10.1016/j.antiviral.2011.10.002] [PMID: 22020302]

[130]   Watanabe S, Rathore AP, Sung C, *et al*. Dose- and schedule-dependent protective efficacy of celgosivir in a lethal mouse model for dengue virus infection informs dosing regimen for a proof of concept clinical trial. Antiviral Res 2012; 96(1): 32-5.
[http://dx.doi.org/10.1016/j.antiviral.2012.07.008] [PMID: 22867971]

[131]   Low JG, Sung C, Wijaya L, *et al*. Efficacy and safety of celgosivir in patients with dengue fever (CELADEN): a phase 1b, randomised, double-blind, placebo-controlled, proof-of-concept trial. Lancet Infect Dis 2014; 14(8): 706-15.
[http://dx.doi.org/10.1016/S1473-3099(14)70730-3] [PMID: 24877997]

[132]   Sung C, Wei Y, Watanabe S, *et al*. Extended evaluation of virological, immunological and pharmacokinetic endpoints of CELADEN: A randomized, placebo-controlled trial of celgosivir in dengue fever patients. PLoS Negl Trop Dis 2016; 10(8): e0004851.
[http://dx.doi.org/10.1371/journal.pntd.0004851] [PMID: 27509020]

[133]   Watanabe S, Chan KW, Dow G, Ooi EE, Low JG, Vasudevan SG. Optimizing celgosivir therapy in mouse models of dengue virus infection of serotypes 1 and 2: The search for a window for potential therapeutic efficacy. Antiviral Res 2016; 127: 10-9.
[http://dx.doi.org/10.1016/j.antiviral.2015.12.008] [PMID: 26794905]

[134]   Caputo AT, Alonzi DS, Marti L, *et al*. Structures of mammalian ER α-glucosidase II capture the binding modes of broad-spectrum iminosugar antivirals. Proc Natl Acad Sci USA 2016; 113(32): E4630-8.
[http://dx.doi.org/10.1073/pnas.1604463113] [PMID: 27462106]

[135]   Warfield KL, Plummer EM, Sayce AC, *et al*. Inhibition of endoplasmic reticulum glucosidases is required for *in vitro* and *in vivo* dengue antiviral activity by the iminosugar UV-4. Antiviral Res 2016; 129: 93-8.
[http://dx.doi.org/10.1016/j.antiviral.2016.03.001] [PMID: 26946111]

[136] Hardes K, Ivanova T, Thaa B, *et al.* Elongated and Shortened Peptidomimetic Inhibitors of the Proprotein Convertase Furin. ChemMedChem 2017; 12(8): 613-20.
[http://dx.doi.org/10.1002/cmdc.201700108] [PMID: 28334511]

[137] Kouretova J, Hammamy MZ, Epp A, *et al.* Effects of NS2B-NS3 protease and furin inhibition on West Nile and Dengue virus replication. J Enzyme Inhib Med Chem 2017; 32(1): 712-21.
[http://dx.doi.org/10.1080/14756366.2017.1306521] [PMID: 28385094]

[138] Peng M, Watanabe S, Chan KW, *et al.* Luteolin restricts dengue virus replication through inhibition of the proprotein convertase furin. Antiviral Res 2017; 143: 176-85.
[http://dx.doi.org/10.1016/j.antiviral.2017.03.026] [PMID: 28389141]

[139] Zhang R, Miner JJ, Gorman MJ, *et al.* A CRISPR screen defines a signal peptide processing pathway required by flaviviruses. Nature 2016; 535(7610): 164-8.
[http://dx.doi.org/10.1038/nature18625] [PMID: 27383988]

[140] Estoppey D, Lee CM, Janoschke M, *et al.* The Natural Product Cavinafungin Selectively Interferes with Zika and Dengue Virus Replication by Inhibition of the Host Signal Peptidase. Cell Reports 2017; 19(3): 451-60.
[http://dx.doi.org/10.1016/j.celrep.2017.03.071] [PMID: 28423309]

[141] Schoggins JW, Wilson SJ, Panis M, *et al.* Corrigendum: A diverse range of gene products are effectors of the type I interferon antiviral response. Nature 2015; 525(7567): 144.
[PMID: 26153858]

[142] Hoffmann HH, Schneider WM, Rice CM. Interferons and viruses: an evolutionary arms race of molecular interactions. Trends Immunol 2015; 36(3): 124-38.
[http://dx.doi.org/10.1016/j.it.2015.01.004] [PMID: 25704559]

[143] Diamond MS, Roberts TG, Edgil D, Lu B, Ernst J, Harris E. Modulation of Dengue virus infection in human cells by alpha, beta, and gamma interferons. J Virol 2000; 74(11): 4957-66.
[http://dx.doi.org/10.1128/JVI.74.11.4957-4966.2000] [PMID: 10799569]

[144] de Veer MJ, Holko M, Frevel M, *et al.* Functional classification of interferon-stimulated genes identified using microarrays. J Leukoc Biol 2001; 69(6): 912-20.
[PMID: 11404376]

[145] Lanford RE, Guerra B, Lee H, Chavez D, Brasky KM, Bigger CB. Genomic response to interferon-alpha in chimpanzees: implications of rapid downregulation for hepatitis C kinetics. Hepatology 2006; 43(5): 961-72.
[http://dx.doi.org/10.1002/hep.21167] [PMID: 16628626]

[146] Sarasin-Filipowicz M, Oakeley EJ, Duong FH, *et al.* Interferon signaling and treatment outcome in chronic hepatitis C. Proc Natl Acad Sci USA 2008; 105(19): 7034-9.
[http://dx.doi.org/10.1073/pnas.0707882105] [PMID: 18467494]

[147] Green AM, Beatty PR, Hadjilaou A, Harris E. Innate immunity to dengue virus infection and subversion of antiviral responses. J Mol Biol 2014; 426(6): 1148-60.
[http://dx.doi.org/10.1016/j.jmb.2013.11.023] [PMID: 24316047]

[148] Muñoz-Jordan JL, Sánchez-Burgos GG, Laurent-Rolle M, García-Sastre A. Inhibition of interferon signaling by dengue virus. Proc Natl Acad Sci USA 2003; 100(24): 14333-8.
[http://dx.doi.org/10.1073/pnas.2335168100] [PMID: 14612562]

[149] Aguirre S, Maestre AM, Pagni S, *et al.* DENV inhibits type I IFN production in infected cells by cleaving human STING. PLoS Pathog 2012; 8(10): e1002934.
[http://dx.doi.org/10.1371/journal.ppat.1002934] [PMID: 23055924]

[150] Angleró-Rodríguez YI, Pantoja P, Sariol CA. Dengue virus subverts the interferon induction pathway via NS2B/3 protease-IκB kinase epsilon interaction. Clin Vaccine Immunol 2014; 21(1): 29-38.
[http://dx.doi.org/10.1128/CVI.00500-13] [PMID: 24173023]

[151] Ashour J, Laurent-Rolle M, Shi PY, García-Sastre A. NS5 of dengue virus mediates STAT2 binding and degradation. J Virol 2009; 83(11): 5408-18.
[http://dx.doi.org/10.1128/JVI.02188-08] [PMID: 19279106]

[152] Mazzon M, Jones M, Davidson A, Chain B, Jacobs M. Dengue virus NS5 inhibits interferon-alpha signaling by blocking signal transducer and activator of transcription 2 phosphorylation. J Infect Dis 2009; 200(8): 1261-70.
[http://dx.doi.org/10.1086/605847] [PMID: 19754307]

[153] Bidet K, Dadlani D, Garcia-Blanco MA. G3BP1, G3BP2 and CAPRIN1 are required for translation of interferon stimulated mRNAs and are targeted by a dengue virus non-coding RNA. PLoS Pathog 2014; 10(7): e1004242.
[http://dx.doi.org/10.1371/journal.ppat.1004242] [PMID: 24992036]

[154] Cobos Jiménez V, Martinez FO, Booiman T, *et al.* G3BP1 restricts HIV-1 replication in macrophages and T-cells by sequestering viral RNA. Virology 2015; 486: 94-104.
[http://dx.doi.org/10.1016/j.virol.2015.09.007] [PMID: 26432022]

[155] Manokaran G, Finol E, Wang C, *et al.* Dengue subgenomic RNA binds TRIM25 to inhibit interferon expression for epidemiological fitness. Science 2015; 350(6257): 217-21.
[http://dx.doi.org/10.1126/science.aab3369] [PMID: 26138103]

[156] Gack MU. Mechanisms of RIG-I-like receptor activation and manipulation by viral pathogens. J Virol 2014; 88(10): 5213-6.
[http://dx.doi.org/10.1128/JVI.03370-13] [PMID: 24623415]

[157] Sulkowski MS, Cooper C, Hunyady B, *et al.* Management of adverse effects of Peg-IFN and ribavirin therapy for hepatitis C. Nat Rev Gastroenterol Hepatol 2011; 8(4): 212-23.
[http://dx.doi.org/10.1038/nrgastro.2011.21] [PMID: 21386812]

[158] Fritz-French C, Tyor W. Interferon-α (IFNα) neurotoxicity. Cytokine Growth Factor Rev 2012; 23(1-2): 7-14.
[http://dx.doi.org/10.1016/j.cytogfr.2012.01.001] [PMID: 22342642]

[159] Kavanagh D, McGlasson S, Jury A, *et al.* Type I interferon causes thrombotic microangiopathy by a dose-dependent toxic effect on the microvasculature. Blood 2016; 128(24): 2824-33.
[http://dx.doi.org/10.1182/blood-2016-05-715987] [PMID: 27663672]

[160] Olagnier D, Peri S, Steel C, *et al.* Cellular oxidative stress response controls the antiviral and apoptotic programs in dengue virus-infected dendritic cells. PLoS Pathog 2014; 10(12): e1004566.
[http://dx.doi.org/10.1371/journal.ppat.1004566] [PMID: 25521078]

[161] Tseng CK, Lin CK, Wu YH, *et al.* Human heme oxygenase 1 is a potential host cell factor against dengue virus replication. Sci Rep 2016; 6: 32176.
[http://dx.doi.org/10.1038/srep32176] [PMID: 27553177]

[162] Es-Saad S, Tremblay N, Baril M, Lamarre D. Regulators of innate immunity as novel targets for panviral therapeutics. Curr Opin Virol 2012; 2(5): 622-8.
[http://dx.doi.org/10.1016/j.coviro.2012.08.009] [PMID: 23017246]

[163] Ireton RC, Gale M Jr. Pushing to a cure by harnessing innate immunity against hepatitis C virus. Antiviral Res 2014; 108: 156-64.
[http://dx.doi.org/10.1016/j.antiviral.2014.05.012] [PMID: 24907428]

[164] Patel DA, Patel AC, Nolan WC, Zhang Y, Holtzman MJ. High throughput screening for small molecule enhancers of the interferon signaling pathway to drive next-generation antiviral drug discovery. PLoS One 2012; 7(5): e36594.
[http://dx.doi.org/10.1371/journal.pone.0036594] [PMID: 22574190]

[165] Silin DS, Lyubomska OV, Ershov FI, Frolov VM, Kutsyna GA. Synthetic and natural immunomodulators acting as interferon inducers. Curr Pharm Des 2009; 15(11): 1238-47.
[http://dx.doi.org/10.2174/138161209787846847] [PMID: 19355963]

[166] Calvert JK, Helbig KJ, Dimasi D, *et al.* Dengue Virus Infection of Primary Endothelial Cells Induces Innate Immune Responses, Changes in Endothelial Cells Function and Is Restricted by Interferon-Stimulated Responses. J Interferon Cytokine Res 2015; 35(8): 654-65.
[http://dx.doi.org/10.1089/jir.2014.0195] [PMID: 25902155]

[167] Yu JS, Wu YH, Tseng CK, *et al.* Schisandrin A inhibits dengue viral replication via upregulating antiviral interferon responses through STAT signaling pathway. Sci Rep 2017; 7: 45171.
[http://dx.doi.org/10.1038/srep45171] [PMID: 28338050]

[168] Yu JS, Tseng CK, Lin CK, *et al.* Celastrol inhibits dengue virus replication via up-regulating type I interferon and downstream interferon-stimulated responses. Antiviral Res 2017; 137: 49-57.
[http://dx.doi.org/10.1016/j.antiviral.2016.11.010] [PMID: 27847245]

[169] Bedard KM, Wang ML, Proll SC, *et al.* Isoflavone agonists of IRF-3 dependent signaling have antiviral activity against RNA viruses. J Virol 2012; 86(13): 7334-44.
[http://dx.doi.org/10.1128/JVI.06867-11] [PMID: 22532686]

[170] Sharma N, Mishra KP, Ganju L. Salidroside exhibits anti-dengue virus activity by upregulating host innate immune factors. Arch Virol 2016; 161(12): 3331-44.
[http://dx.doi.org/10.1007/s00705-016-3034-1] [PMID: 27581807]

[171] Tsai WL, Cheng JS, Shu CW, *et al.* Asunaprevir evokes hepatocytes innate immunity to restrict the replication of hepatitis C and dengue virus. Front Microbiol 2017; 8: 668.
[http://dx.doi.org/10.3389/fmicb.2017.00668] [PMID: 28473813]

[172] Chiang C, Beljanski V, Yin K, *et al.* Sequence-specific modifications enhance the broad-spectrum antiviral response activated by RIG-I agonists. J Virol 2015; 89(15): 8011-25.
[http://dx.doi.org/10.1128/JVI.00845-15] [PMID: 26018150]

[173] Pryke KM, Abraham J, Sali TM, *et al.* A novel agonist of the TRIF pathway induces a cellular state refractory to replication of Zika, Chikungunya, and dengue viruses. MBio 2017; 8(3): e00452-17.
[http://dx.doi.org/10.1128/mBio.00452-17] [PMID: 28465426]

[174] Fusco DN, Pratt H, Kandilas S, *et al.* HELZ2 is an IFN effector mediating suppression of dengue virus. Front Microbiol 2017; 8: 240.
[http://dx.doi.org/10.3389/fmicb.2017.00240] [PMID: 28265266]

[175] Corrêa G, de A Lindenberg C, Fernandes-Santos C, *et al.* The purinergic receptor P2X7 role in control of Dengue virus-2 infection and cytokine/chemokine production in infected human monocytes. Immunobiology 2016; 221(7): 794-802.
[http://dx.doi.org/10.1016/j.imbio.2016.02.003] [PMID: 26969484]

[176] Lima-Junior RS, Mello CdaS, Siani AC, Valente LM, Kubelka CF. Uncaria tomentosa alkaloidal fraction reduces paracellular permeability, IL-8 and NS1 production on human microvascular endothelial cells infected with dengue virus. Nat Prod Commun 2013; 8(11): 1547-50.
[PMID: 24427938]

[177] Fialho LG, da Silva VP, Reis SR, *et al.* Antiviral and Immunomodulatory Effects of Norantea brasiliensis Choisy on Dengue Virus-2. Intervirology 2016; 59(4): 217-27.
[http://dx.doi.org/10.1159/000455855] [PMID: 28329744]

[178] Mello CD, Valente LM, Wolff T, *et al.* Decrease in Dengue virus-2 infection and reduction of cytokine/chemokine production by Uncaria guianensis in human hepatocyte cell line Huh-7. Mem Inst Oswaldo Cruz 2017; 112(6): 458-68.
[http://dx.doi.org/10.1590/0074-02760160323] [PMID: 28591408]

[179] Sood R, Raut R, Tyagi P, *et al.* Cissampelos pareira Linn: Natural Source of Potent Antiviral Activity against All Four Dengue Virus Serotypes. PLoS Negl Trop Dis 2015; 9(12): e0004255.
[http://dx.doi.org/10.1371/journal.pntd.0004255] [PMID: 26709822]

[180] Wolf D, Goff SP. Host restriction factors blocking retroviral replication. Annu Rev Genet 2008; 42: 143-63.

[http://dx.doi.org/10.1146/annurev.genet.42.110807.091704] [PMID: 18624631]

[181]   Fink J, Gu F, Ling L, *et al.* Host gene expression profiling of dengue virus infection in cell lines and patients. PLoS Negl Trop Dis 2007; 1(2): e86.
[http://dx.doi.org/10.1371/journal.pntd.0000086] [PMID: 18060089]

[182]   Jiang D, Weidner JM, Qing M, *et al.* Identification of five interferon-induced cellular proteins that inhibit west nile virus and dengue virus infections. J Virol 2010; 84(16): 8332-41.
[http://dx.doi.org/10.1128/JVI.02199-09] [PMID: 20534863]

[183]   Hinson ER, Cresswell P. The antiviral protein, viperin, localizes to lipid droplets via its N-terminal amphipathic alpha-helix. Proc Natl Acad Sci USA 2009; 106(48): 20452-7.
[http://dx.doi.org/10.1073/pnas.0911679106] [PMID: 19920176]

[184]   Helbig KJ, Carr JM, Calvert JK, *et al.* Viperin is induced following dengue virus type-2 (DENV-2) infection and has anti-viral actions requiring the C-terminal end of viperin. PLoS Negl Trop Dis 2013; 7(4): e2178.
[http://dx.doi.org/10.1371/journal.pntd.0002178] [PMID: 23638199]

[185]   Perreira JM, Chin CR, Feeley EM, Brass AL. IFITMs restrict the replication of multiple pathogenic viruses. J Mol Biol 2013; 425(24): 4937-55.
[http://dx.doi.org/10.1016/j.jmb.2013.09.024] [PMID: 24076421]

[186]   Diamond MS, Farzan M. The broad-spectrum antiviral functions of IFIT and IFITM proteins. Nat Rev Immunol 2013; 13(1): 46-57.
[http://dx.doi.org/10.1038/nri3344] [PMID: 23237964]

[187]   Brass AL, Huang IC, Benita Y, *et al.* The IFITM proteins mediate cellular resistance to influenza A H1N1 virus, West Nile virus, and dengue virus. Cell 2009; 139(7): 1243-54.
[http://dx.doi.org/10.1016/j.cell.2009.12.017] [PMID: 20064371]

[188]   Chan YK, Huang IC, Farzan M. IFITM proteins restrict antibody-dependent enhancement of dengue virus infection. PLoS One 2012; 7(3): e34508.
[http://dx.doi.org/10.1371/journal.pone.0034508] [PMID: 22479637]

[189]   John SP, Chin CR, Perreira JM, *et al.* The CD225 domain of IFITM3 is required for both IFITM protein association and inhibition of influenza A virus and dengue virus replication. J Virol 2013; 87(14): 7837-52.
[http://dx.doi.org/10.1128/JVI.00481-13] [PMID: 23658454]

[190]   Zhu X, He Z, Yuan J, *et al.* IFITM3-containing exosome as a novel mediator for anti-viral response in dengue virus infection. Cell Microbiol 2015; 17(1): 105-18.
[http://dx.doi.org/10.1111/cmi.12339] [PMID: 25131332]

[191]   Helbig KJ, Eyre NS, Yip E, *et al.* The antiviral protein viperin inhibits hepatitis C virus replication via interaction with nonstructural protein 5A. Hepatology 2011; 54(5): 1506-17.
[http://dx.doi.org/10.1002/hep.24542] [PMID: 22045669]

[192]   Szretter KJ, Brien JD, Thackray LB, Virgin HW, Cresswell P, Diamond MS. The interferon-inducible gene viperin restricts West Nile virus pathogenesis. J Virol 2011; 85(22): 11557-66.
[http://dx.doi.org/10.1128/JVI.05519-11] [PMID: 21880757]

[193]   Jiang D, Weidner JM, Qing M, *et al.* Identification of five interferon-induced cellular proteins that inhibit west nile virus and dengue virus infections. J Virol 2010; 84(16): 8332-41.
[http://dx.doi.org/10.1128/JVI.02199-09] [PMID: 20534863]

[194]   Lu MY, Liao F. Interferon-stimulated gene ISG12b2 is localized to the inner mitochondrial membrane and mediates virus-induced cell death. Cell Death Differ 2011; 18(6): 925-36.
[http://dx.doi.org/10.1038/cdd.2010.160] [PMID: 21151029]

[195]   Dai J, Pan W, Wang P. ISG15 facilitates cellular antiviral response to dengue and west nile virus infection in vitro. Virol J 2011; 8: 468.
[http://dx.doi.org/10.1186/1743-422X-8-468] [PMID: 21992229]

[196] Tay MY, Fraser JE, Chan WK, *et al.* Nuclear localization of dengue virus (DENV) 1-4 non-structural protein 5; protection against all 4 DENV serotypes by the inhibitor Ivermectin. Antiviral Res 2013; 99(3): 301-6.
[http://dx.doi.org/10.1016/j.antiviral.2013.06.002] [PMID: 23769930]

[197] Giovannoni F, Damonte EB, García CC. Cellular promyelocytic leukemia protein is an important dengue virus restriction factor. PLoS One 2015; 10(5): e0125690.
[http://dx.doi.org/10.1371/journal.pone.0125690] [PMID: 25962098]

[198] Pan XB, Han JC, Cong X, Wei L. BST2/tetherin inhibits dengue virus release from human hepatoma cells. PLoS One 2012; 7(12): e51033.
[http://dx.doi.org/10.1371/journal.pone.0051033] [PMID: 23236425]

CHAPTER 3

Synergistic Interaction Between Plant Products and Antibiotics Against Potential Pathogenic Bacteria

Banasri Hazra[1,*], Sutapa Biswas Majee[2], Subhalakshmi Ghosh[1] and Dhruti Avlani[2]

[1] *Department of Pharmaceutical Technology, Jadavpur University, Kolkata 700032, India*

[2] *Division of Pharmaceutics, NSHM Knowledge Campus, Kolkata-Group of Institutions, Kolkata 700053, India*

Abstract: The emergence of multi-drug resistant pathogenic bacteria, coupled with a decline in discovery of new drugs, has gradually steered the world to the doorstep of post-antibiotic era as trivial infections often become untreatable with the existing antibiotics. Therefore, design and development of new therapeutic strategies would be of paramount importance, primarily by interfering with mechanisms leading to drug resistance. Accordingly, researchers are aiming at the restoration of activity of existing antibiotics by using resistance modifying agents (RMA), and looking for suitable secondary plant metabolites to function as RMAs.

Plant-derived RMAs are believed to rejuvenate the action of conventional antibiotics *via* unique mechanisms, as for example, by acting upon bacterial efflux pumps, enhancing membrane permeability, and inhibiting the synthesis of proteins responsible for bacterial resistance. However, due to the lack of adequate pharmacological data, these phytochemicals are yet to be approved for clinical use, despite the upcoming prospect of their therapeutic application.

This chapter focuses on the relevant screening strategies to characterise new RMAs from plant constituents exhibiting resistance modifying activity against pathogenic bacteria. Also, the respective mode of synergistic interaction of these agents has been discussed in view of their potential application to supplement the conventional antibiotics against drug-resistant bacterial infections.

Keywords: Antimicrobial resistance, Antibiotic adjuvant, Efflux pump inhibitor, FICI, Isobologram, Plant-derived RMA, Pathogenic bacteria, Phytochemical, Resistance modifying agent, Synergistic interaction.

* Corresponding author Banasri Hazra: BG 172, Salt Lake City, Kolkata – 700091, India; Tel: +91 9330871566; E-mail: banasri@gmail.com; banasrihazra@yahoo.co.in

Atta-ur-Rahman & M. Iqbal Choudhary (Eds.)

INTRODUCTION

The clinical acceptance of penicillin, followed by its industrial production in the 1940s, was hailed as the greatest landmark in the history of antimicrobial chemotherapy. This discovery heralded the era of antibiotics as a new class of therapeutics was developed from bacterial and fungal metabolites hidden in natural reservoirs. Since then, the antibiotics have revolutionized medical practice, and hence, considered to be miracle drugs of the 20th century [1]. The bandwagon of antibiotics progressed more or less smoothly over the next few decades until the momentum received unforeseen jolts from reports on drug resistant *Salmonella* emanating from the clinics during 1990s. In those days, it was rather unexpected that a few patients did not respond to therapy with ciprofloxacin, the synthetic drug that had been successfully introduced into the clinic [2]. This was indeed a surprise as many Enterobacteriaceae are susceptible to ciprofloxacin, and it often remains the drug of choice to treat salmonellosis even to this day. However, that is how the prophetic warning sounded by Sir Alexander Fleming in his Nobel award lecture delivered in 1945 came to be true. He had the foresight to predict the ominous possibility of misusing penicillin at sub-lethal dosage and creating resistant microbes with a fatal outcome [3]. In fact, the phenomenon of antimicrobial resistance ensued mainly due to unbridled application of these life-saving medicines in combating microbial infections not only in humans, but also in agriculture, animal husbandry and poultry farms. In 1994, the Time Magazine had aptly expressed the mounting worldwide concern about antimicrobial resistance and emerging infections as "Revenge of the killer microbes" [4]. In the long run, 'multidrug resistant' (MDR) bacteria have evolved to classify a host of resistance patterns associated with the therapeutic failures occurring in numerous clinics around the world [5]. Hence, the European Centre for Disease Prevention and Control (ECDC), and CDC in Atlanta, USA, jointly proposed that the definition of MDR would be the "acquired non-susceptibility to at least one agent in three or more antimicrobial categories" [CDC; 6].

In order to counteract the propagation of microbial drug resistance, a major way forward is to develop compound(s) to be used as adjuvant, or resistance modifying agent (RMA) that acts in concert with the known conventional antibiotics, thus enhancing their activity against resistant isolates. The strategy of resistance modifying activity implies that an antimicrobial agent could be co-administered with an inhibitor or adjuvant that deactivates the bacterial resistance mechanism. This will ultimately lead to the desired bacteriostatic / bactericidal effect, with the RMA acting in synergistic unison with the conventional antibiotics to increase its efficacy by suppressing bacterial resistance mechanisms, partially or completely, thereby enhancing the sensitivity of bacterial strains exhibiting intrinsic resistance against the antibiotic [7]. However, most of these

RMAs are non-antibiotic molecules themselves, devoid of inhibitory activity against the target bacteria.

Looking for healing power in plants continues to be a historical practice since the time of Hippocrates and earlier [8]. Till this day, the kingdom of plants acts like a springboard to usher in medicinal products, hence, considered to be a superb pool for novel drugs and unexplored antimicrobials to be enlisted in modern pharmacopoeia in due course. Therefore, in order to face the challenge of the 'superbugs' in 'post-antibiotic' era it is imperative to augment the regime of antimicrobial therapeutics as well as to look for RMAs by exploring the scope of complementary and alternative medicines derived from herbal resources. Currently, a growing trend is observed to undertake research on traditional medicinal plants based on ethno-medicinal data relating to management of microbial diseases. Thus, a number of screening studies rooted in sound ecological principles have been conducted on plants as prospective source for antimicrobial agents, and many of these phytochemicals could be exploited to develop prospective therapeutic candidates as well as RMAs [9 - 20].

Presently we are seized of the putative role of plant derived secondary metabolites to ameliorate the problem caused by the growing resistance observed in microbial cells against standard antibiotic treatment. Truly, the mechanisms of such resistance are complex and often multi-factorial, and secondary metabolites isolated as pure compounds or given as whole plant extracts have been found to modify antibiotic resistance through multi-fold strategies. In fact, plant-derived adjuvants, in comparison to their synthetic counterparts, are characterized by their structural uniqueness, possessing distinctive functional groups and chiral centres [21]. Therefore, it has been found that co-administration of these natural products reversed the resistance and restored the efficacy of multiple antibiotics in multidrug resistant strains in a synergistic manner [22 - 28]. Actually, a good number of reviews covering discovery of plant-products with antimicrobial activity, and application of phytochemicals as resistance modifying agents / antibiotic adjuvants are available in the literature [9, 21, 29 - 32]. However, it is necessary to compile the outcomes with an added focus on the current developments in the light of relevant mechanisms of antibiotic resistance.

In this article, a general overview has been given on secondary metabolites belonging to different chemical classes which have shown promising results in terms of various mechanisms to tackle the resistant pathogenic bacteria (Table **2**). Plant products exhibiting efflux pump inhibitory activity against *S. aureus,* Mycobacteria and other pathogenic bacteria have been presented in Table **3**. Effect of selected phytochemicals on bacterial cell membrane permeability and their ability to enhance the efficacy of conventional antibiotics have been compiled in Table **4**. Examples of plant products interfering with bacterial protein synthesis are given in Table **5**. Inhibition of biofilm formation in several bacterial species by plant compounds or extracts thereby helping to overcome resistance has been exemplified in Table **6**.

Here, it begs to be mentioned that most of these observations are based on *in vitro* studies involving either standard bacterial culture, or clinical isolates of resistant strains obtained from patient samples. Reports on *in vivo* assessment of phytochemicals for their antimicrobial properties, or clinical evaluation of phytochemical RMAs–antibiotic combination therapies are sparsely available in the literature. There still exists a huge lacuna in corroborating the *in vitro* findings on animal models; thus, in the industrial set-up, only a few selected candidates reached the stage of pre-clinical drug trial for anti-infective activity [33, 21]. Nevertheless, we have added a few recent instances of *in vivo* studies at the end of the present article.

BACTERIAL RESISTANCE TOWARDS CLINICAL ANTIBIOTICS

Background

Antimicrobial resistance is the ability of a microorganism (bacteria/ virus/ parasite) to resist the effect of drugs, chemicals, or other agents designed to cure the infection caused by the microbe, and to stop the drug from working against it. It is understandable that bacteria have evolved over millions of years to adopt sophisticated mechanisms of drug resistance in order to avoid getting killed by antimicrobial molecules present in the surrounding environment. As a result, standard treatments become ineffective; infections persist and also spread to others [34]. In fact, the inhibitory molecules / antibiotics have been fished out from nature, and modified /imitated / formulated to develop drugs for our own protection from bacterial infection. Resistance to these drugs as observed in clinical settings are typically recognised to be the expression of "acquired resistance" in a bacterial population that was originally susceptible to the antimicrobial compound.

Actually, the development of such acquired resistance might be caused either by the mutations in chromosomal genes or due to the acquisition of external genetic determinants of resistance, likely obtained from intrinsically resistant organisms present in the environment. Readers interested to get exhaustive explanation of the multi-layered events leading to antibiotic resistance mechanism are directed to consult state-of-the-art reviews articles in this field [35 - 39].

Development of bacterial resistance to an antibiotic leads to a concomitant rise in its minimum inhibitory concentration (MIC) value, thereby limiting its efficacy for the treatment. Recently, in January 2018, European Committee on Antimicrobial Susceptibility Testing (EUCAST) has released the rational document for interpretation of MICs and zone diameters for key pathogens against different classes of currently relevant clinical antibiotics (Table **1**).

Table 1. Antimicrobial agents linked to EUCAST rationale documents for the treatment of *Enterobacteriaceae*, *Pseudomonas aeruginosa*, *Acinetobacter baumannii* and *Campylobacter jejuni* infections (European Committee of Antimicrobial Susceptibility Testing. Breakpoint tables for interpretation of MICs and zone diameters. Version 8.0, 2018).

Antimicrobial Agent	MIC Breakpoint (mg/L) for Susceptibility			
	Enterobacteriaceae	*P. aeruginosa*	*A. baumannii*	*C. jejuni*
Penicillin				
Amoxicillin	≤8	-	ND	ND
Piperacillin	≤8	≤16	ND	ND
Piperacillin-tazobactam	≤8	≤16	ND	ND
Cephalosporin				
Cefotaxime	≤1	-	ND	ND
Ceftaroline	≤0.5	-	ND	ND
Ceftazidime	≤1	≤8	ND	ND
Ceftobiprole	≤0.25	IE	ND	ND
Cefepime	≤1	≤8	ND	ND
Carbapenem				
Doripenem	≤1	≤1	ND	ND
Ertapenem	≤0.5	IR	IR	ND
Imipenem	≤2	≤4	≤2	ND
Meropenem	≤2	≤2	≤2	ND
Monobactam				
Aztreonam	≤1	≤1	IR	ND
Fluoroquinolone				
Ciprofloxacin	≤0.25	≤0.5	≤1	0.5
Levofloxacin	≤0.5	≤1	ND	ND
Moxifloxacin	≤0.25	-	ND	ND
Ofloxacin	≤0.25	-	ND	ND
Aminoglycoside				
Amikacin	≤8	≤8	≤8	ND
Gentamicin	≤2	≤4	≤4	ND
Netilmicin	≤2	≤4	ND	ND
Tobramycin	≤2	≤4	≤4	ND
Macrolide				
Erythromycin	-	-	ND	4
Tetracycline				
Doxycycline	-	-	ND	ND
Minocycline	-	-	ND	ND
Tetracycline	-	-	ND	2
Tigecycline	≤1	IR	ND	ND

(Table 1) contd.....

Antimicrobial Agent	MIC Breakpoint (mg/L) for Susceptibility			
	Enterobacteriaceae	*P. aeruginosa*	*A. baumannii*	*C. jejuni*
Miscellaneous agents				
Colistin	≤2	≤2	≤2	ND
Trimethoprim-Sulfamethoxazole	≤2	-	ND	ND

MIC = Minimum inhibitory concentration
ND = Not defined
IR = Intrinsic resistance
'-' indicates that susceptibility testing is not recommended as the species is a poor target for therapy with the agent.
"IE" indicates that there is insufficient evidence that the organism or group is a good target for therapy with the agent.

However, the resistant bacteria would no longer be inhibited at the normal dosage regimen of the antibiotic [40]. Likewise, multiple drug resistance is defined as the resistance to two or more drugs, or drug classes [41]. Of particular concern are the six most widely prevalent nosocomial ESKAPE pathogens, *viz. Enterococcus faecium, Staphylococcus aureus, Klebsiella pneumoniae, Acinetobacter baumannii, Pseudomonas aeruginosa* and *Enterobacter* spp. which have high levels of resistance and frequently "escape" eradication by antibiotics [7]. In addition to these, *Mycobacterium tuberculosis, Candida albicans*, malarial parasites and human immunodeficiency virus (HIV) also appear to be insurmountable obstacles in modern clinical setting [29].

However, ever-increasing instances of multidrug resistant bacteria failing to respond to even second-line antibiotics started building up the pressure, and presented a challenge to the medical and pharmaceutical fraternity in general. In this context the title of a book *"Magic Bullets, Lost Horizons"* rhetorically summed up the current predicament of drug resistance that might prove to be one of the greatest threats to public health in the 21st century [42].

Right now, drug resistance is a major healthcare concern and clinical problem around the globe [34]. In the most recalcitrant situations, the increase in patient morbidity and mortality is attributed to recurrent infections and hospitalization with longer stays, eventually raising the suffering as well as the cost of treatment. Notwithstanding this alarming scenario it is unfortunate that introduction of newer antibiotics by pharmaceutical industry has been thwarted by the financial risk involved in the venture, leading to a nearly exhausted development pipeline [43]. In fact, the period from the 1960s to the 2000s is known as the "Innovation Gap" when hardly any new class of antibiotic got introduced to the clinics [44 - 46]. Also, many well-established drugs had to be discontinued due to rapidly acquired resistance even before due recovery of their development costs. This led to the contraction of funding for antibiotic research, and the gap between the clinical need and supply of innovative antibiotics started widening day by day.

In the survey data from Infectious Diseases Society of America, Boucher *et al.* had rightly observed an emerging scenario of 'bad bugs, no drugs' [47]. Nevertheless, in the current millennium, new antibiotics like linezolid, daptomycin, bedaquiline and baxdela have emerged [48]. At present, several new molecular entities with the potential to treat serious bacterial infections are undergoing approval to enter the clinics [49]. Notwithstanding the advent of potential candidates in the development pipeline, a cautionary bell has been sounded on the likely emergence of fresh antibiotic-resistant strains which would yet again nullify the ostensible progress [50]. This is seemingly the vindication of Paul Ehrlich's prophetic statement that *"drug resistance follows the drug like a faithful shadow"* [51].

Mechanisms and Associated Factors

The major biochemical mechanisms for antibiotic resistance involve energy-dependent antibiotic efflux pumps causing extrusion of the antibiotic from the active site, modification of target accessibility including creation of permeability barrier, production of hydrolytic or modifying enzymes, alteration of targets such that they are no longer susceptible to antibacterial action, and biofilm formation, as represented in the cartoon below (Fig. **1**).

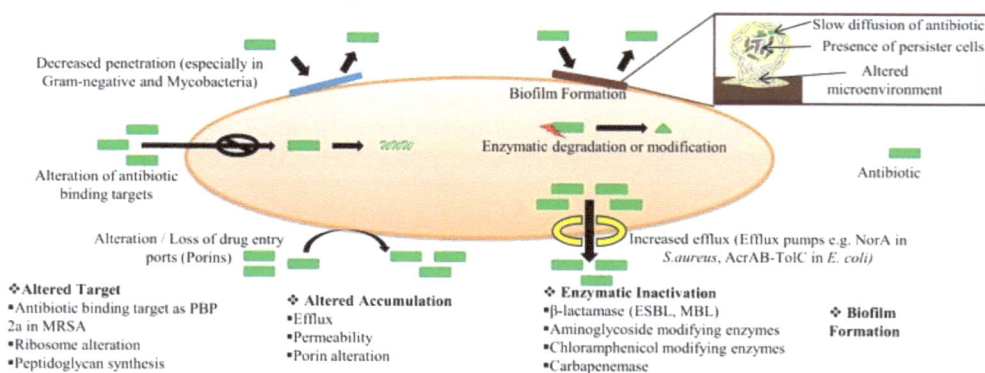

Fig. (1). Antibiotic resistance mechanisms.

Therefore, in order to search for new RMAs, it is important to elucidate the specific mechanism(s) adopted by the bacteria to become resistant to an antibiotic. In this article, we have tried to organise the information on the mode of action reported for the plant-derived RMAs by various investigators in Tables **2-6**. Additional discussion on the implication of each of these mechanisms with reference to prospective phytochemicals has been presented below in a section on **phytochemicals and relevant bacterial resistance mechanisms**.

SCREENING STRATEGIES TO CHARACTERISE PLANT PRODUCTS WITH POTENTIAL RESISTANCE MODIFYING ACTIVITY

Numerous studies were conducted worldwide to explore plant-derived secondary metabolites for their ability to modulate antibiotic resistance towards clinically used conventional antibiotics in pathogenic bacteria. Such compounds may possess inherent antibacterial activity at higher doses, or may not have such activity at all. Further, combination therapy of phytochemicals with conventional antibiotics has shown synergistic reduction of the MIC of antibiotics against drug-resistant micro-organisms by involving multiple targets implicated in resistance towards several classes of antibiotics [21, 30, 52]. The efficacy of combination of secondary metabolite with antibiotic can be assessed using the micro-dilution checkerboard, time-kill curves, and agar well diffusion method for determination of %RIZD (relative zone inhibition diameter) [53, 54].

The modulation assay is a quick and easy method to identify potential efflux pump inhibitors against Gram-positive and Gram-negative bacteria. Serial doubling dilutions of extract or phytochemical assumed to be a substrate for an efflux transporter, is added and microtitre plates are then interpreted in the same manner as MIC determinations [55]. Evaluation of efflux inhibitory activity can be done by measuring decrease in fluorescence intensity due to suppression of efflux pump substrate, ethidium bromide (EtBr) or Rhodamine 6G in bacterial cells by proposed efflux pump inhibitor. This study is relevant especially during assessment of inhibition of proton motive force-driven multidrug efflux pump. Parallel studies may also be conducted to demonstrate increase in accumulation of fluorescent substrates inside the cells due to efflux inhibition by the inhibitor molecule. For example, Hoechst 33342(H33342) accumulation assay is performed to evaluate the effect of efflux pump inhibitors on the activity of MexAB-OprM efflux pumps as in study of conessine as a novel multidrug efflux pump inhibitor in *P. aeruginosa* [56]. However, some times, false results have been obtained by ethidium bromide assay owing to quenching effects of matrix components. A new mass spectrometry-based efflux pump inhibition assay has been developed for evaluating efflux pump inhibitory activity of crude extract of the botanical *Hydrastis canadensis* and pure flavonoids in situations where optical interference precludes the application of fluorescence–based assays [57, 58]. Inhibition of *A. baumannii* efflux pumps has also been studied spectrofluorimetrically by measuring accumulation of EtBr, an indicator of the AdeABC efflux pump inhibition, and Pyronin Y, which is an indicator of the AdeIJK efflux pump inhibition [59].

The influence of plant-derived secondary metabolite /RMA on bacterial membrane integrity can be followed by using LIVE/DEAD BacLight Bacterial Viability kits (mixture of the green fluorescent dye SYTO 9 and propidium iodide). The kinetics of propidium iodide intracellular penetration is studied by measuring the relative fluorescence units, in terms of the SYTO 9 fluorescence at 481 nm and 510 nm in a microplate reader [60]. Ability of phytochemical to permeabilize outer membrane of bacteria can be evaluated by 1-N-phenylnaphthylamine (NPN) uptake assay. NPN is a membrane potential-sensitive, uncharged lipophilic fluorescent probe that shows strong fluorescence upon exposure to a hydrophobic environment as in cell membranes. The efficacy of plant extract or phytochemical is monitored at 37 °C intermittently for 1 h using a Varioskan Flash spectral scanning multimode reader. If the extract is unable to enhance cell membrane permeability, there will be no effect on the level of NPN accumulation in bacterial isolates [56, 59]. Nusslein *et al.* used a spectrofluorimetric method to investigate the cytoplasmic membrane permeabilizing properties of the plant extracts [61]. Similarly, activities of extracts of *C. citrinus* and *V. adoensis*on bacterial cell membranes were studied using disC3-5 [3, 3'-dipropylthiadicarbocyanine iodide] [62]. Assessment of membrane permeability and extent of cell damage can be visually examined and confirmed by Scanning Electron Microscopy, Transmission Electron Microscopy and Confocal Fluorescence Microscopy [63 - 65]. The damage to the cytoplasm membrane can be quantified by potassium leakage from bacterial cells, using a flame photometer. In this method, the rise in potassium ion concentration in the supernatant due to leakage induced by phytochemical-antibiotic combination is measured [66, 67]. Calcium ion mobilisation assay has also been carried out fluorimetrically in *S. aureus* cells treated with mixture of gentamicin sulfate and *Ginkgo biloba* polyprenols [68]. Inhibitory effect on biofilm formation can be determined through mass quantification by crystal violet assay where spectrophotometric measurements are carried out at 540 nm [69]. Recently, secondary metabolites with synergistic activities could be identified by adopting metabolomics approach on vast number of combinations of plant chemical and antibiotics at various concentration levels [70].

ASSESSMENT OF SYNERGISTIC INTERACTION BETWEEN ANTIBIOTIC AND A PHYTOCOMPOUND AGAINST RESISTANT BACTERIA

Fractional Inhibitory Concentration Index (FICI)

The fractional inhibitory concentration (FIC) and fractional inhibitory concentration index (FICI) are used to evaluate the extent of synergistic interaction by using the following equations:

$$\text{FIC (antibiotic)} = \frac{\text{MIC (antibiotic) in combination with phytocompound}}{\text{MIC (antibiotic) alone}}$$

$$\text{FIC (phytocompound)} = \frac{\text{MIC (phytocompound) in combination with antibiotic}}{\text{MIC (phytocompound) alone}}$$

$$\text{FICI} = \text{FIC (antibiotic)} + \text{FIC (phytocompound)}$$

An FIC value of ≤ 0.5 indicates synergism, while an 'additive effect' is defined by a value observed in the range of $0.5 <$ to ≤ 1. FICI of $1 <$ to ≤ 2 indicates 'indifference' and value greater than 2 signifies 'antagonism' as defined by Mackay *et al.* [71]. It has been observed that caffeic acid, quercetin, ellagic acid and epigallocatechin gallate exhibited resistance modulating activity in ~15–38% of the ESBL-type and KPC-type carbapenemase-producing *K. pneumoniae* clinical isolates with evidences of synergistic interaction (FICI value of ≤ 0.5) with antibiotics like ciprofloxacin, gentamicin and tetracycline. Here, reserpine, a phytochemical, was used as a positive control [63]. Potentiation studies on another plant-derived RMA, *viz.*, kaempferol 3-O-α-L-(2,4-bis-E-p-coumaroyl) rhamnoside with ciprofloxacin against *S. aureus* 1199B showed a 4-fold reduction in MIC of ciprofloxacin, as corroborated by FIC index of 0.19, whereas reserpine, the positive control, exhibited FICI of 0.37 in the same experiment [72].

Modulation Factor (MF)

Evaluation of the ability of phytochemicals to potentiate the effect of conventional antibiotics and its ability to reverse antibiotic resistance in bacterial strains can be assessed by another parameter called modulation factor (MF) [73]. The modulation factor (MF) was used to quantify the effect of the inhibitors on the MIC of antibiotics and EtBr. The MF reflects the reduction of MIC values of a given antibiotic in the presence of the efflux inhibitor (the test phytochemical) and was considered to be significant with $MF \geq 4$ (four-fold reduction) [74]. The MF of pinocembrin, isolated from *A. calcarata,* has been found to be 8 when effect on ethidium bromide efflux was studied at sub-inhibitory concentration of 62.5 μg/ml [73]. Similarly, modulation of antimicrobial resistance of different antibiotics against various strains of *Campylobacter jejuni* by (-)-α-pinene has also been expressed in terms of modulation factor [60].

Isobologram

A method of representing the results of combination studies by the use of an isobologram has been advocated in this regard, so that additive and non-additive interactions could be observed graphically [75, 76]. This method was employed to demonstrate the resistance modifying property of a methanolic extract of pomegranate fruit pericarp [PGME]. PGME in combination with ciprofloxacin was tested on 29 different clinical isolates of extended-spectrum-β-lactamase (ESBL)-producing *E. coli* and *K. pneumoniae* or *metallo-β-lactamase* (MBL)-producing *P. aeruginosa* using a 96-well microtitre plate. The reference strains used were *E. coli* ATCC 35218, *K. pneumoniae* ATCC 700603 and *P. aeruginosa* ATCC 27853. An isobologram illustrating the synergistic effect of ciprofloxacin-PGME combination on one of the tested clinical isolates (E16) of ESBL-producing *E. coli* is presented as an example in Fig. (**2**) [76]. Growth inhibition data were calculated and plotted in a graph using respective doses (μg/ml) of plant extract and antibiotic as rectangular coordinates (X and Y). The straight line joining the points of maximum concentrations of the two components of the combination is called the 'line of additivity'. This line provides a convenient means for visually distinguishing between additive from non-additive interactions on the basis of whether or not the experimental curve falls on this line (additive), below this line (synergistic) or above this line (antagonistic) [77].

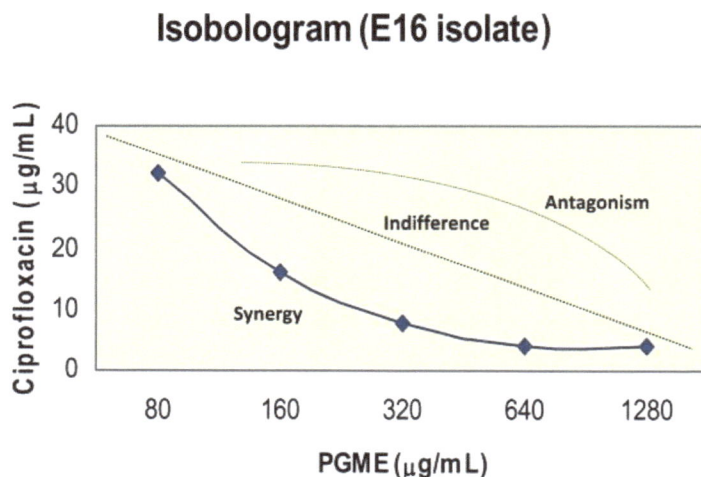

Fig. (**2**). Isobologram illustrating the synergistic effect of ciprofloxacin-PGME combination on an ESBL-producing strain of *E. coli*.

SEARCH FOR PLANT-DERIVED SECONDARY METABOLITES WITH PROSPECTIVE RESISTANCE MODIFYING ACTIVITY

Key Early Studies Pertaining to Discovery of RMAs from Plants

Antibiotic resistance has evolved in bacteria over the millennia of fighting a chemical war, first with each other, and then with fungi and plants [78]. The phenomenon could be explained when multidrug resistance pumps were discovered in bacteria [79 - 82]. New insight on drug resistance was generated by deliberating upon the role of these membrane proteins acting as efflux pumps to extrude a variety of chemically unrelated antimicrobial agents from the cell. For example, clinical resistance to synthetic quinolones in *Pseudomonas aeruginosa* is largely due to the expression of the MexAB–OprM pump [83]. Accordingly, the ubiquitous multidrug resistance pumps could confer the bacteria with effective defence mechanisms to survive the assault from antimicrobial agents. Particularly, synthetic hydrophobic cations such as quaternary ammonium antiseptics like benzalkonium chloride, and ethidium bromide, were found to be preferred substrates of such MDR pumps. At this point, a group of cationic berberine alkaloids was identified as natural substrates of MDR pumps that fuelled the evolution of RMAs from plants [84]. As it became apparent that microbial efflux pumps could render the plant-derived toxins essentially ineffective, therefore, it was presumed that the plants might contain efflux pump inhibitors (EPI) in order to effectively utilise the berberine alkaloids to its own benefit. This concept was confirmed by the presence of 5′-methoxyhydnocarpin (5′-MHC) in *Berberis fremontii*, a Native American traditional medicinal plant with antimicrobial and other medicinal properties. It was shown that efflux of berberine from pathogenic *Staphylococcus aureus* expressing the NorA MDR pump that confers resistance to quinolones and antiseptics was completely inhibited by 5′-MHC [85, 86]. This observation provided a clear example of synergy described at a molecular level between medicinal plant components acting in conjunction with berberine alkaloids to provide the plant with effective defence mechanism. The seminal discovery paved the way to search for plant-derived EPIs like 5′-MHC which did not show antimicrobial activity *per se* [55, 87, 88]. In addition, this resolved the conundrum about the fact that most of the plant-derived antimicrobial compounds reportedly exhibited MICs in the range of 100-1000 µg/ml, making them too weak to fight with the plant pathogens unless helped by the RMAs present in the same plant. The alkaloid reserpine was the first such compound which is used as a positive RMA for the screening studies searching for plant-derived EPIs [89, 90].

Recent Studies

Now, based on the aforesaid background information, we will try to provide a comprehensive review of recent information published on plant-derived secondary metabolites which have shown promising results in terms of modulation of antibiotic resistance *via* various mechanisms against resistant pathogenic bacteria (Table **2**). In this Table, the plant-derived compounds and extracts are shown along with the drug-resistant bacteria selected for the study. FICI values and mode of action are also provided wherever reported by the respective investigators. Chemical structures of selected phytochemicals are compiled in Fig. (**3**).

Table 2. Plant-derived secondary metabolites with prospective resistance modifying activity.

Secondary Metabolite [Class of Compound]	Occurrence (Plant and Plant Part)	Test Bacteria	Synergistic Interaction [FICI]	Probable Mode of Action	Special Comments	Ref.
Apigenin[Flavonoid]	*Cytisus striatus* (Hill) Rothm. (Leguminosae) (Leaf)	*S. aureus* 1199B *S. aureus* M116 *S. aureus* RWW337 *S. aureus* RWW50	CIP [0.38; against SA M116 and SA RWW337] ERY [0.38; against SA M116]	Inhibits efflux pump Affects membrane permeability	Synergistic effect with CIP and ERY not observed in strains other than those mentioned EtBr accumulation improved	[70]
Boeravinone B[Rotenoid]	*Boerhaavia diffusa* (Nyctaginaceae) (Root)	*S. aureus* 1199B *S. aureus* MT 23142 Methicillin-resistant *S. aureus* 15187	CIP [---]b NOR [---]b	Dual inhibitor of NorA efflux pump of *S. aureus* and human P-glycoprotein Reduces biofilm formation Reduces intracellular invasion of bacteria	EtBr efflux prevented Binds to the Ile 23 and Glu 222 residues of the Nor A efflux pump through strong hydrogen bonding formed by phenolic hydroxyl groups and thus block the interaction of substrate quinolones with the efflux binding cavity Observed to interact with P-gp at the verapamil binding site, particularly with the residues Met69, Phe72, Tyr307, Tyr310, Phe314, Leu332, Phe335, Phe336, Leu339, Phe728, Phe759, Phe957, Phe978, and Val982 through hydrophobic Π– Π interactions	[91]
Caffeic acid[Polyphenol]	----a	ESBL-type and KPC-type carbapenemase-producing *K. pneumoniae*	CIP [0.38]	Inhibits efflux-mediated extrusion of antibiotic	Intracellular accumulation of CIP found to be 17μg per 2 X 10⁸ bacterial cells, when tested in KpE 8 Reported to demonstrate synergistic activity with SDZ and GENTA against a reference strain of *P. aeruginosa.*	[63]
Carvacrol[Monoterpene]	*Origanum* sp. (Labiatae) (Whole herb)	*C. violaceum* *S. aureus* *S. enterica* *P. aeruginosa* *L. monocytogenes* Erythromycin-resistant *Streptococcus pyogenes*	ERY [0.25-0.50]	Exhibits anti-quorum sensing activity observed in *C. violaceum* Exhibits anti-biofilm activity observed in all test strains except *P. aeruginosa* Increases bacterial membrane permeability, causes membrane disruption and destabilisation Reduces proton motive force	Inhibits microbial and fungal toxin production Exhibits anti-inflammatory, analgesic, anti-arthritic, anti-allergic, anti-carcinogenic, anti-diabetic, cardio-protective, gastro-protective, hepato-protective, and neuro-protective properties Increased sensitivity to CLM and SMX for strain H3380, and STREP and SMX for strain 43 of *S. typhimurium* DT104 Synergy (FICI ≤ 0.5) found in 21 out of 32 strains tested from checkerboard assay and confirmed in17 out of 23 strains using 24-h time-kill curves. Strains where synergy was detected included 6 *erm*(TR)/iMLS, 5/6 *erm*(B)/iMLS, 2/8 *erm*(B)/cMLS, and 8/12 *mef*(A)/M isolates	[21, 92-95]

(Table 2) contd.....

Secondary Metabolite [Class of Compound]	Occurrence (Plant and Plant Part)	Test Bacteria	Synergistic Interaction [FICI]	Probable Mode of Action	Special Comments	Ref.
Cinchonain[Flavonolignan]	*Secondatia floribunda* A. DC (Apocynaceae) (Stalk's inner bark and heartwood)	*S. aureus* ATCC 12692 *E. coli* ATCC 25922	AMI [---]*b* NEO [---]*b*	Affects cellular membrane fluidity Interferes with activity of enzymes involved in replication, transcription and repair	-	[96]
Combretum zeyheri extract[Alkaloid]	*Combretum zeyheri* (Combretaceae) (Leaf)	*Mycobacterium smegmatis*, mc² 155	CIP [---]*b*	Inhibits efflux pump	Efflux of ciprofloxacin from the cells inhibited to the same extent as reserpine, however, no improvement observed in drug accumulation inside the cells	[16]
Conessine[Alkaloid]	*Holarrhena antidysenterica* (Roth) Wall. ex A.DC.	a.*P. aeruginosa* K1455 b. Clinical isolate of *A. baumannii*	a.CXM [---]*b* LEVO [---]*b* RIF [---]*b* TET [---]*b* b. NOVO [≤ 0.5] RIF [≤ 0.5]	a.Competitive inhibition and/or blocking access to the substrate binding site of MexAB-OprM pump Binding pocket different from that of PAβN b. Interferes with AdeIJK pump	a.Potential to be active against homologous resistance–nodulation–division (RND) family in other Gram-negative pathogens May act on other intrinsic resistance determinants	a.[56] b.[59]
Curcumin [Phenyl-propanoid]	----*a*	a. *S. aureus* SA-1199B *S. aureus* XU212 *S. aureus* RN4220 *S. aureus* Mupr b. *P. aeruginosa* PA01 c. MDR-strain of *P. aeruginosa*	a.- b.- c. PIP [---]*b* LEVO [---]*b* MER [---]*b*	a.Inhibits NorA efflux pump b. Inhibits adherence of the bacteria to polypropylene surfaces in *P. aeruginosa* PA01	a. Mimics hydrophobic interactions as well as H-bonding interactions of CIP with Nor A efflux pump. Additional interaction reported with the Ser299 residue c. Could result in weak restoration of the activity of PIP, MER and LEVO versus the MDR strain of *P. aeruginosa in vitro* but treatment of *G. mellonella* larvae infected with the MDR strain with curcumin-LEVO/PIP resulted in improved therapeutic benefit compared to either of the agents alone	a.[97] b.[98, 99] c.[99]
Daidzein[Isoflavone]	*Cytisus striatus* (Hill) Rothm. (Leguminosae) (Leaf)	*S. aureus* 1199B	CIP [---]*b*	Inhibits efflux pump	-	[70]
Diospyrin[Naphthoquinone]	*Diospyros montana* Roxb. (Ebenaceae) (Stem bark)	*Mycobacterium aurum* A+	CIP [---]*b*	Inhibits efflux pump	Probably acts as pseudosubstrate for efflux pump	[100]
Epigallocatechin-3-gallate (EGCG)[Polyphenol]	*Punica granatum* Linn. (Punicaceae) (Fruit)	ESBL-type and KPC-type carbapenemase-producing *K. pneumoniae*	a. CIP [0.25] b. TET [---]*b*	a.Inhibits efflux-mediated extrusion of antibiotic.Swells up bacterial cellInduces partial disruption of cell membraneInhibits quorum sensingDestroys biofilm activity	a.In bacterialcells pre-treated with EGCG, ~17-fold greater CIP accumulation observed in comparison with the untreated controlMore pertinent inhibitor of efflux pumps than reserpine	[19, 63]
Essential oil	*Eucalyptus camaldulensis* Dehnh. (Myrtaceae) (Leaf)	MDR-*Acinetobacter baumannii*	CIP [---]*b* GENTA [---]*b* PMX [---]*b*	Affects bacterial cell membrane structure	Spatulenol, cryptone, p-cymene, 1,8-cineole, terpinen-4-ol, β-pinene present Bacterial count reduced under detection limit after 6h of incubation	[101]

(Table 2) contd.....

Secondary Metabolite [Class of Compound]	Occurrence (Plant and Plant Part)	Test Bacteria	Synergistic Interaction [FICI]	Probable Mode of Action	Special Comments	Ref.
Essential oil[Terpenoid]	*Salvia sp.* *Matricana recutita*	Methicillin-resistant *Staphylococcus epidermidis* clinical strains	OXA [≤ 0.3]	Damages cell wall Interferes with peptidoglycan synthesis	Essential oil contains terpenoids like 1,8-cineole, β-thujone, camphor, borneol, p-cymene Carnosol, obtained from crude extract of *Salvia officinalis* lowered MIC of aminoglycosides in vancomycin-resistant *Enterococci*	[102, 103]
Essential oil[Terpenoid]	*Zingiber cassumunar* Roxb (Zingiberaceae) (Rhizome)	Extensively-drug resistant *Acinetobacter baumannii*	GENTA [---]b AMI [---]b DOX [---]b TET [---]b CIP [---]b	Affects cell membrane	Main components are sabinene, terpinene-4-ol and terpinene Modified morphology of *A. baumannii* after treatment with the essential oil is an adaptive response to stress and toxic substances	[104]
Galangin [Flavonoid]	*Alpinia calcarata* Roscoe (Zingiberaceae) (Rhizome) *Alpinia officinarum* Hance (Zingiberaceae) (Rhizome)	a. *S. aureus* SA 1199B b. MRSA (MJMC001, MJMC002, MJMC004), *S. aureus* SA1199B, RN4220 and XU212 c. *Stenotrophomonas maltophilia*	a. NOR [0.12-0.28] b. β-lactam antibiotics	a. Inhibits Nor A as well as other efflux pumps present in *S. aureus* SA 1199 b.Interacts with penicillinase Causes cytoplasmic membrane damage Inhibits protein synthesis Induces changes in PBP2a c. Inhibits the L1 metallo-β-lactamase	a. Observed modulatory effect better than standard EPIs, reserpine and verapamil. Demonstrated good modulatory activity with EtBr. Non-specific modulator of efflux pump	a. [73] b. [105] c. [106]
Gallic acid and gallates [Phenolic acid]	*Camelliasinensis*(L.) Kuntze (Theaceae) (Leaf)	NorA over-expressing *S. aureus* strain	NOR [---]b OXA [---]b TET [---]b	Increases membrane permeability Inhibits Tet K and Tet B efflux pump Inhibits β-lactamase Inhibits PBP2a synthesis Reacts with peptidoglycan	-	[12]
Genistein[Isoflavone]	*Cytisus striatus* (Hill) Rothm. (Leguminosae) (Leaf and flower)	*S. aureus* 1199B *S. aureus* M116 *S. aureus* RWW337 *S. aureus* RWW50	CIP [0.5; against SA M116] [0.38; against SA RWW337] ERY [---]b	Inhibits efflux pump Affects membrane permeability	Synergistic effect with CIP observed in other strains tested but FICI values not given. Synergistic effect with ERY not observed in other strains tested EtBr accumulation improved Exhibits synergistic effect with anticancer drugs Inhibits drug accumulation in MRP-over-expressing cells	[70, 107]
Grape pomace extract	Grape pomace of Cabernet Sauvignan var. *Vitisvinifera*L. (Vitaceae)	a.MRSA b.Clinical isolates of multidrug-resistant *E. coli*	a. NAL, NOR, CIP, CLM, TET, LEVO, OXA [0.047-0.063] b. NAL, NOR, CIP, CLM, TET, LEVO, OXA [0.031-0.281]	Inhibits synthesis of proteins and peptidoglycans Disrupts cell membrane integrity Increases permeability of outer and inner membrane	Extract rich in phenolic compounds such as quercetin, gallic acid, protocatechuic acid and luteolin. Also contains terpenes *e.g.* uvaol, β-amirin, palmitic acid, eicosanol, scualene and estearic acid which could also contribute to the synergy	[108]

(Table 2) contd.....

Secondary Metabolite [Class of Compound]	Occurrence (Plant and Plant Part)	Test Bacteria	Synergistic Interaction [FICI]	Probable Mode of Action	Special Comments	Ref.
Imperatorin [Coumarin]	*Metrodorea mollis* Taub. (Rutaceae) *Pilocarpus spicatus* A.St.-Hil. (Rutaceae)	*S. aureus*	ERY [---]*b* NOR [---]*b* TET [---]*b*	Inhibits efflux pump	-	[27]
Kaempferol [Flavonoid]	*Alpinia calcarata* Roscoe (Zingiberaceae) (Rhizome) *Alpinia officinarum* Hance (Zingiberaceae) (Rhizome)	*S. aureus* SA 1199B	NOR [0.15]	Inhibits Nor A efflux pump Interacts with penicillinase Causes cytoplasmic membrane damage Inhibits protein synthesis Induces changes in PBP2a Inhibits the L1 metallo-β-lactamase	Observed modulatory effect better than standard EPIs, reserpine and verapamil.	[73]
Linoleic acid [Fatty acid]	*Portulaca oleracea* L. (Portulacaceae) (Whole herb)	*S. aureus* RN 4220/pUL5054 *S. aureus* APH2'-AAC6' *S. aureus* -APH3' *S. aureus* -ANT4'	ERY [0.38]	Increases membrane permeability of bacterial cells Interferes with activity of MsrA pump Inhibits bacterial enoyl-acyl carrier protein reductase	Inactive as EPI for other tested resistant strains of *S. aureus*	[109]
Luteolin [Flavonoid]	Grape pomace of Caberne Sauvignan var. *Vitisvinifera*L. (Vitaceae)	a. Amoxicilli–resistant *E.coli* (DMST 20661, 20662, 20970, 20971) b. *Streptococcus pyogenes*	a. AMO [< 0.47] b. CAZ [0.37]	a.Inhibits activity of few ESBL Inhibits synthesis of proteins and peptidoglycans Disrupts cell membrane integrity Increases permeability of outer and inner membrane Inhibits enzymes participating in synthesis of folic acid Increases fatty acid and nucleic acid content b.Same mechanisms as in a	Enhanced the activity of IMP, CEPH, ME, CET, in the order as mentioned against clinical isolates of MRSA at 500 µg/ml	a. [110] b. [111, 112]
Luteolin-quercetin [Flavonoid]	----*a*	MRSA clinical isolates	IMI [---]*b* CET [---]*b*	Causes significant leakage of intracellular potassium ions, proteins Alters cytoplasmic membrane permeability	-	[67]
Maple syrup extract [Phenol-rich]	North American maple tree *Acer saccharum* Marsh. (Sapindaceae) (Sap) *Acer rubrum* L. (Sapindaceae) (Sap)	*E.coli* CFT073	CIP [0.38]	Increases outer membrane permeability Inhibits multidrug efflux pumps Inhibits biofilm formation Down-regulates genes associated with resistance to multiple drugs and biofilm formation	Extract contains gallic acid, catechol, catechaldehyde, syringaldehyde, vanillin and 3-hydroxybenzoic acid Synergistic effect observed at sub-lethal concentrations Low synergistic activity observed in *P. aeruginosa* PA01, *P. aeruginosa* PA14	[113]

(Table 2) contd.....

Secondary Metabolite [Class of Compound]	Occurrence (Plant and Plant Part)	Test Bacteria	Synergistic Interaction [FICI]	Probable Mode of Action	Special Comments	Ref.
Morin-rutin-quercetin [Flavonoid]	----a	MRSA clinical isolates	IMI [0.45] CET [0.44] CEPH [0.50] MET [0.50]	Causes significant leakage of intracellular potassium ions Damages cytoplasmic membrane Rutin reported to possess anti-biofilm potential against *Streptococcus suis*	Morin is an isomer of quercetin Maximum synergistic effect observed with three flavonoids in combination in comparison to either of the flavonoids alone or combination of any two of them AMP, AMO showed additive effect with the three flavonoids in combination	[66, 114]
Nerolidol [Sesquiterpene]	*Piper claussenianum* (Miq.) C. DC. (Piperaceae) (Leaf)	a. *S. aureus* b. *E. coli*	a. AMO / CLAV [---]b CIP [---]b GENTA [---]b ERY [---]b VAN [---]b b. AMO / CLAV [---]b IMI [---]b	Damages cell membrane and causes leakage of potassium ions Increases outer membrane permeability Exhibits anti-biofilm effect	Synergistic activity exhibited by *cis*-nerolidol and the racemic mixture of *cis*- and *trans*-isomers (1:1) Susceptibility of *E. coli* ATCC 25922 to polymyxin B also enhanced	[115]
Oleic acid [Fatty acid]	*Portulaca oleracea* L. (Portulacaceae) (Whole herb)	*S. aureus* RN 4220/pUL5054 *S. aureus* APH2'-AAC6' *S. aureus* -APH3' *S. aureus* -ANT4'	ERY [0.38]	Increases membrane permeability of bacterial cells Interferes with activity of MsrA pump	Not active against the growth of RN4220 when used alone. Inactive as EPI for other tested resistant strains of *S. aureus*	[110]
Palmitoleic acid [Fatty acid]	*Portulaca oleracea* L. (Portulacaceae) (Whole herb)	*S. aureus* RN 4220/pUL5054 *S. aureus* APH2'-AAC6' *S. aureus* -APH3' *S. aureus* -ANT4'	ERY [0.09]	Exhibits rapid membrane depolarisation and disruption of macro-molecular synthesis on the bacterial cells Reduces the level of D-alanine modification Affected strain lacks major surface protein IsdA	Highly potent growth inhibitor against RN4220	[110]
α-Pinene [Monoterpene]	*Alpinia katsumadai* Hayala (Zingiberaceae) (Seed)	*Campylobacter jejuni*	CIP [---]b ERY [---]b TC [---]b	Disrupts membrane integrity Interferes with several metabolic pathways, specially those involved in response to heat shock	At low concentration antimicrobial efflux inhibited through targeting of the main efflux system CmeABC and another, not yet characterised, efflux protein, Cj1687	[60]

(Table 2) contd.....

Secondary Metabolite [Class of Compound]	Occurrence (Plant and Plant Part)	Test Bacteria	Synergistic Interaction [FICI]	Probable Mode of Action	Special Comments	Ref.
Pinostrobin [Flavonoid]	----*a*	Methicillin-resistant *S. aureus*(SA 1199B) Laboratory derived mutant strain of *P.aeruginosa* Laboratory derived mutant strain of *E. coli*	CIP [----]*b*	More effective against efflux pumps of MRSA, interacts efficiently with MFS class of efflux pump such as NorB, NorC, Mde A etc Exhibits anti-biofilm effects in *S. aureus* by interfering with quorum sensing mechanism Enhances membrane permeability in *E. coli*	Reported to be inhibitor for voltage gated sodium channel in mammalian brain	[74]
Polyprenol [Isoprenoid]	*Ginkgo biloba* L. (Ginkgoaceae) (Leaf)	*S. aureus*	GENTA sulfate [0.5]	Destabilizes membrane Loosens membrane structure by removal of magnesium ions Increases ion permeability	Reported to reduce the dose and frequency of some classes of antibiotics *in vitro*, when administered in form of microemulsion with globules in specified diameter range	[68]
Quercetin [Flavonoid]	----*a*	*Streptococcus pyogenes* (DMST 30653, 30654, 30655)	CAZ [0.27]	Disrupts cytoplasmic membrane integrity Alters membrane permeability Inhibits β-lactamase Inhibits peptidoglycan synthesis	Synergy also observed between quercetin and ERY, GENTA, IMI, LEVO, OXA, VAN, against MRSA strains, between quercetin and AMO, OXA against penicillin-resistant *S. aureus* and vancomycin-intermediate *S.aureus* respectively	[66, 111]
Resveratrol [Stilbene]	*Nauclea pobeguiinii* (Pobég. ex Pellegr.) Merr. ex E.M.A. Petit(Rubiaceae)[Bark]	*E. coli* AG102, *E. coli* AG100ATet *Enterobacter aerogenes* CM64 *K. pneumonia* KP55 *P.aeruginosa* PA124 *Providencia stuartii* PS2636	CIP [0.03-0.5] CLM [0.03-0.5 except *E. coli* AG102] KANA [0.03-0.5 except *Providencia stuartii* PS2636] STREP [0.25-0.5 except *E.coli* AG102 and *Providencia stuartii* PS2636] TET [0.06-0.5 except *Enterobacter aerogenes* CM64 and *E. coli* AG102]	Inhibits efflux pump	No synergistic effect obtained with beta-lactams CPM and AMO	[25]

a : --- indicates where the phytochemical has been purchased in pure form

b : [---] indicates where parameter other than FICI has been reported

List of abbreviations for antibiotics. AMI : Amikacin; AMO : Amoxicillin; CAZ : Ceftazidime; CEPH : Cephradine; CET : Ceftriaxone; CIP : Ciprofloxacin; CLAV : Clavulanic acid; CLM : Chloramphenicol; CPM : cefepime; CXM : Cefotaxime; DOX : Doxycycline; ERY : Erythromycin; GENTA : Gentamicin; IMI : Imipenem; KANA : Kanamycin; LEVO : Levofloxacin; MER: Meropenem; MET : Methicillin; NAL : Nalidixic acid; NEO : Neomycin; NOR : Norfloxacin; NOVO : novobiocin; OXA : Oxacillin; PIP : Piperacillin; PMX : Polymyxin B; RIF : Rifampicin; SDZ : Sulfadiazine; SMX : Sulfamethoxazole; STREP :

Streptomycin; SXT : Trimethoprim-sulfamethoxazole; TC : Triclosan; TET: Tetracycline; VAN: Vancomycin.
Other abbreviations. ESBL : Extended-spectrum β- lactamase; MBL : metallo-β-lactamase; MRSA : Methicillin-resistant *S. aureus*; PBP : Penicillin-binding protein

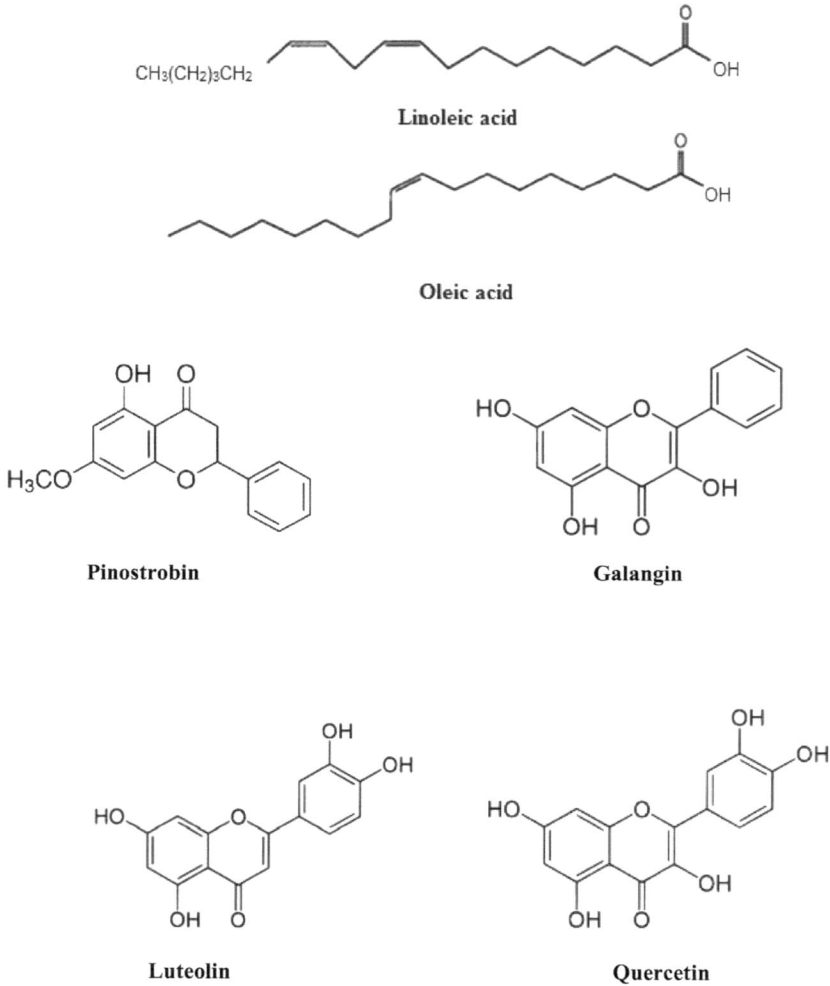

Linoleic acid

Oleic acid

Pinostrobin

Galangin

Luteolin

Quercetin

Fig. 3 contd.....

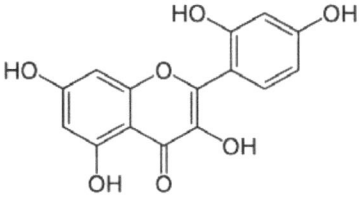

Morin

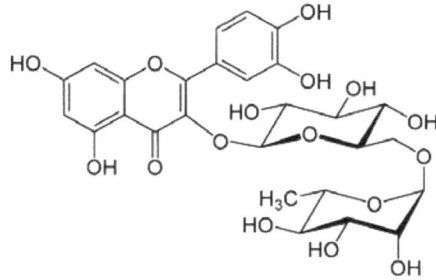

Rutin

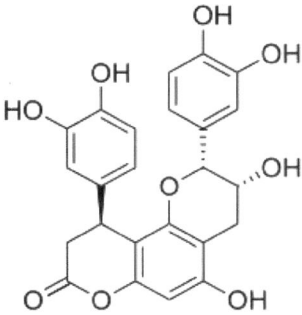

Cinchonain

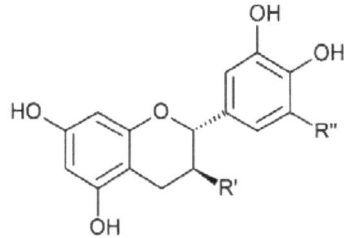

R' = OH; R" = H - Epicatechin
R' = OH; R" = OH - Epigallocatechin
R' = gallate ester; R" = H - Epicatechin gallate
R' = gallate ester; R" = OH - Epigallocatechin gallate

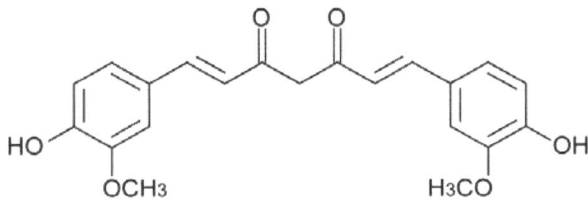

Curcumin

Fig. 3 contd.....

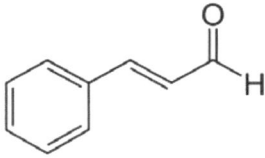

Cinnamaldehyde

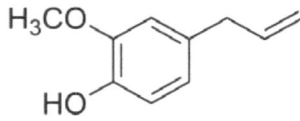

Eugenol

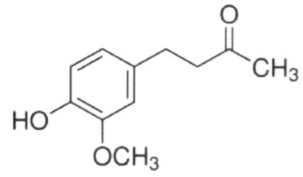

Zingerone

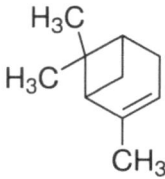

α-Pinene

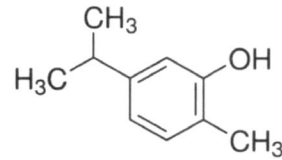

Carvacrol

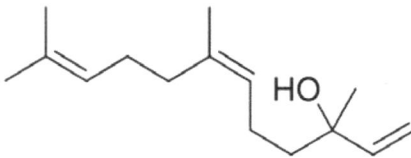

Nerolidol

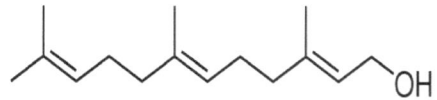

Farnesol

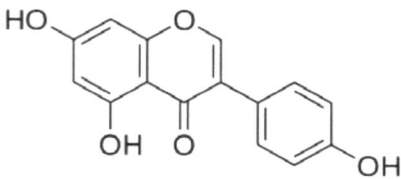

Genistein

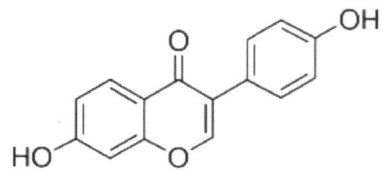

Daidzein

Fig. 3 contd.....

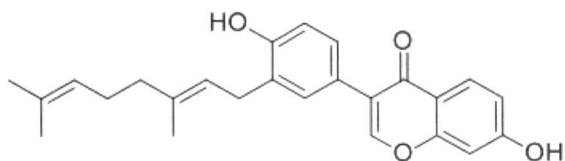

Corylifol A

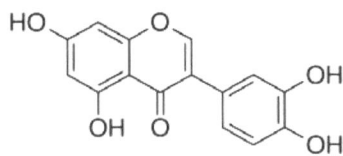

Orobol

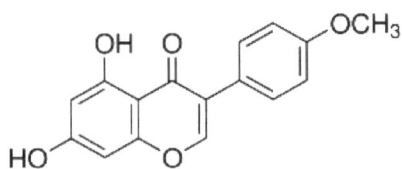

Biochanin A

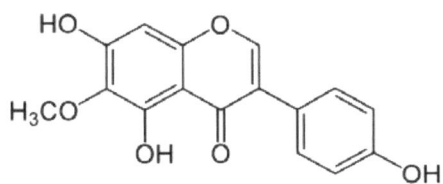

Tectorigenin

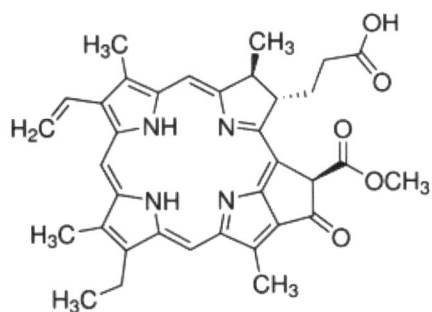

Pheophorbide a

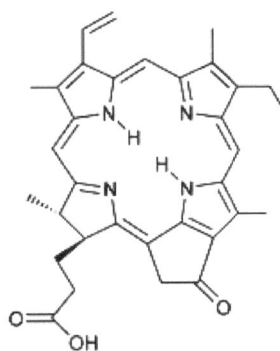

Pyropheophorbide a

Fig. 3 contd.....

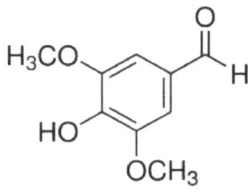

Syringaldehyde

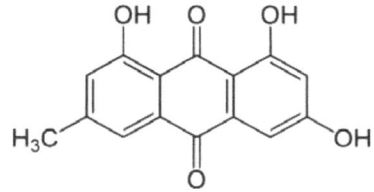

Emodin

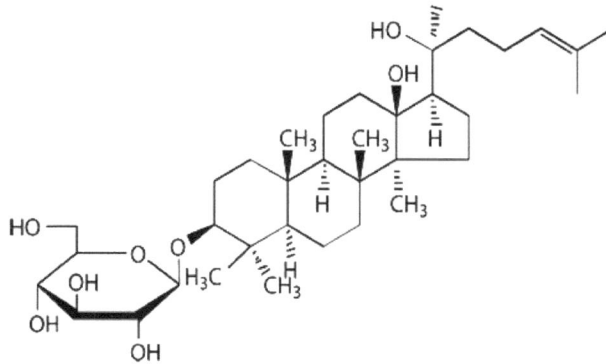

Ginsenoside 20(S)-Rh2

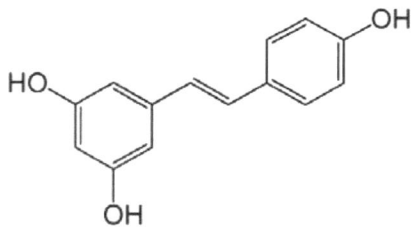

Resveratrol

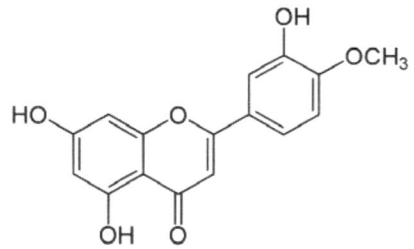

Diosmetin

Fig. 3 contd.....

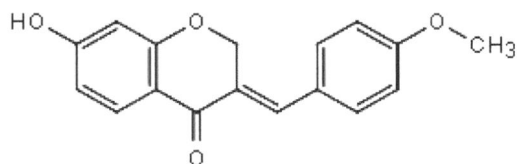

Bonducellin

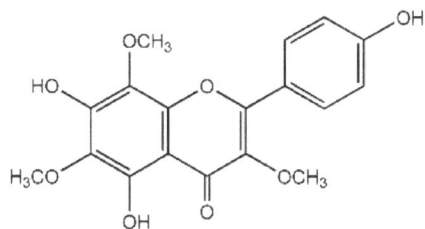

Sarothrin

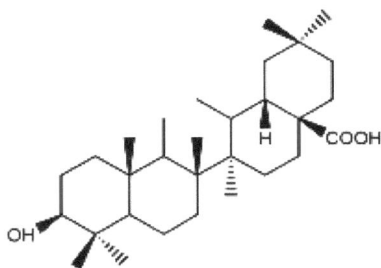

Oleanolic acid

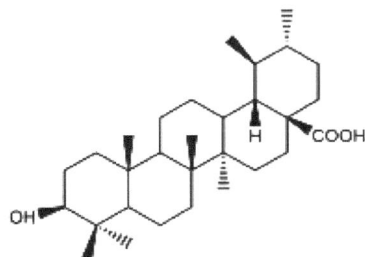

Ursolic acid

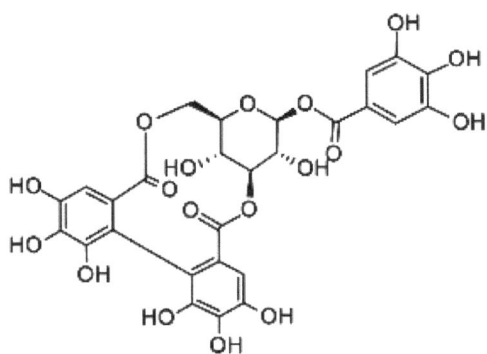

Corilagin

Fig. 3 contd.....

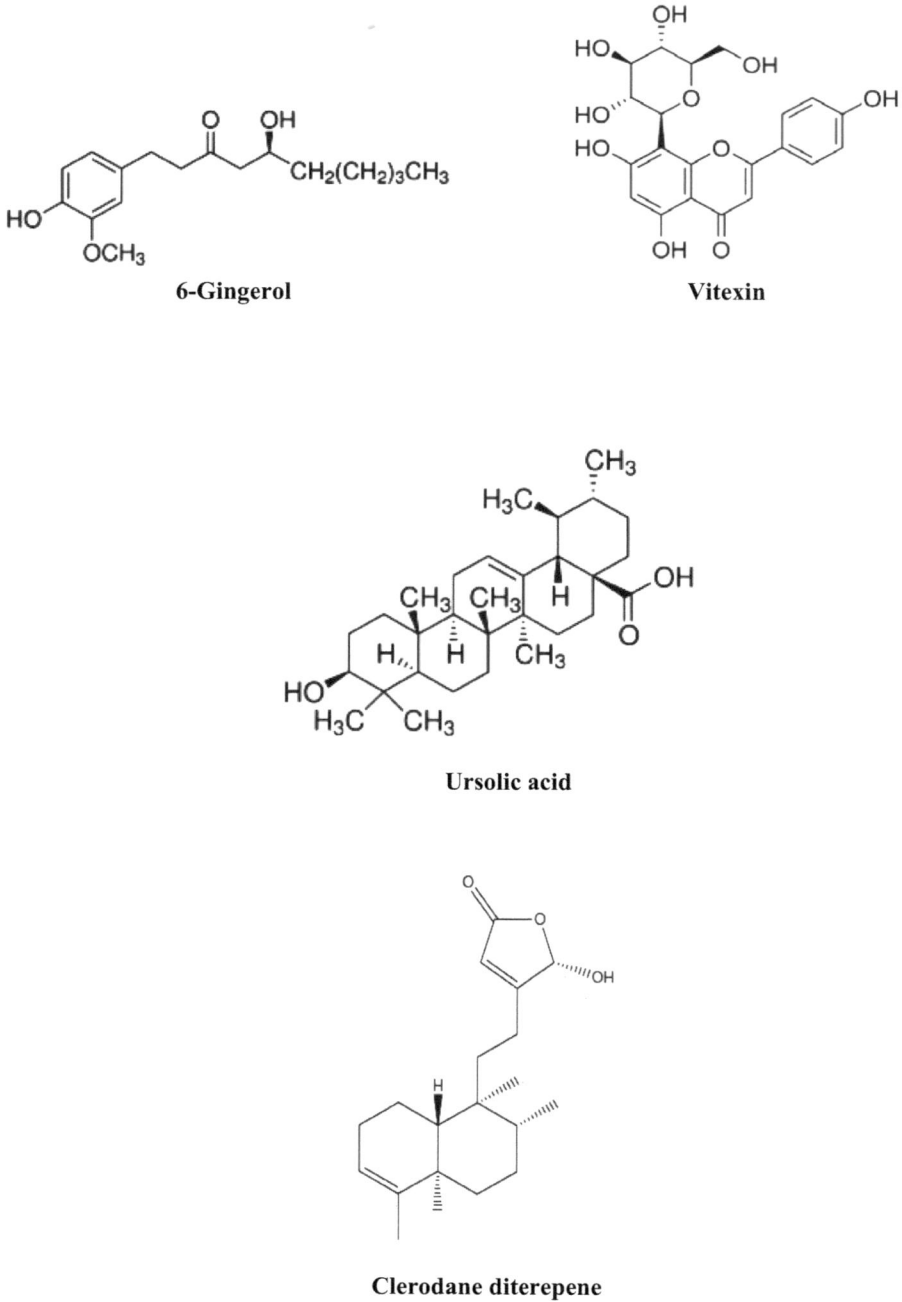

6-Gingerol

Vitexin

Ursolic acid

Clerodane diterepene

Fig. (3). Chemical structures of selected phytocompounds.

PHYTOCHEMICALS AND RELEVANT BACTERIAL RESISTANCE MECHANISMS

A complete understanding of the mechanisms by which bacteria become resistant to antibiotics is of paramount importance to design novel strategies to counter the resistance threat. Therefore, we would like to present some of the research undertaken on plant products acting as prospective RMAs to overcome antibiotic resistance in pathogenic bacteria through involvement of five major mechanistic pathways as has been depicted in Fig. (**1**) above:

  i. Efflux pump inhibition
 ii. Bacterial cell membrane permeabilisation,
iii. Protein synthesis inhibition
 iv. Enzymatic inactivation
  v. Biofilm formation inhibition.

Efflux Pump Inhibition

Efflux pumps (EP) are membrane transport proteins consisting of either 12 or 14 transmembrane helices. EPs - found in both Gram-positive and Gram-negative bacteria as well as eukaryotic organisms - are involved in extrusion of xenobiotics, antibiotics and toxic molecules from the cell without causing any structural degradation of the molecule. The expulsion process results in sub-optimal intracellular concentration of antibiotic in the bacterial cell. Thus, the MIC can only be achieved at a much higher dosage due to lowering of the efficacy of the antibiotic in question, although all EPs do not confer clinically relevant levels of antimicrobial resistance [116]. Again, over-expression of EPs leads to development of multidrug resistance against different classes of antibiotics in various clinical isolates of pathogenic strains and reduced susceptibility of the bacteria to the antibiotics [29, 32, 72]. This mechanism of resistance affects a wide range of antimicrobial classes including protein synthesis inhibitors, fluoroquinolones, β-lactams, carbapenems and polymyxins. Efflux of the antibiotic from the cell creates a favourable and selective environment for resistant species with mutations and alterations in drug targets [117]. EPs thus can be considered to play a crucial role in ensuring survival of the species and determining pathogenicity and virulence of the micro-organism.

EPs may be either substrate-specific [*e.g.* TetK efflux pump in *S. aureus* for tetracycline], or the same pump can work on multiple substrates and thus responsible for transport of multiple low- molecular-weight, structurally unrelated molecules, out of the cells, as evident in MDR pathogens [*e.g.* intrinsic and acquired resistance in *E. coli* to multiple antibiotics *viz.* β-lactams, cephalosporins, fluoroquinolones, macrolides, fusidic acid, novobiocin, chloramphenicol, rifampicin is attributed to tripartite AcrAB-TolC efflux pump] [118]. The genes encoding multidrug efflux pumps and those encoding specific drug efflux pumps are located on transferable genetic elements or plasmids, respectively [119].

Efflux pump transporters can be classified into five major families depending upon the source of energy, amino acid sequence analogies, predicted secondary protein structures, identified 3D crystal protein structures, and phylogenetic relationships [120]:

a. Major facilitator superfamily (MFS) [*e.g.* NorA, NorB, NorC, QacA, QacB, LmrS efflux pumps in *S. aureus*, Bmr efflux pump in *Bacillus subtilis*],
b. Resistance–nodulation-division (RND) [*e.g.* AcrAB-TolC efflux pump in *E. coli*, MexAB-OprM efflux pump in *P. aeruginosa*],
c. Small multidrug resistance (SMR) [*e.g.* QacG, QacH, QacJ efflux pumps in *S. aureus*; AceI pump in *A. baumannii*, EmrE in *E. coli*],
d. Multidrug and toxic efflux (MATE) [*e.g.* MepA pump in *S. aureus*, YdhE pump in *E. coli*] and
e. ATP-binding cassette (ABC) [*e.g.* MacB pump in *E. coli*; Sav1866 efflux pump in *S. aureus*].

The first three families include H^+/drug antiporters, whereas the fourth one includes H^+/drug and Na^+/drug antiporters. Since, they depend on exchange of protons or sodium ions as the source of their energy, and hence, called proton motive force (PMF). ABC group of efflux pumps utilise energy derived from hydrolysis of ATP to facilitate drug transport [116, 121]. Nearly 50% of efflux pumps belong to MFS family and are active in Gram-positive bacteria. AcrB efflux pump of *E. coli* and MexB pump of *P. aeruginosa*, are associated with two other classes of proteins, the outer membrane channel such as TolC of *E. coli* and OprM of *P. aeruginosa*, belonging to the OMF (outer membrane factor) family of proteins. For Gram-negative bacteria and Mycobacteria, the structure of the EP and thus, the efflux mechanism and substrate specificity are different from those in Gram-positive bacteria. Pumps of tripartite RND family take active role in resistance to antibiotics in Gram-negative bacteria [29, 74, 122 - 125].

Out of more than 40 suggested transporters in *E. coli*, overproduction of only AcrAB-TolC has demonstrated clinically significant fluoroquinolone resistance, although AcrAB-TolC, MdfA, and NorE are reported to modify fluoroquinolone MICs when expressed with their own promoters in laboratory growth media. Again, plasmid-borne efflux pump gene *qepA* was found in a small percentage of *E. coli* isolates, conferring resistance to both fluoroquinolones and aminoglycosides. Over-expression of *mdfA* or *norE* causes variable increase in

MICs of ciprofloxacin and norfloxacin, but with no effect on levofloxacin. On the other hand, overexpression of *acrAB,* and either *mdfA* or *norE* synergistically increases fluoroquinolone MICs. It is to be noted that deletion of *acrAB* only decreases MIC of fluoroquinolones. It is assumed that *acrAB* is normally expressed at higher levels than *mdfA* and *norE,* and thus masks their contributions [126]. Regulation of *acrAB* expression occurs at multiple levels, locally by AcrR and globally by SoxS and MarA. Over-expression of *soxS*, caused by mutation in *soxR* or *marA,* due to mutation in *marR*, or from mutations in *acrR* lead to enhanced activity of the AcrAB efflux pump, all of which inactivate the suppressor protein [127]. Two different crystal structures have been proposed for *E. coli* MdfA, one in complex with acetylcholine and the other with reserpine, which are substrate and inhibitor of vesicular neurotransmitter transporters (VNT), respectively, indicating different binding sites of these two molecules [128]. Other postulated mechanisms for resistance to quinolones in *E. coli* include mutations in *gyr*A gene (amino acid codon Ser-83 and Asp-87), mutations in the *par*C gene (amino acid codon Ser-80 and Glu-84), plasmid-mediated DNA gyrase and topoisomerase IV protection, *etc* [129, 130].

The genome of *P. aeruginosa* is predicted to encode four clinically relevant RND MDR efflux pumps such as MexAB-OprM, MexCD-OprJ, MexEF-OprN and MexXY-OprM, which are found to be up-regulated in drug-resistant clinical isolates. Phe-Arg-β-naphthylamide (PAβN, also named MC-207) is a model inhibitor of *P. aeruginosa* RND efflux pumps [131]. Antibiotic resistance in *Campylobacter jejuni* is mediated by two different RND-type efflux pumps, namely, CmeABC and CmeDEF, of which the first one is responsible for conferring intrinsic and acquired resistance to a large number of antibiotics such as fluoroquinolones and macrolides and also pure phenolic compounds and phenolic extracts obtained from plant sources [132, 133]. Resistance to macrolide is increased by interplay of CmeABC with 23S rRNA targe*t al*terations, or ribosomal protein modifications [134].

Apart from affecting antibiotic transport out of the cells, broad spectrum efflux pumps can also facilitate development of other resistance mechanisms such as secretion of antibiotic degrading enzymes *e.g.* extended spectrum β-lactamases and mutation of antibiotic targets. In *P. aeruginosa*, efflux pumps are reported to be linked to down-regulation of quorum-sensing (QS) signals and biofilm formation. Therefore, a substance with efflux pump modulatory activity can also inhibit biofilm formation [29, 32]. Although limited structural homology exists between efflux pumps in mammalian and bacterial cells, substrate overlap has been observed and reserpine, verapamil and piperine have been found to inhibit efflux pumps in both mammalian and bacterial cells [117].

Since, efflux pumps are ubiquitous across microbial population and are mediators of antibiotic resistance, design, development and characterisation of potent efflux pump inhibitors or efflux pump modulators represent a promising and powerful strategy in, modulation of pump activity, enhancing antibiotic uptake, modification of / reduction in intrinsic antibiotic resistance, restoration of antibiotic susceptibility and reduction of emergence of new recalcitrant strains. Efflux pump inhibitors (EPI) can be used as adjuvants in combination with conventional and initially ineffective antibiotics to elicit synergistic effect and optimize therapy regimen in control and containment of infections caused by pathogenic drug-resistant bacteria [29, 116]. A lipid-soluble protonophore, carbonyl cyanide *m*-chlorophenylhydrazone (CCCP) is one of the earliest identified inhibitors of NorA efflux pump. It acts as a potent uncoupler of electron transfer from ATP synthesis and works by blocking formation of the electrochemical proton gradient generated during electron transport by the respiratory chain carriers [135]. Addition of CCCP increased the uptake of ofloxacin in *S. aureus* strains that were highly resistant to methicillin [136].

Genome analysis of *S. aureus* reveals that out of 30 genes which can act as transporter proteins for different drugs, 17 can encode multidrug–resistant efflux pumps. They include the chromosomally encoded NorA, NorB, NorC, MdeA and SdrM as well as the plasmid-encoded QacA/B pumps. A new RND pump, FarE, from *S. aureus* has been identified and contributes to fatty acid resistance via transport of arachidonic and linoleic acids [121]. Over-expression of Nor A and MdeA in clinical isolates occurs due to mutations in *norA* and *mdeA* promoter regions, respectively. NorA expression is also controlled by a two-component regulator, ArlSR as its deletion from *S. aureus* results in constitutive expression of norA [120]. The NorA efflux pump confers resistance to hydrophilic fluoroquinolones, reserpine, verapamil, quaternary ammonium compounds, and dyes like ethidium bromide (EtBr), rhodamine and acridines. Resistance to hydrophobic quinolones is attributed to NorB and NorC pumps. NorB and NorC are negatively regulated by MgrA [120]. The plasmid- borne *qac* genes (*qacA*, *-B*, and *-C*), encoding QacA/B pumps confer resistance to quaternary ammonium compounds (Qac) and other cationic biocides. These genes have been detected in clinical isolates whereas, other plasmid-borne *qac* genes (*qacG*, *-H*, and *-J*) have been found to occur in food-borne and veterinary isolates of *S. aureus* [119]. Another plasmid-encoded efflux pump is TetA(K) conferring high resistance to tetracycline class of antibiotics. Other chromosome-encoded efflux pumps that are present include LmrS, MsrA, MefA, MdeA and Tet38 which confer resistance to multiple drugs, resistance of variable degree to erythromycin or only to tetracycline [117, 137]. LmrS is a MFS efflux pump with drug/H^+ antiporter activity, which can extrude multiple, structurally unrelated antimicrobial compounds. LmrS in *S. aureus* is homologous to putative lincomycin resistance proteins of *Bacillus* spp., *Lactobacillus* spp., and *Listeria* spp. Similarly, MdeA is homologous to EmrB of *E. coli*, LmrB of *B. subtilis* and FarB of *Neisseria gonorrhoeae*. Tet38 confers resistance to tetracyclines and some fatty acids and promotes bacterial colonization of skin and helps in survival in abscess environment [121]. Efflux pump inhibitors like CCCP and reserpine were found to act as efflux substrates at low concentrations and reduced the MICs of only some LmrS antimicrobial substrates. But at comparatively higher concentrations they may indirectly inhibit the pump by collapsing the proton gradient [119].

Apart from efflux pump mediated antibiotic resistance in *S. aureus*, other possible mechanisms for resistance to 4-quinolones include alterations or point mutations of DNA gyrase *(gyrA)* and alterations in the *cfx-ofx* locus conferring low-level resistance to the quinolones. DNA gyrase is a tetrameric protein consisting of A and B subunits encoded by the *gyrA* and *gyrB* genes, respectively. In a study by Tanaka, resistance to ofloxacin, levofloxacin, ciprofloxacin, sparfloxacin, tosufloxacin and norfloxacin in 14 clinical isolates of methicillin-resistant *S. aureus* was attributed to Ser→Leu substitution and Glu→Lys substitution caused by alteration at codons 84 and 88, respectively, and silent mutation at codon 86 in eight test strains [136].

The emergence of MDR- and extremely drug-resistant XDR- mycobacterial infections poses a serious challenge to global healthcare system, resulting in higher percentages of mortality and socioeconomic burdens in developing nations. There is a dire need to introduce new innovative strategies, from identification of new targets to discovery of novel chemical scaffolds to design of novel therapeutic regimens. Multidrug resistance in *M. tuberculosis* is associated with constitutive or inducible expression of efflux systems. The efflux pumps belonging to the ABC (ATP-binding cassette) class, encoded by *Rv1218c*, and the SMR (small multidrug resistance) class, encoded by *Rv3065*, seem to play significant roles in extruding different antibiotics. Other efflux pumps encoded by *Rv0849* and *Rv1258c* contribute less to efflux of chemical moieties [138]. *Rv1258c* is a secondary transporter belonging to the Major Facilitator Superfamily (MFS) of efflux pumps and is structurally analogous to MefA, a 12-membrane spanning MFS pump involved in macrolide resistance in *Streptococcus pneumoniae*. *Rv1258c* is transcriptionally induced, following residence in macrophage, and is supposed to act as a virulence factor induced in the intracellular environment encountered by the mycobacteria [139]. The complexity of the problem has further increased due to reports of bedaquiline-resistant mycobacterial strains. Low-level bedaquiline resistance and clofazimine cross-resistance are attributed to mutations in the *rv0678* gene encoding the MmpL5 efflux pump repressor. The surge of resistance to this potent anti-mycobacterial drug has emphasized the need for searching novel efflux pump inhibitors which can be employed as adjuvants in tuberculosis therapy [140, 141].

Mycobacterium smegmatis mc^2 155 (wild type) is a non-pathogenic, rapidly growing strain of Mycobacteria and is considered as a model system for study of efflux pump activity as well as identification of EPIs for Mycobacteria [142, 143]. Genes encoding putative drug efflux pumps and responsible for intrinsic resistance in *Mycobacterium smegmatis* have been identified as LfrA, LfpA, PstB, Mmr, *etc.* Other well-studied genes expressing EPs include Rv1145, Rv1146, Rv1877, Rv2846c and Rv3065. It has been observed that the deletion of LfrA (strain XZL1675) and mmr homologue enhanced the susceptibility of the strains to EtBr, acriflavine and fluoroquinolones [144].

The EPIs of plant origin have been found to co-exist with antimicrobial principles as in case of berberine and 5′-methoxy hydnocarpin. The latter phytochemical has been identified as an effective EPI for NorA pump of *S. aureus* [86]. Most of the EPIs discovered so far have been found to be small molecules effective against *S. aureus* and studies on EPI against Mycobacteria are in nascent stage [29, 32]. There are several reports of EPI effect of plant secondary metabolites or plant extracts against clinically used antibiotics as well as antibiotics of natural origin in *C. jejuni*, *P. aeruginosa*, *K. pneumoniae*, and *E. coli*, all of which have been included in Table **3**.

Alteration of Bacterial Cell Membrane Permeability

The outer membrane in Gram-negative bacteria is an important barrier that provides protection against toxic compounds, including antibiotics and host innate immune molecules such as cationic antimicrobial peptides. Thus, major functions of the outer membrane are to facilitate development of antimicrobial resistance and to interpret bacterial membrane-damaging signals. Several instances of Gram-negative bacteria with resistance to commonly used antibiotics, *viz.* quinolones, colistins (polymyxins), carbapenems, cephalosporins, and other β-lactam antibiotics, are being reported [174]. Resistance to specific antibiotics such as β-lactams develops due to alterations in barrier properties resulting from changes in the hydrophobic characteristics of the membrane or null mutations in porins. For example, resistance to imipenem for *Acinetobacter baumanii* has been attributed to loss of porin transport channels. Similarly, clinical resistance to tobramycin in uncharacterised *Pseudomonas aeruginosa* isolates from individuals with cystic fibrosis might be due to loss of outer membrane permeability of the antibiotic. Therefore, the need for new antibiotics for resistant Gram-negative bacteria could be partially overcome by introduction of compounds that target the outer membrane barrier and improve the penetration of antibiotics across the outer membrane. Alteration of the outer membrane barrier can thus enhance antibiotic

Table 3. Efflux pump inhibitory activity of plant-derived secondary metabolites.

Secondary Metabolite [Class of Compound]	Occurrence (Plant and Plant Part)	Pump(s) Affected	Potentiates the Action of / Enhances the Uptake of	Comments	Ref.
Against *S. aureus*				-	
Acacetin [Flavonoid]	*Sidastrum micranthum* (A. St.-Hil.) Fryxell (Malvaceae) (Aerial part)	NorA in *S. aureus* 1199B TetK in *S. aureus* IS-58 MsrA in *S. aureus* RN4220 /pUL5054	NOR TET ERY		[145]
Blackberry pomace extract [Phenolic acid]	*Rubus fruticosus* (Rosaceae) (---)	NorA, NorB, NorC, MdeA, SdrM, and SepA	MET	Protocatechuic, coumaric, vanillic, caffeic, and gallic acids present Reduces MRSA biofilm formation on plastic surface Down-regulates the expression of methicillin resistance (mecA) Reduces MRSA adherence to and invasion into human skin keratinocyte Hek001 cells Induces anti-apoptosis and anti-autophagy pathways through over-expression of Bcl-2 gene and down-regulation of TRADD and Bax genes in Hek001 cells	[146]
Capsaicin [Phenylpropanoid]	*Capsicum spp.* (Solanaceae) (Chili pepper)	Nor A	CIP	Reduces the invasiveness and virulence of *S. aureus* Significantly reduces the emergence of CIP-resistant mutants of *S. aureus*	[117]

(Table 3) contd.....

		Nor A	NOR	Down-regulates MFS and MATE family efflux genes such as *nor* A, *nor* B, *nor* C, *mde* A and *mep* A Lowers microbial burden of lung, liver, kidney, spleen and blood in Swiss albino female mice infected with *S. aureus*	[147]
Clerodane diterpene 16 α-hydroxycleroda-3,13(14)- *Z* -dien-15,16-olide [Terpenoid]	*Polyalthia longifolia* (Sonn.) Thwaites (Annonaceae) (Leaf)				
Diosmetin [Flavonoid]	----[a]	Nor A MsrA in *S. aureus* RN4220/pUL5054	a.CIP b.ERY	Suppresses pyruvate kinase activity of MRSA in a dose-dependent manner Leads to ATP deficiency inside bacterial cell leading to antimicrobial effects	[148]
Emodin [Anthraquinone]	*Aloe saponaria* (Aiton) Haw. (Latex)	---	CLM	Exhibits synergistic activity also with PAβN	[149, 150]
Essential oil	*Chenopodium ambrosioides* L. (Chenopodiaceae) (Leaf)	TetK	TET	Main component is α-terpinene	[151]
Essential oil	*Origanum vulgare* L. (Lamiaceae) (---)	TetK	TET	Exhibits synergistic effect due to carvacrol and thymol Thymol alters periplasmic proteins and citrate metabolic pathway	[152] [153]
Ginsenoside 20(S)-Rh2 [Saponin]	----[a]	Nor A	CIP	Inhibits NorA mediated efflux of pyroninY, NorA substrate Increases the rate (Km reduced) and extent (higher AUC value) of CIP entering into the bacteria	[154]

(Table 3) contd.....

Hesperetin [Flavonoid]	----[a]	Nor A	NOR	-	[155]
Kaempferol 3-O-α-L-(2,4-*bis*-E-p-coumaroyl)-rhamnoside [Flavonoid]	*Persea lingue* Nees (Lauraceae) (Leaf)	Nor A	CIP	Acts by targeting topo-isomerase IV	[72]
7,4'-di-O-methyl-isoscutellarein [Flavonoid]	*Sidastrum micranthum* (A. St.-Hil.) Fryxell (Malvaceae) (Aerial part)	NorA in *S. aureus* 1199B TetK in *S. aureus* IS-58 MsrA in *S. aureus* RN4220/pUL5054	NOR TET ERY	-	[145]
4', 5'-ODCQA (peracetyl derivative of 5'- O-caffeoylquinic acid (5'-OQCA) [Phenylpropanoid]	*Artemisia absinthium* (Asteraceae) (Leaf)	NorA QacA	BER CIP NOR LEVO	Potentiates action of erythromycin in *E. coli* 5'-OQCA inhibits biofilm formation	[156]
Oxychelerythrine [Benzophenanthridine alkaloid]	*Zanthoxylum capense* (Thunb.) Harv. (Rutaceae) (Root)	NorA	ERY OXA TET	Promotes moderate accumulation of EtBr inside bacterial cells, comparable to that of verapamil May interact with cell membrane in a manner similar to berberine	[157]
Oxynitidine [Benzophenanthridine alkaloid]	*Zanthoxylum capense* (Thunb.) Harv. (Rutaceae) (Root)	NorA	TET	Promotes moderate accumulation of EtBr inside bacterial cells, comparable to that of verapamil May interact with cell membrane in a manner similar to berberine	[157]
Pheophorbide a, Pyropheophorbide a [Chlorophyll catabolite]	----[a]	MDR efflux pump other than NorA is affected in *S.aureus* ATCC 29213	ERY	Inhibits LmrS, MdeA pumps in *B. subtilis*	[137]
Syringaldehyde [Phenolic aldehyde]	*Pilosocereus pachycladus* F. Ritter (Cactaceae) (Stem)	NorA	NOR TET	Affects TetK tetracycline efflux pump	[158]

(Table 3) contd.....

Tannic acid [Tannin]	----[a]	Nor A	NOR	Reported to reduce the membrane integrity in target organisms and to alter the structure and function of membrane-embedded proteins. Also reported to cause direct disturbance of the microbial metabolism by inhibiting oxidative phosphorylation	[159]
4',5,6,7-tetramethoxyflavone	*Praxelis clematidea* R.M. King & Robinson (Asteraceae) (Aerial Part)	NorA	NOR	-	[160]
Against *Mycobacterium smegmatis* mc²155					
1'-S-1'–acetoxyeugenolacetate [Phenylpropanoid]	*Alpinia galanga* (Zingiberaceae) (Rhizome)	-	EtBr	Enhances accumulation and inhibits efflux of EtBr in a dose-dependent manner. Better modulator as compared to standard EPIs reserpine, verapamil, chlorpromazine and CCCP	[144]
Bonducellin [Homoisoflavonoid]	*Caesalpinia digyna* Rottler (Leguminosae) (Root)	-	EtBr	-	[161]
trans, trans-1,7—diphenyl hepta-4,6-diene-3-one [Diarylheptanoid]	*Alpinia katsumadai* Hayala (Zingiberaceae) (Seed)	-	RIF EtBr	-	[162]
4-[2-(5-butylfuran-2-yl)ethyl]-2-methoxyphenol [Phenol]	*Aframomum melegueta* (Roscoe) K. Schum. (Zingiberaceae) (Seed)	-	RIF	-	[163]

(Table 3) contd.....

6-paradol [Ketone]	*Aframomum melegueta* (Roscoe) K. Schum. (Zingiberaceae) (Seed)	-	INH RIF	-	[163]
Pinocembrin [Flavonoid]	*Alpinia katsumadai* Hayala (Zingiberaceae) (Seed)	-	ETHAM EtBr	EtBr efflux inhibition comparable to CCCP	[162]
rac-6-dihydroparadol [Ketone]	*Aframomum melegueta* (Roscoe) K. Schum. (Zingiberaceae) (Seed)	-	RIF	-	[163]
Sarothrin (Flavonoid)	*Alkanna orientalis* (Boraginaceae) (Leaf and flower)	-	---[b]	-	[164]
Against *Campylobacter jejuni*					
Carnosic acid [Phenol]	----[a]	CmeABC	PAβN CCCP	Only 4-fold difference in MICs when tested in absence of any of the mentioned control EPIs	[132]
Ferulic acid [Phenol]	----[a]	CmeABC	PAβN CCCP	Only 4-fold difference in MICs when tested in absence of any of the mentioned control EPIs	[132]
Rosemary extract	*Rosemarinus officinalis* L.		PAβN	≥ 64-fold difference in MIC	[132]
Sinapinic acid [Phenol]	----[a]	CmeABC	PAβN CCCP	Only 4-fold difference in MICs when tested in absence of any of the mentioned control EPIs	[132]
Syringic acid [Phenol]	----[a]	CmeABC	PAβN CCCP	Only 4-fold difference in MICs when tested in absence of any of the mentioned control EPIs	[132]
Against *P. aeruginosa*					
Callistemon citrinus extract	*Callistemon citrinus*(Curtis) Skeels (Myrtaceae) (Leaf)	MexXY-OprM MexCD-Opr	RH 6G	-	[165]
Berberis vulgaris extract	*Berberis vulgaris* L. (Berberidaceae) (Root and rhizome)	MexAB-OprM	CIP	-	[166]

(Table 3) contd.....

Against *E. coli*					
1,2,6-tri-O-galloyl-β-D-glucopyranose [Gallotannin]	*Terminalia chebula* (Gaertn.)Retz. (Combretaceae) (Fruit)	-	GENTA TMP	Enhances accumulation of EtBr	[167]
Levisticum officinale extract	*Levisticum officinale* W.D.J.Koch (Apiaceae) (Leaf and branch)	-	CIP	Similar effect also observed with falcarindiol isolated from chloroform extract of the leaves	[168]
Sophora alopecuroides extract	*Sophora alopecuroides* (Leguminosae) (Seed)	AcrAB–TolC	CIP	Can lower the MIC of CIP in biofilm-producing high-resistance *P. aeruginosa* isolates with overexpression of *mexA* and also destroy the integrity of biofilm Mode of action slightly different from that of PAβN IC$_{50}$ value (50% cytotoxic concentration) of total alkaloid in the extract in BHK21 (Baby hamster kidney fibroblasts) cells reported to be 36 mg/mL	[169]
Against *K. pneumonia*					
Berberine [Alkaloid]	----^{a}	AcrAB-TolC AcrR	CIP	CIP uptake increased probably *via* channel formation in bacterial membranes	[170]
Eucalyptus robusta extract	*Eucalyptus robusta* (Myrtaceae) (Leaf and bark)	-	CIP CLM ERY NOR TET STREP	-	[171]
Mangifera indica extract	*Mangifera indica* L. (Anacardiaceae) (Leaf)	-	CLM ERY TET	-	[172]
Punigratane [Alkaloid]	*Punica granatum* L. (Punicaceae) (Rind)	-	NOR	-	[173]

----^{a}: purified phytochemical procured from commercial source
----^{b}: synergistic activity not investigated
Abbreviations: BER: Berberine; ETHAM: Ethambutol; RH6G: Rhodamine 6G; RIF: Rifampicin; TMP: Trimethoprim

susceptibility for resistant organisms [174]. The existence of synergistic relationship between transmembrane efflux pump and the cell membrane barrier creates an additional obstacle in the path of effective control of Gram-negative pathogens and can accelerate the development of antimicrobial resistance [175]. Low permeability of outer membrane and expression of efflux pumps confer intrinsic resistance to novobiocin in *A. baumannii*. Permeability enhancers facilitate reversible lowering or removal of the permeability barrier and allow easy access to the antibiotic to its target site. Pores may be formed in the membranes resulting in leakage of intracellular contents like potassium, calcium ions, *etc*. Plant compounds or secondary metabolites containing a steroid or triterpenoid aglycone attached to one or more sugar chains can permeabilise bacterial membranes. This would lead to loss in rigidity and mechanical integrity of the membranes and will thus increase sensitivity to antibiotic [59, 61]. In Table **4**, some plant extracts and a flavonoid of plant origin have been included to demonstrate the effect of phytochemicals on bacterial cell membrane permeabilisation and/or reversal of antibiotic resistance.

Table 4. Increased membrane permeability in drug–resistant bacterial strains by secondary metabolites of plant origin.

Secondary Metabolite [Class of Compound]	Occurrence (Plant and Plant Part)	Test Bacteria	Synergistic Interaction	Ref.
Callistemon citrinus extract	*Callistemon citrinus* (Linn.) (Myrtaceae) (Leaf)	*S. aureus* *P. aeruginosa*	---[a]	[61]
Holarrhena antidysenterica extract	*Holarrhena antidysenterica* (Roth) Wall. ex A.DC. (Apocynaceae) (Stem bark)	MDR-*Acinetobacter baumannii* XDR-*Acinetobacter baumannii*	NOVO	[59]
Poincianella pyramidalis extract	*Poincianella pyramidalis* (Tul.) LP Queiroz (Fabaceae) (---)	*S. aureus* *P. aeruginosa* *E. coli*	GENTA	[176]
Syzygium cumini Extract	*Syzygium cumini* (L.) Skeels (Myrtaceae) (Seed)	*B. subtilis*	---[a]	[64]

(Table 3) contd.....

Secondary Metabolite [Class of Compound]	Occurrence (Plant and Plant Part)	Test Bacteria	Synergistic Interaction	Ref.
5,7,3′,4′-tetramethoxyflavone [Flavonoid]	*Murraya paniculata* (Linn.) JACK (Rutaceae) (Leaf)	*E. coli* ATCC 25922 *S. aureus* ATCC 12692 *S. aureus* ATCC 358	AMI GENTA NEO KANA	[177]
Vernonia adoensis extract	*Vernonia adoensis* Sch.Bip. ex Walp. (Asteraceae) (Leaf)	*S. aureus*	---^{a}	[61]

----^{a}: synergistic activity not investigated
Abbreviations for antibiotics. KANA: Kanamycin; NOVO: Novobiocin

Protein Synthesis Inhibition

A common survival strategy for bacteria against deleterious effects of antibiotics is to bypass the action of the antibiotic by interfering with their target site. This may be achieved by protection or modification of the target site to reduce affinity for the antibiotic molecule. Target changes induced by bacteria may consist of point mutations in the genes encoding the target site, enzymatic alterations of the binding site (*e.g.* addition of methyl groups), and/or replacement or bypass of the original target. Examples of clinical relevance include methicillin resistance in *S. aureus* due to the acquisition of an exogenous PBP and vancomycin resistance in enterococci through modifications of the peptidoglycan structure mediated by the *van* gene clusters [35].

One of the primary mechanisms for resistance to β-lactam antibiotics in *S. aureus* is the acquisition of a gene encoding a modified penicillin-binding protein (PBP), known as PBP 2a, found in MRSA and coagulase-negative staphylococci [178 - 180]. A characteristic feature of PBP 2a is that it is intrinsically resistant to inhibition by β-lactams and maintains its activity in the presence of antibiotic concentrations which inhibit most endogenous PBP enzymes, thus substituting for their functions in cell wall synthesis and allowing growth in the presence of the β-lactam inhibitors [178]. PBP2a is under allosteric control, whereas PBP is not. PBP2a is encoded by the *mecA* gene, which is carried on a distinct mobile genetic element, staphylococcal chromosome cassette (SCC*mec*). Complete expression of the gene is controlled by unique three-component arrangement of *mecR1-mec--mecR2* regulatory gene, comprising of a sensor protein (MecR1) and a repressor (MecI). SCC*mec* is present in MRSA but absent in methicillin-susceptible *S. aureus* (MSSA) [181]. The genes *mecR1* and *mecI* are located within the upstream region of the *mecA* gene. In presence of β-lactam antibiotic such as methicillin, *mecR1* is activated which encodes for the inducing protein, MecR1 and PBP 2a production is stimulated. PBP 2a has low affinity for all β-lactams, including penicillins, cephalosporins (except for last generation compounds) and carbapenems. Role of PBP-2a in cell wall biosynthesis is well-defined but it has not been directly implicated in drug resistance. The protein acts as transpeptidase in *S. aureus*, enabling cross-linking of N-acetylmuramyl-pentapeptide with pentaglycine in the developing cell wall, and plays an active role in growth of micro-organism. Apart from the genes mentioned above responsible for endowing micro-organism with methicillin resistance, another gene, *femA* gene is also reported to be involved, not through its participation in PBP 2a synthesis but through a role in synthesis of cell wall components of *S. aureus* [182]. Susceptibility to oxacillin and nafcillin in two common clinical isolates of community acquired-MRSA (CA-MRSA) strains is controlled by the gene encoding PBP 4. They are positive for *mecA* and PBP 2a. Deletion of the gene encoding PBP 4 introduced into hospital acquired MRSA (HA-MRSA) demonstrated negligible effect on oxacillin MICs. Although PBP 4 exhibits low affinity for most β-lactams, cefoxitin, a semisynthetic β-lactam, efficiently acylates PBP 4 and is synergistic with oxacillin in killing CA-MRSA strains [178]. Plant compounds such as flavonoids interfere with the activity of PBP-2a when the peptidoglycan synthesis in bacteria is impeded and integrity of the cell membrane is disrupted, as manifested by loss/leakage of intracellular potassium ions detected by flame photometry. In this manner, flavonoids ultimately cause lowering of MIC of conventional antibiotics and amplify their therapeutic efficacy [67]. In Table **5**, some examples of plant extracts or plant-derived secondary metabolites have been presented targeting cell wall synthesis by interfering with the action of PBP.

Table 5. Protein synthesis inhibition by phytochemicals.

Secondary Metabolite [Class of Compound]	Occurrence (Plant and Plant Part)	Test Bacteria	Synergistic Interaction	Ref.
Corilagin [Tannin]	*Acalypha wilkesiana* Mull. Arg. (Euphorbiaceae) (Whole plant)	MRSA	AMP	[183]
Duabanga grandiflora extract	*Duabanga grandiflora* (Lythraceae) (Leaf)	MRSA	AMP	[184]

(Table 5) contd.....

Secondary Metabolite [Class of Compound]	Occurrence (Plant and Plant Part)	Test Bacteria	Synergistic Interaction	Ref.
Oleanolic acid [Triterpenic acid]	*Vitellaria paradoxa* C.F. Gaertn (Sapotaceae) (Leaf and twigs)	MRSA	AMP OXA NAF	[185]
1-(piperidin-1-yl)-4-propoxythioxanthone [Thioxanthone]	*Cratoxylum maingayi* Dyer (Hypericaceae) (Stem bark)	MRSA	AMP OXA	[186]
Ursolic acid [Triterpenic acid]	*Vitellaria paradoxa* C.F. Gaertn (Sapotaceae) (Leaf and twigs)	MRSA	AMP OXA NAF	[185]
Ursolic acid - Oleanolic acid [Triterpenic acid]	*Chamaedora tepejilote* (Arecaceae) (Whole plant) *Lantana hispida* (Verbenaceae) (Whole plant)	*M. tuberculosis* H37Rv	-	[187]

Abbreviation for antibiotic. NAF: Nafcillin

Enzymatic Inhibition

Antibiotic degradation or inactivation can occur by any of the following mechanisms-enzymatic hydrolysis, group transfer reactions or redox reactions. Enzyme-catalysed antibiotic inactivation is of prime concern because of its ability to induce resistance to antibiotics. Several detoxifying enzymes such as β-lactamases, esterases, aminoglycoside acetyltransferases, kinases *etc.* take active part in the catalytic reactions which result in alteration of various target binding sites such as *mec* genes in *S. aureus*, van genes in *Enterococci* and some efflux pump systems (TetA, Qac *etc.*). Structures most susceptible to hydrolysis include esters and amides. Antibiotics are hydrolysed by the respective enzymes in presence of water as a co-substrate and excreted out of the bacterial cell even before their entry. Numerous reports of antibiotic resistance due to degradation by extended-spectrum-β-lactamases (ESBL) in *S. aureus* and *Enterobacteriaceae* are actually complicating the situation [32, 50]. Subgroup 2b (molecular class A) of Group 2 β- lactamases comprises of broad-spectrum β-lactamases, such as TEM-1, TEM-2, SHV-1, and ROB-1, which can hydrolyze penicillins and broad-spectrum cephalosporins. Subgroup 2be represents ESBLs *e.g.*, variants of TEM and SHV families and CTX-M type enzymes, which can also inactivate oxyimino cephalosporins and monobactams. Most currently known ESBLs belong to the

TEM, SHV, CTX-M, or OXA families of β-lactamases whereas, less common ESBLs include BEL-1, BES-1, SFO-1, TLA-1, TLA-2, and members of the PER and VEB enzyme families [188]. Plasmid-borne ESBL, especially those belonging to the CTX-M family are responsible for incidences of resistance to third-generation cephalosporins in *Enterobacteriaceae*. Carbapenemase-producing strains of *P. aeruginosa, A. baumannii* and *Klebsiella pneumoniae* have emerged globally over the last decade. VIM- and NDM-type metallo-betalactamases, OXA-48 and KPC appear to threaten the existence of carbapenems as effective antimicrobial agents in the near future. Apart from bearing resistance determinants for β-lactams and carbapenems in ESBL- and carbapenemase-encoding plasmids, they also confer resistance to other antimicrobial classes, such as aminoglycosides (aminoglycoside-modifying enzymes or 16S rRNA methylases) and fluoroquinolones (Qnr, AAC(6')-Ib-cr or efflux pumps), accounting to multidrug resistance in *Enterobacteriaceae*. MDR in non-fermenting Gram-negative bacteria, such as *Pseudomonas aeruginosa, Acinetobacter baumannii* and *Stenotrophomonas maltophilia*, may be attributed to occurrence of sequential chromosomal mutations, leading to the overproduction of intrinsic β-lactamases, hyper-expression of efflux pumps, target modifications and permeability alterations. Resistance to aminoglycosides in *Enterobacteriaceae* is due to aminoglycoside-modifying enzymes (AMEs) such as aminoglycoside phosphotransferase, aminoglycoside nucleotidyltransferase, and aminoglycoside acetyltransferase [189 - 191]. *In E. coli*, there are evidences of existence of TEM-1 *β*-lactamase, ESBLs, carbapenemases, or plasmid-mediated quinolone resistance (PMQR) mechanisms. Other mechanisms such as ribosomal methylases affecting aminoglycoside or plasmid mediated fosfomycin resistance, occuring in association with ESBL and/or carbapenemase production are yet to be elucidated. Most ESBLs among *Escherichia coli* clinical isolates in the UK were encoded by transformable plasmids, majority of which were diverse multiresistant IncF types possessing multiple addiction systems. However, β-lactam resistance in either non-ESBL-producing single drug resistamt or MDR *E. coli* isolates is more likely to be mediated by nontransferrable TEM β-lactamase enzymes carried by transposons, which are then integrated into the chromosomal DNA [127]. The spread of $bla_{CTX-M-15}$, harbouring bla_{OXA-1} and *aac(6')-Ib-cr*, and often transferring trimethoprim and tetracycline resistance can be attributed not just to clonal expansion, but also to the horizontal dissemination of related plasmids. A recent study on drug resistance mechanisms in *E. coli* in a hospital setting in China showed the presence of isolates with multiple resistant genes, including carbapenemase (bla_{KPC-2}), ESBL ($bla_{CTX-M-3}$, $bl_{aCTX-M-14}$, $bla_{CTX-M-55}$), and quinolone (*qnrA, qnrB, qnrC, qnrD, qnrS* and *aac(6')-Ib-cr*) resistance genes [129]. Other degrading and modifying enzymes such as active-site serine carbapenemases, plasmid-encoded class C cephalosporinases and acquired metallo-β-lactamases have also been reported to exist in different bacterial strains [21]. Tetracyclines prevent the binding of aminoacyl-tRNA to the A-site on 30S ribosome and their activity is blocked by acetyltransferases which have been detected in *S. aureus*, *Enterococcus faecalis* and *Streptococcus pneumoniae* [60]. Many plant extracts as well as pure compounds such as extracts from *Garcinia lucida* and *Bridelia micrantha* epigallocatechin gallate have demonstrated significant inhibitory effect on β-lactamases with subsequent enhancement of bacterial sensitivity towards penicillin and augmentation of antimicrobial efficacy of ampicillin and sulbactam against MRSA [36]. Farnesol is another plant-derived triterpenoid which can reduce the secretion and activity of β-lactamase in MRSA. Ursolic acid, a plant-derived triterpenoid exhibited significant activity against *S. aureus* and *B. cereus*. The strategy of co-administering an inhibitor of antibiotic-degrading enzyme of synthetic origin, such as β-lactamase inhibitor, has been long known to restore the activity of the antibiotic; and the same strategy is expected to show potential with plant secondary metabolites. Synergistic effect has been observed during co-administration of triterpenoids with both ampicillin and tetracycline in *S. aureus* and *B. cereus* [154]. In fact, the ability of amoxapine to resensitize MRSA *S. aureus* strain ATCC 43300 to oxacillin in both agar diffusion and broth microdilution assays has been demonstrated in a latest study [192]. Since amoxapine also reduced the bacterial cleavage of nitrocefin in a dose-dependent manner, it could be assumed to exert its adjuvant effects through suppression of β-lactamase activity.

Biofilm Formation Inhibition

Bacterial strains lacking a genetic basis for resistance might exhibit significant resistance to antibiotics especially if they are present in a sessile state. This has been observed with *P. aeruginosa* strains which do not have the multidrug-resistant efflux pumps but show resistance to ciprofloxacin when present in films [32]. Biofilm resistance has been implicated as a major obstacle in treatment of many commonly occurring diseases such as dental caries, mastitis, otitis media, endocarditis, chronic wounds and osteomyelitis. In the US, nearly 17 million new biofilm infections are reported every year, of which 550,000 cases become fatal [193]. Efficacy of antibiotics is not only threatened by continuing emergence of pathogens resistant to these agents but also by the formation of biofilms by some bacterial strains. Resistance acquisition is an evolutionary strategy devised by bacteria to enhance their chances of survival whereas biofilm formation is an inherent characteristic of the strain and is a very common form of microbial organization. It contributes to chronicity of persistent infections associated with implantable medical devices. Characteristics of biofilm are significantly different from those of free-living (planktonic) micro-organisms in terms of morphology, physiology and genetic constitution. Mutation occurs more frequently in biofilm-forming species and horizontal gene transmission is much higher. Biofilms are produced by bacteria themselves during their growth and consist of persistent, structured communities of microbial cells enclosed in surface-associated matrix of extracellular polymeric substances. The matrix contains ions, nutrients and extracellular degrading enzymes such as lactamases, proteases and polysaccharidases. They promote cellular adhesion to both living and non-living surfaces. They act as diffusion barriers to penetration of conventional antibiotics, reduce their sensitivity, can escape the host's innate immunity system and require higher doses for eradication compared to planktonic bacteria. Unusually high dose not only increases risk of toxicity but may also aggravate occurrence of antibiotic resistance. A small percentage of biofilm–based bacteria remain active even after exposure to high dose of antibiotic. Thus, bacteria become 10-1000-fold more resistant to antibiotics due to biofilm formation. Accessible mature biofilms can be inactivated and removed by suitable agents or various approaches can be employed or molecules can be designed or isolated from renewable natural sources targeting various stages of biofilm development. These compounds can change the bacterial phenotype without any genetic alteration to avoid development of resistance. Plant polyphenolics are examples of natural compounds endowed with numerous functions which facilitate modification of bacterial behavior through effects on bacterial motility, surface adhesion, biofilm formation, quorum sensing etc. Therefore, these types of molecules can be employed as resistance modifying agents where they can improve interaction of antibiotic with the target located inside the bacterial biofilm [9, 113]. Thus, any plant secondary metabolite which can act as anti-adhesive compound will be effective in preventing biofilm formation and facilitate bacterial clearance from host system [193, 194]. Phytochemicals of diverse structure can be exploited to develop biofilm inhibitors with multiple targets of action. Since the efflux pumps play a crucial role in determining tolerance level of bacterial biofilms to antibiotics, administration of EPIs alone or as adjuvants to conventional antibiotics, or co-administration of EPI with metal-chelating agent can attenuate bacterial resistance in biofilm-forming species. There is a report of biofilm inactivation in *S. aureus* and *E. faecalis* by administration of caffeoylquinic acid extracted from *A. absinthium* and moxifloxacin at sub-MIC [32]. Table **6** illustrates a few phytochemicals showing ability to inhibit biofilm formation in bacterial strains and also some compounds showing synergistic effect with classical antibiotics in biofilm-forming species.

Table 6. Biofilm formation inhibition by plant products.

Secondary Metabolite [Class of Compound]	Occurrence (Plant and Plant Part)	Test Bacteria	Synergistic Interaction	Special Remarks	Ref.
Curcumin	---[a]	*S. epidermidis*	Cinnamaldehyde	Both disrupted the bacterial membrane as manifested by permeability studies on *E.coli* ML-35p	[195]
Eugenol	---[a]	*P. aeruginosa*	---[b]	Competitive binding of eugenol to quorum sensing, QS receptor (LasR) occurs leading to significant repression of QS associated genes besides the virulence factor (VF) genes	[23, 95, 196]
6-gingerol [Non-volatile oil]	---[a]	*P. aeruginosa*	---[b]	Molecular binding observed between 6-gingerol and the QS receptor LasR Diminished virulence factors *viz.* exoprotease, rhamnolipid, and pyocyanin	[197]
Quercus cerris extract	*Quercus cerris* L. (Fagaceae) (Leaf, fruit and stem)	Methicillin-resistant *S. aureus*	---[b]	-	[198]
Vitexin [Flavone]	*Vitex peduncularis* (Wall.) (Verbenaceae) (Leaf)	*Pseudomonas aeruginosa*	AZT GENTA	Binding to ligand binding pockets of two QS proteins, LasA and LuxR affinity	[199]
Zingerone [Ketone]	---[a]	*P. aeruginosa* PA01	CIP	Inhibited production of extracellular polysaccharide, alginate Decreased cell surface hydrophobicity Inhibited bacterial attachment and colonization	[200, 201]

----[a]: purified phytochemical procured from commercial source
----[b]: synergistic activity not investigated; **Abbreviation for antibiotic.** AZT: Azithromycin

ADDITIONAL STRATEGIES FOR SCREENING AND DEVELOPMENT OF PLANT PRODUCTS AS ADJUVANTS IN ANTIMICROBIAL THERAPY

Mostly, plant-derived secondary metabolites can destroy the structure of bacterial cell membrane, thereby altering the integrity of membrane and leading to improved penetration and increased influx of the antibiotics into bacterial cells. Thus, better interaction with their targets of action can impede the vital enzymes involved in DNA replication, transcription and translation in bacteria. In this way, synergistic interaction takes place to enhance the susceptibility of bacteria and considerably lowers the MICs of extant antibiotics to bring them back into action. This would be an important strategy to combat spreading of antibiotic resistance by extending the life span of our current repertoire of antibiotics [52, 202, 203].

In Vivo Validation

For the discovery and development of novel antimicrobial agents, plant extracts / compounds are generally screened to assess their efficacy and potential toxicity, *in vitro*. Eventually, successful candidates must be evaluated in animal models for their potential application in humans. Commonly, murine models are used for studying microbial infections *in vivo*. However, there are ethical, budgetary and logistical hurdles associated with the use of rodents as infection models. Lately, an insect called *Galleria mellonella* (honeycomb moth) from the order *Lepidoptera* and the family Pyralidae has become popular as a surrogate host to study microbial infections, and as a screening platform for antibiotics. Although *G. mellonella* infection model is still in its infancy, but a lot of articles appeared on this topic in PubMed, of which >200 were published during 2014-2015 alone. In some of the studies, survival in *G. mellonella* was strongly correlated with survival in mice [204]. Experiments on combinations of antibiotics with novel compounds / plant products have shown synergism when administered to infected *G. mellonella* larvae. For example, combination of curcumin with antibiotics such as piperacillin or levofloxacin restored the efficacy of the antibiotics and reduced the level of *in vivo* infection with a MDR strain of *P. aeruginosa* in *G. mellonella* larvae [97]. Supplementation with carvacrol exerted protective effect on antibiotic-induced gut dysbiosis, reduced *Clostridium difficile* infection and lowered the clinical symptoms of diarrhoea in C57BL/6 mice. It effectively induced a favorable shift in the composition of the gut microbiome without reducing the microbiota diversity [204]. Kaempferol 3-O-α-L-(2,4-*bis*-E-p-coumaroyl)-rhamnoside, a plant-derived flavonoid investigated as a RMA, was found to be non-toxic on intramuscular administration in mice, and, hence, could be assumed to be safe for topical application [72]. Administration of ginsenoside 20(S)-Rh2 to ciprofloxacin-treated mice with peritonitis caused by *S. aureus* doubled the survival rate in comparison to ciprofloxacin alone. The beneficial effect was not produced by enhanced plasma concentration of ciprofloxacin, as observed from pharmacokinetic data [154]. Significant reduction in systemic staphylococcal burden was observed in lungs, liver, kidney, spleen and blood of Swiss albino mice on administration of a combination of norfloxacin with clerodane diterpene. No increase in pro-inflammatory cytokines could be detected in the blood levels of septic shock mouse model, nor was any mortality reported [147]. Grape pomace extract-antibiotic combination proved to be non-toxic for HeLa cell lines at concentrations investigated to assess synergistic effect, and thus can be safely used in animal models for further study [108]. Acute toxicity studies on oral administration of hydro-ethanolic extract of *Murraya paniculata* leaves revealed no change in haematological parameters of mice, nor any indication of CNS / ANS toxicity. Also, no significant microscopic changes to indicate acute toxicity was observed in histopathological study [177]. Similarly, 6-gingerol was found to be safe as mortality rate in mice infected with *P. aeruginosa* decreased after treatment with this compound [197]. In another study, vitexin - a polyphenolic group of phytochemicals -was found to cause moderate attenuation in biofilm forming capability of *P. aeruginosa* at sub-MIC doses. Again, the combination of vitexin with either azithromycin or gentamicin showed synergistic antibiofilm activity, while maximum attenuation was observed with the combination of vitexin (110 µg/ml) and gentamicin (2.5 µg/ml) *in vitro*. Thereafter, a mouse model was used to evaluate the *in vivo* anti-biofilm activity of vitexin alone and in combination with antibiotics against catheter associated infection by *P. aeruginosa* [199]. It could be inferred that combination of vitexin with azithromycin or gentamicin will not allow the organism to develop MDR as vitexin will potentiate the anti-biofilm activity of these antibiotics against *P. aeruginosa*.

Standardisation of Botanical Extracts

Recently, several reports have indicated that complex botanical extracts are superior to a single phytochemical compound in terms of antibiotic adjuvant activity against different bacterial species [108, 205 - 207]. In fact, it is likely that a plant extract composed of a cocktail of interacting compounds would simultaneously hit multiple pharmacological targets that are beyond the reach of any drug based on a single compound, and thereby provide a clue to develop a novel combination therapy. But, unfortunately, in most cases, the lack of complete pharmacokinetic / pharmacodynamic profiles with regard to the toxicological aspect impeded the safe entry of these botanical extracts for clinical trial in humans. Recently, WHO has passed a mandate to develop innovative scientific methods for discovery, validation, characterization and standardization of multi-component botanical therapeutics as offshoots of traditional / anecdotal systems for their acceptance into mainstream medicine [208]. Therefore, complex botanical compositions that would meet the FDA standards for safety and efficacy are eligible for an alternative pathway for regulatory approval as "botanical drugs", distinct from dietary supplements. These are standardized to the level of marker compounds, and, once approved, must be regulated like other single compound pharmaceuticals [208, 209].

iChip Technology

Traditionally, discovery of antibiotics has been conducted by screening of microorganism extracts for putative antimicrobial activity. Presently, an innovative approach called iChip has been designed for *in situ* cultivation of novel micro-organisms that would not grow under normal laboratory conditions. The iChip utilises a system composed of hundreds of miniature diffusion chambers, each loaded with a single cell. The diffusion system allows the cells on the iChip - made of a polyoxymethylene thermoplastic plate- to interact with naturally occurring nutrients and environmental factors. This technique helps to get access to a greater diversity of microorganisms from natural sources like underground soils, and could be a 'game changer' for discovering new antibiotics [210]. Thus, iChip, allowed isolation of an antibiotic from soil microbes to get a novel drug, namely, teixobactin with significant potency against Gram-positive bacteria, like *Staphylococcus aureus* including MRSA, *Streptococcus pneumonia* and *Mycobacterium tuberculosis* [211]. Teixobactin was also effective in curing experimental infections of MRSA in mice. However, clinical trials must be carried out for teixobactin to ensure its safe application in patients [212].

CONCLUDING REMARKS

Currently, the emergence of antimicrobial resistance has posed the toughest challenge for healthcare professionals around the world in the brink of the so-called 'post-antibiotic era' [6]. Infectious 'superbugs' have been characterised in community- and hospital-acquired Gram-positive and Gram-negative pathogens, particularly methicillin-resistant *Staphylococcus aureus* (MRSA), penicillin-resistant *Streptococcus pneumoniae*, multidrug-resistant tuberculosis (MDR-TB), or vancomycin-resistant *Enterococcus spp.* which are increasingly refusing to respond to existing medicines, thereby creating a virtual maelstrom in the public health domain. In the meantime, pharmaceutical companies focused more on broad-spectrum agents to widen the potential market resulting in an overall drop in approvals for new antibiotics over the last 30 years [213]. Thus, our arsenal of antibiotics that could effectively deal with bacterial infections is rapidly dwindling in the face of bacteria expressing multidrug resistance. As the demand for new antibiotics increased, several technologically advanced approaches such as genomics and high-throughput screening were launched in the 1990s for creating optimised versions of existing antibiotics, and designing synthetic molecules for activity against microorganisms. Unfortunately, these steps did not produce extraordinary success, leading to the realisation that without the discovery of a reliable lead/target pair, the chances of acquiring novel antibiotics are rather slim.

Again, with the discovery of bacterial efflux pumps, it became apparent that efflux pumps are able to extrude structurally diverse compounds, including antibiotics used in a clinical setting, to render them therapeutically ineffective. Hence, antibiotic resistance can develop rapidly through changes in the expression of efflux pumps, including changes to some antibiotics considered to be drugs of last resort. It is therefore imperative that new antibiotics, resistance-modifying agents and, more specifically, efflux pump inhibitors (EPIs) are characterised. The use of bacterial resistance modifiers such as EPIs could facilitate the re-introduction of therapeutically ineffective antibiotics back into clinical use such as ciprofloxacin, and might even suppress the emergence of MDR strains. The resistance-modifying activities of many new chemical classes of EPIs derived from natural sources warrant further studies to assess their potential as leads for clinical development. Further, as a therapeutic strategy, molecules that target the cell membrane or cell walls are most likely to synergize with conventional antibiotics or antiseptics by weakening the cell envelope and increasing cellular permeability [214]. In fact, microbial natural products are often endowed with ability to enter bacterial cells and interact with relevant target(s).

Hence, in the present scenario, natural product screening would be a fruitful strategy to discover pathogen-specific drug leads for designing novel antibiotics. Therefore, efforts are going on to study naturally occurring drug scaffolds with wide structural diversity, isolated from various geographical locations, with a view to combating antimicrobial resistance jointly with classical antibiotics by deploying multiple modes of action. The rich history of medical traditions has developed under the influence of diverse cultures over millennia. Today, such traditions are still alive in the folk medical practices of indigenous people all over the world. It is essential to take a cue from ethnopharmacology in order to open up the bountiful resource of pathogen-specific drug leads awaiting discovery in the realm of natural biodiversity facing oblivion, before it is too late.

CONSENT FOR PUBLICATION

Not applicable.

CONFLICT OF INTEREST

The authors declare no conflict of interest, financial or otherwise.

ACKNOWLEDGEMENTS

The authors gratefully acknowledge the technical support and helpful suggestion provided by Dr. Anirban Mandal of the Department of Botany, Calcutta University, and Dr. Diganta Dey of M/S Ashok Laboratory Clinical Testing Centre Pvt. Ltd., Kolkata, India.

ABBREVIATIONS

ANS	Autonomic nervous system
AREC	Amoxicillin-resistant *E. coli*
CCCP	Carbonylcyanide m-chlorophenylhydrazone
CDC	Centre for Disease Prevention and Control
CNS	Central nervous system
DNA	Deoxyribonucleic acid
EP	Efflux pump
EPI	Efflux pump inhibitor
ESBL	Extended-spectrum β-lactamase
EtBr	Ethidium bromide
FDA	Food and Drug Administration
FICI	Fractional inhibitory concentration index
HIV	Human immunodeficiency virus
MBL	Metallo-β-lactamase
MDR	Multidrug resistant
MF	Modulation factor
MIC	Minimum inhibitory concentration
MRP	Multidrug resistance-associated protein
MRSA	Methicillin-resistant *Staphylococcus aureus*
NMP	1-(1-Naphthylmethyl)-piperazine
NPN	1-N-phenylnaphthylamine
PAβN	Phe-arg-β-naphthylamide
PBP	Penicillin binding protein
PGME	Pomegranate methanolic extract
QS	Quorum sensing
RIZD	Relative inhibition zone diameter

RMA	Resistance modifying agent
RNA	Ribonucleic acid
RND	Resistance–Nodulation-Division
TB	Tuberculosis
VF	Virulence factor
WHO	World Health Organization
XDR	Extensively drug resistant

REFERENCES

[1]   Arseculeratne SN, Arseculeratne G. A re-appraisal of the conventional history of antibiosis and Penicillin. Mycoses 2017; 60(5): 343-7.
[http://dx.doi.org/10.1111/myc.12599] [PMID: 28144986]

[2]   Piddock LJV, Whale K, Wise R. Quinolone resistance in salmonella: clinical experience. Lancet 1990; 335(8703): 1459.
[http://dx.doi.org/10.1016/0140-6736(90)91484-R] [PMID: 1972228]

[3]   Fleming A. Penicillin. Available from: http://www.nobelprize.org/nobel_prizes/ medicine/laureates/1945/fleming-lecture.pdf [cited 24th January 2017].

[4]   Revenge of the killer microbes: Are we losing the war against infectious diseases. Time Magazine, 12th September, 1994.

[5]   Magiorakos AP, Srinivasan A, Carey RB, *et al.* Multidrug-resistant, extensively drug-resistant and pandrug-resistant bacteria: an international expert proposal for interim standard definitions for acquired resistance. Clin Microbiol Infect 2012; 18(3): 268-81.
[http://dx.doi.org/10.1111/j.1469-0691.2011.03570.x] [PMID: 21793988]

[6]   Antibiotic resistance threats in the United States. CDC 2013. [updated: 10th April 2017]. Available from: www.cdc.gov/drugresistance/threat-report-2013/

[7]   Roger FG, Greenwood D, Norbby SR, Whitley RJ. Antibiotic and chemotherapy: The problem of resistance. 8th Ed. Churchill Livingstone 2003; pp. 25-47.

[8]   Edelsein L. The genuine works of Hippocrates. Bull Hist Med 1945; 7: 236-48.

[9]   Silva LN, Zimmer KR, Macedo AJ, Trentin DS. Plant natural products targeting bacterial virulence factors. Chem Rev 2016; 116(16): 9162-236.
[http://dx.doi.org/10.1021/acs.chemrev.6b00184] [PMID: 27437994]

[10]   Nazzaro F, Fratianni F, De Martino L, Coppola R, De Feo V. Effect of essential oils on pathogenic bacteria. Pharmaceuticals (Basel) 2013; 6(12): 1451-74.
[http://dx.doi.org/10.3390/ph6121451] [PMID: 24287491]

[11]   Kim S, Lee H, Lee S, Yoon Y, Choi KH. Antimicrobial action of oleanolic acid on Listeria mono-cytogenes, Enterococcus faecium, and Enterococcus faecalis. PLoS One 2015; 10(3): e0118800. [11p].
[http://dx.doi.org/10.1371/journal.pone.0118800] [PMID: 25756202]

[12]   Reygaert WC. The antimicrobial possibilities of green tea. Front Microbiol 2014; 5: 434. [8p].
[http://dx.doi.org/10.3389/fmicb.2014.00434] [PMID: 25191312]

[13]   Garmanaa AN, Sukandara EY, Fidriannya I. Activity of several plant extracts against drug-sensitive and drug resistant microbes. Proceedings of the international seminar on natural product medicines. 2012. Procedia Chem 2014; 13: 164-9.

[14]   Ginovyan M, Petrosyan M, Trchounian A. Antimicrobial activity of some plant materials used in Armenian traditional medicine. BMC Complement Altern Med 2017; 17(1): 50. [9p].

[http://dx.doi.org/10.1186/s12906-017-1573-y] [PMID: 28095835]

[15] Newman DJ, Cragg GM. Natural products as sources of new drugs from 1981 to 2014. J Nat Prod 2016; 79(3): 629-61.
[http://dx.doi.org/10.1021/acs.jnatprod.5b01055] [PMID: 26852623]

[16] Nyambuya T, Mautsa R, Mukanganyama S. Alkaloid extracts from *Combretum zeyheri* inhibit the growth of *Mycobacterium smegmatis*. BMC Complement Altern Med 2017; 17(1): 124.
[http://dx.doi.org/10.1186/s12906-017-1636-0] [PMID: 28228097]

[17] Carter DA, Blair SE, Cokcetin NN, *et al.* Therapeutic manuka honey: No longer so alternative. Front Microbiol 2016; 7: 569.
[http://dx.doi.org/10.3389/fmicb.2016.00569] [PMID: 27148246]

[18] Quave CL. Antibiotics from nature: Traditional medicine as a source of new solutions for combating antimicrobial resistance. AMR Control 2016.

[19] Dey D, Ray R, Hazra B. Antimicrobial activity of pomegranate fruit constituents against drug-resistant Mycobacterium tuberculosis and β-lactamase producing Klebsiella pneumoniae. Pharm Biol 2015; 53(10): 1474-80.
[http://dx.doi.org/10.3109/13880209.2014.986687] [PMID: 25858784]

[20] Dey D, Ray R, Hazra B. Antitubercular and antibacterial activity of quinonoid natural products against multi-drug resistant clinical isolates. Phytother Res 2014; 28(7): 1014-21.
[http://dx.doi.org/10.1002/ptr.5090] [PMID: 24318724]

[21] Abreu AC, McBain AJ, Simões M. Plants as sources of new antimicrobials and resistance-modifying agents. Nat Prod Rep 2012; 29(9): 1007-21.
[http://dx.doi.org/10.1039/c2np20035j] [PMID: 22786554]

[22] Garvey MI, Rahman MM, Gibbons S, Piddock LJ. Medicinal plant extracts with efflux inhibitory activity against Gram-negative bacteria. Int J Antimicrob Agents 2011; 37(2): 145-51.
[http://dx.doi.org/10.1016/j.ijantimicag.2010.10.027] [PMID: 21194895]

[23] Aelenei P, Miron A, Trifan A, Bujor A, Gille E, Aprotosoaie AC. Essential oils and their components as modulators of antibiotic activity against Gram-negative bacteria. Medicines (Basel) 2016; 3(3): 19. [34p].
[http://dx.doi.org/10.3390/medicines3030019] [PMID: 28930130]

[24] Fankam AG, Kuiate JR, Kuete V. Antibacterial and antibiotic resistance modifying activity of the extracts from *Allanblackia gabonensis, Combretum molle and Gladiolus quartinianus* against Gram-negative bacteria including multi-drug resistant phenotypes. BMC Complement Altern Med 2015; 15: 206. [12p].
[http://dx.doi.org/10.1186/s12906-015-0726-0] [PMID: 26122102]

[25] Seukep JA, Sandjo LP, Ngadjui BT, Kuete V. Antibacterial and antibiotic-resistance modifying activity of the extracts and compounds from *Nauclea pobeguinii* against Gram-negative multi-drug resistant phenotypes. BMC Complement Altern Med 2016; 16: 193. [8p].
[http://dx.doi.org/10.1186/s12906-016-1173-2] [PMID: 27386848]

[26] Barreto HM, Lima I, Coelho K, *et al.* Effect of Lippia origanoides H.B.K. essential oil in the resistance to aminoglycosides in methicillin resistant *Staphylococcus aureus*. Eur J Integr Med 2014; 6: 560-4.
[http://dx.doi.org/10.1016/j.eujim.2014.03.011]

[27] Madeiro SA, Borges NH, Souto AL, de Figueiredo PT, Siqueira-Junior JP, Tavares JF. Modulation of the antibiotic activity against multidrug resistant strains of coumarins isolated from Rutaceae species. Microb Pathog 2017; 104: 151-4.
[http://dx.doi.org/10.1016/j.micpath.2017.01.028] [PMID: 28109770]

[28] Wink M, Ashour ML, El-Readi MZ. Secondary metabolites from plants inhibiting ABC transporters and reversing resistance of cancer cells and microbes to cytotoxic and antimicrobial agents. Front Microbiol 2012; 3: 130. [12p].

[http://dx.doi.org/10.3389/fmicb.2012.00130] [PMID: 22536197]

[29] Prasch S, Bucar F. Plant derived inhibitors of bacterial effux pumps: an update. Phytochem Rev 2015. [14p].
[http://dx.doi.org/10.1007/s11101-015-9436-y]

[30] Upadhyay A, Upadhyaya I, Kollanoor-Johny A, Venkitanarayanan K. Combating pathogenic microorganisms using plant-derived antimicrobials: a minireview of the mechanistic basis. BioMed Res Int 2014; 2014: 761741. [18 p].
[http://dx.doi.org/10.1155/2014/761741] [PMID: 25298964]

[31] Ohene-Agyei T, Mowla R, Rahman T, Venter H. Phytochemicals increase the antibacterial activity of antibiotics by acting on a drug efflux pump. MicrobiologyOpen 2014; 3(6): 885-96.
[http://dx.doi.org/10.1002/mbo3.212] [PMID: 25224951]

[32] Borges A, Abreu AC, Dias C, Saavedra MJ, Borges F, Simões M. New perspectives on the use of phytochemicals as an emergent strategy to control bacterial infections including bio☐lms. Molecules 2016; 21(7): 877. [41p].
[http://dx.doi.org/10.3390/molecules21070877] [PMID: 27399652]

[33] Harvey AL. Natural products in drug discovery. Drug Discov Today 2008; 13(19-20): 894-901.
[http://dx.doi.org/10.1016/j.drudis.2008.07.004] [PMID: 18691670]

[34] WHO. Antimicrobial Resistance Fact sheet http://www.who.int/mediacentre/factsheets/fs194/en/

[35] Munita JM, Arias CA. Mechanisms of antibiotic resistance. Microbiol Spectr 2016; 4(2)
[PMID: 27227291]

[36] Manson JM, Hancock LE, Gilmore MS. Mechanism of chromosomal transfer of *Enterococcus faecalis* pathogenicity island, capsule, antimicrobial resistance, and other traits. Proc Natl Acad Sci USA 2010; 107(27): 12269-74.
[http://dx.doi.org/10.1073/pnas.1000139107] [PMID: 20566881]

[37] Thomas CM, Nielsen KM. Mechanisms of, and barriers to, horizontal gene transfer between bacteria. Nat Rev Microbiol 2005; 3(9): 711-21.
[http://dx.doi.org/10.1038/nrmicro1234] [PMID: 16138099]

[38] Poole K. Overcoming antimicrobial resistance by targeting resistance mechanisms. J Pharm Pharmacol 2001; 53(3): 283-94.
[http://dx.doi.org/10.1211/0022357011775514] [PMID: 11291743]

[39] Richardson LA. Understanding and overcoming antibiotic resistance. PLoS Biol 2017; 15(8): e2003775. [5p].
[http://dx.doi.org/10.1371/journal.pbio.2003775] [PMID: 28832581]

[40] Kumarasamy KK, Toleman MA, Walsh TR, *et al.* Emergence of a new antibiotic resistance mechanism in India, Pakistan, and the UK: a molecular, biological, and epidemiological study. Lancet Infect Dis 2010; 10(9): 597-602.
[http://dx.doi.org/10.1016/S1473-3099(10)70143-2] [PMID: 20705517]

[41] Gill EE, Franco OL, Hancock RE. Antibiotic adjuvants: diverse strategies for controlling drug-resistant pathogens. Chem Biol Drug Des 2015; 85(1): 56-78.
[http://dx.doi.org/10.1111/cbdd.12478] [PMID: 25393203]

[42] Amyes SGB. Magic bullets, lost horizons: the rise and fall of antibiotics. London: Taylor & Francis 2001.
[http://dx.doi.org/10.4324/9780203303009]

[43] Spellberg B, Miller LG, Kuo MN, Bradley J, Scheld WM, Edwards JE Jr. Societal costs versus savings from wild-card patent extension legislation to spur critically needed antibiotic development. Infection 2007; 35(3): 167-74.
[http://dx.doi.org/10.1007/s15010-007-6269-7] [PMID: 17565458]

[44] Fischbach MA, Walsh CT. Antibiotics for emerging pathogens. Science 2009; 325(5944): 1089-93.
[http://dx.doi.org/10.1126/science.1176667] [PMID: 19713519]

[45] Walsh C. Where will new antibiotics come from? Nat Rev Microbiol 2003; 1(1): 65-70.
[http://dx.doi.org/10.1038/nrmicro727] [PMID: 15040181]

[46] Silver LL. Challenges of antibacterial discovery. Clin Microbiol Rev 2011; 24(1): 71-109.
[http://dx.doi.org/10.1128/CMR.00030-10] [PMID: 21233508]

[47] Boucher HW, Talbot GH, Bradley JS, *et al.* Bad bugs, no drugs: no ESKAPE! An update from the
Infectious Diseases Society of America. Clin Infect Dis 2009; 48(1): 1-12.
[http://dx.doi.org/10.1086/595011] [PMID: 19035777]

[48] https://www.accessdata.fda.gov/drugsatfda_docs/label/2017/208610s000,208611s000lbl.df

[49] Jarvis LM. FDA approvals hit a 20-year high in 2017, with cancer and rare-disease drugs dominating
the list of new medicines. Chem Eng News 2018; 22(January) https://cen.acs.org/
articles/96/web/2018/01/banner-year-new-drugs.html

[50] Wright GD. Antibiotics adjuvants: Rescuing antibiotics from resistance. Trends Microbiol 2016;
24(11): 862-71.
[http://dx.doi.org/10.1016/j.tim.2016.06.009] [PMID: 27430191]

[51] Wax RG, Lewis K, Salyers AA, Taber H. Bacterial resistance to antimicrobials 2nded. Boca Raton,
Florida: CRC Press, Taylor & Francis 2008.

[52] Sanhueza L, Melo R, Montero R, Maisey K, Mendoza L, Wilkens M. Synergistic interactions between
phenolic compounds identified in grape pomace extract with antibiotics of different classes against
Staphylococcus aureus and *Escherichia coli*. PLoS One 2017; 12(2): e0172273. [15p].
[http://dx.doi.org/10.1371/journal.pone.0172273] [PMID: 28235054]

[53] Abreu AC, Serra SC, Borges A, Saavedra MJ, Salgado AJ, Simões M. Evaluation of the best method
to assess antibiotic potentiation by phytochemicals against *Staphylococcus aureus*. Diagn Microbiol
Infect Dis 2014; 79(2): 125-34.
[http://dx.doi.org/10.1016/j.diagmicrobio.2014.03.002] [PMID: 24717959]

[54] Aboulmagd E, Al-Mohammed HI, Al-Badry S. Synergism and post antibiotic effect of green tea
extract and imipenem against methicillin-resistant *Staphylococcus aureus*. Microbiol J 2011; 3: 89-96.

[55] Stavri M, Piddock LJV, Gibbons S. Bacterial efflux pump inhibitors from natural sources. J
Antimicrob Chemother 2007; 59(6): 1247-60.
[http://dx.doi.org/10.1093/jac/dkl460] [PMID: 17145734]

[56] Siriyong T, Srimanote P, Chusri S, *et al.* Conessine as a novel inhibitor of multidrug efflux pump
systems in *Pseudomonas aeruginosa*. BMC Complement Altern Med 2017; 17(1): 405. [7p].
[http://dx.doi.org/10.1186/s12906-017-1913-y] [PMID: 28806947]

[57] Brown AR, Ettefagh KA, Todd D, *et al.* A mass spectrometry-based assay for improved quantitative
measurements of efflux pump inhibition. PLoS One 2015; 10(5): e0124814. [12p].
[http://dx.doi.org/10.1371/journal.pone.0124814] [PMID: 25961825]

[58] Maesaki S, Marichal P, Vanden Bossche H, Sanglard D, Kohno S. Rhodamine 6G efflux for the
detection of CDR1-overexpressing azole-resistant Candida albicans strains. J Antimicrob Chemother
1999; 44(1): 27-31.
[http://dx.doi.org/10.1093/jac/44.1.27] [PMID: 10459807]

[59] Siriyong T, Chusri S, Srimanote P, Tipmanee V, Voravuthikunchai SP. Holarrhena antidysenterica
extract and its steroidal alkaloid, conessine, as resistance-modifying agents against extensively drug-
resistant *Acinetobacter baumannii*. Microb Drug Resist 2016; 22(4): 273-82.
[http://dx.doi.org/10.1089/mdr.2015.0194] [PMID: 26745443]

[60] Kovač J, Šimunović K, Wu Z, *et al.* Antibiotic resistance modulation and modes of action of (-)-
α-pinene in *Campylobacter jejuni*. PLoS One 2015; 10(4): e0122871. [14p].

[http://dx.doi.org/10.1371/journal.pone.0122871] [PMID: 25830640]

[61]   Nüsslein K, Arnt L, Rennie J, Owens C, Tew GN. Broad-spectrum antibacterial activity by a novel abiogenic peptide mimic. Microbiology 2006; 152(Pt 7): 1913-8.
[http://dx.doi.org/10.1099/mic.0.28812-0] [PMID: 16804167]

[62]   Chitemerere TA, Mukanganyama S. Evaluation of cell membrane integrity as a potential antimicrobial target for plant products. BMC Complement Altern Med 2014; 14: 278. [8p].
[http://dx.doi.org/10.1186/1472-6882-14-278] [PMID: 25078023]

[63]   Dey D, Ghosh S, Ray R, Hazra B. Polyphenolic secondary metabolites synergize the activity of commercial antibiotics against clinical isolates of β-lactamase-producing Klebsiella pneumonia. Phytother Res 2016; 30(2): 272-82.
[http://dx.doi.org/10.1002/ptr.5527] [PMID: 26668123]

[64]   Yadav AK, Saraswat S, Sirohi P, *et al.* Antimicrobial action of methanolic seed extracts of Syzygium cumini Linn. on Bacillus subtilis. AMB Express 2017; 7(1): 196. [10p].
[http://dx.doi.org/10.1186/s13568-017-0500-4] [PMID: 29098477]

[65]   Cao X, Meng L, Zhang N, Zhou Z. Microscopic examination of polymeric monoguanidine, hydrochloride-induced cell membrane damage in multidrug-resistant Pseudomonas aeruginosa. Polymers (Basel) 2017; 9(9): 398. [13p].
[http://dx.doi.org/10.3390/polym9090398]

[66]   Amin MU, Khurram M, Khattak B, Khan J. Antibiotic additive and synergistic action of rutin, morin and quercetin against methicillin resistant Staphylococcus aureus. BMC Complement Altern Med 2015; 15: 59. [12p].
[http://dx.doi.org/10.1186/s12906-015-0580-0] [PMID: 25879586]

[67]   Usman Amin M, Khurram M, Khan TA, *et al.* Effects of luteolin and quercetin in combination with some conventional antibiotics against methicillin-resistant Staphylococcus aureus. Int J Mol Sci 2016; 17(11): 1947. [16 p].
[http://dx.doi.org/10.3390/ijms17111947] [PMID: 27879665]

[68]   Tao R, Wang C, Ye J, Zhou H, Chen H. Polyprenols of *Ginkgo biloba* enhance antibacterial activity of five classes of antibiotics. BioMed Res Int 2016; 2016: 4191938. [8p].
[http://dx.doi.org/10.1155/2016/4191938] [PMID: 27642597]

[69]   Monte J, Abreu AC, Borges A, Simões LC, Simões M. Antimicrobial activity of selected phytochemicals against Escherichia coli and Staphylococcus aureus and their biofilms. Pathogens 2014; 3(2): 473-98.
[http://dx.doi.org/10.3390/pathogens3020473] [PMID: 25437810]

[70]   Abreu AC, Coqueiro A, Sultan AR, *et al.* Looking to nature for a new concept in antimicrobial treatments: isoflavonoids from Cytisus striatus as antibiotic adjuvants against MRSA. Sci Rep 2017; 7(1): 3777. [16p].
[http://dx.doi.org/10.1038/s41598-017-03716-7] [PMID: 28630440]

[71]   Mackay ML, Milne K, Gould IM. Comparison of methods for assessing synergic antibiotic interactions. Int J Antimicrob Agents 2000; 15(2): 125-9.
[http://dx.doi.org/10.1016/S0924-8579(00)00149-7] [PMID: 10854808]

[72]   Holler JG, Christensen SB, Slotved HC, *et al.* Novel inhibitory activity of the Staphylococcus aureus NorA efflux pump by a kaempferol rhamnoside isolated from Persea lingue Nees. J Antimicrob Chemother 2012; 67(5): 1138-44.
[http://dx.doi.org/10.1093/jac/dks005] [PMID: 22311936]

[73]   Randhawa HK, Hundal KK, Ahirrao PN, *et al.* Efflux pump inhibitory activity of ⬜avonoids isolated from Alpinia calcarata against methicillin-resistant Staphylococcus aureus. Biologia 2016; 71(5): 484-93.
[http://dx.doi.org/10.1515/biolog-2016-0073]

[74]   Christena LR, Subramaniam S, Vidhyalakshmi M, *et al.* Dual role of pinostrobin-a flavonoid nutraceutical as an efflux pump inhibitor and antibiofilm agent to mitigate food borne pathogens. RCS Adv 2015; 5: 61881. [7p].

[75]   Dey D, Debnath S, Hazra S, Ghosh S, Ray R, Hazra B. Pomegranate pericarp extract enhances the antibacterial activity of ciprofloxacin against extended-spectrum β-lactamase (ESBL) and metallo-- -lactamase (MBL) producing Gram-negative bacilli. Food Chem Toxicol 2012; 50(12): 4302-9. [http://dx.doi.org/10.1016/j.fct.2012.09.001] [PMID: 22982804]

[76]   Dey D. Antibacterial and antitubercular activity of selected plant products against multidrug resistant clinical isolates PhD Dissertation Jadavpur University 2015; page 116

[77]   Tallarida RJ, Porreca F, Cowan A. Statistical analysis of drug-drug and site-site interactions with isobolograms. Life Sci 1989; 45(11): 947-61. [http://dx.doi.org/10.1016/0024-3205(89)90148-3] [PMID: 2677570]

[78]   Lewis K. Multidrug resistance: Versatile drug sensors of bacterial cells. Curr Biol 1999; 9(11): R403-7. [http://dx.doi.org/10.1016/S0960-9822(99)80254-1] [PMID: 10359693]

[79]   Rouch DA, Cram DS, DiBerardino D, Littlejohn TG, Skurray RA. Efflux-mediated antiseptic resistance gene qacA from Staphylococcus aureus: common ancestry with tetracycline- and sugar-transport proteins. Mol Microbiol 1990; 4(12): 2051-62. [http://dx.doi.org/10.1111/j.1365-2958.1990.tb00565.x] [PMID: 2089219]

[80]   Neyfakh AA, Bidnenko VE, Chen LB. Efflux-mediated multidrug resistance in Bacillus subtilis: similarities and dissimilarities with the mammalian system. Proc Natl Acad Sci USA 1991; 88(11): 4781-5. [http://dx.doi.org/10.1073/pnas.88.11.4781] [PMID: 1675788]

[81]   Lomovskaya O, Lewis K. Emr, an *Escherichia coli* locus for multidrug resistance. Proc Natl Acad Sci USA 1992; 89(19): 8938-42. [http://dx.doi.org/10.1073/pnas.89.19.8938] [PMID: 1409590]

[82]   Ahmed M, Borsch CM, Taylor SS, Vázquez-Laslop N, Neyfakh AA. A protein that activates expression of a multidrug efflux transporter upon binding the transporter substrates. J Biol Chem 1994; 269(45): 28506-13. [PMID: 7961792]

[83]   Li XZ, Nikaido H, Poole K. Role of mexA-mexB-oprM in antibiotic efflux in *Pseudomonas aeruginosa*. Antimicrob Agents Chemother 1995; 39(9): 1948-53. [http://dx.doi.org/10.1128/AAC.39.9.1948] [PMID: 8540696]

[84]   Hsieh PC, Siegel SA, Rogers B, Davis D, Lewis K. Bacteria lacking a multidrug pump: a sensitive tool for drug discovery. Proc Natl Acad Sci USA 1998; 95(12): 6602-6. [http://dx.doi.org/10.1073/pnas.95.12.6602] [PMID: 9618458]

[85]   Neyfakh AA, Borsch CM, Kaatz GW. Fluoroquinolone resistance protein NorA of Staphylococcus aureus is a multidrug efflux transporter. Antimicrob Agents Chemother 1993; 37(1): 128-9. [http://dx.doi.org/10.1128/AAC.37.1.128] [PMID: 8431010]

[86]   Stermitz FR, Lorenz P, Tawara JN, Zenewicz LA, Lewis K. Synergy in a medicinal plant: antimicrobial action of berberine potentiated by 5'-methoxyhydnocarpin, a multidrug pump inhibitor. Proc Natl Acad Sci USA 2000; 97(4): 1433-7. [http://dx.doi.org/10.1073/pnas.030540597] [PMID: 10677479]

[87]   Gibbons S, Oluwatuyi M, Kaatz GW. A novel inhibitor of multidrug efflux pumps in Staphylococcus aureus. J Antimicrob Chemother 2003; 51(1): 13-7. [http://dx.doi.org/10.1093/jac/dkg044] [PMID: 12493782]

[88]   Gibbons S. Phytochemicals for bacterial resistance-strengths, weaknesses and opportunities. Planta Med 2008; 74(6): 594-602.

[http://dx.doi.org/10.1055/s-2008-1074518] [PMID: 18446673]

[89] Gibbons S, Udo EE. The effect of reserpine, a modulator of multidrug efflux pumps, on the *in vitro* activity of tetracycline against clinical isolates of methicillin resistant *Staphylococcus aureus* (MRSA) possessing the tet(K) determinant. Phytother Res 2000; 14(2): 139-40.
[http://dx.doi.org/10.1002/(SICI)1099-1573(200003)14:2<139::AID-PTR608>3.0.CO;2-8] [PMID: 10685116]

[90] Michalet S, Cartier G, David B, *et al.* N-caffeoylphenalkylamide derivatives as bacterial efflux pump inhibitors. Bioorg Med Chem Lett 2007; 17(6): 1755-8.
[http://dx.doi.org/10.1016/j.bmcl.2006.12.059] [PMID: 17275293]

[91] Singh S, Kalia NP, Joshi P, *et al.* Boeravinone B, A novel dual inhibitor of NorA bacterial efflux pump of Staphylococcus aureus and human P-glycoprotein, reduces the biofilm formation and intracellular invasion of bacteria. Front Microbiol 2017; 8: 1868.
[http://dx.doi.org/10.3389/fmicb.2017.01868] [PMID: 29046665]

[92] Friedman M. Chemistry and multibeneficial bioactivities of carvacrol (4-isopropyl 2-methylphenol), a component of essential oils produced by aromatic plants and spices. J Agric Food Chem 2014; 62: 7652-70.

[93] Magi G, Marini E, Facinelli B. Antimicrobial activity of essential oils and carvacrol, and synergy of carvacrol and erythromycin, against clinical, erythromycin-resistant Group A Streptococci. Front Microbiol 2015; 6: 165. [7p].
[http://dx.doi.org/10.3389/fmicb.2015.00165] [PMID: 25784902]

[94] Johny A K, Hoagland T, Venkitanarayanan K. Effect of subinhibitory concentrations of plant-derived molecules in increasing the sensitivity of multidrug-resistant Salmonella enterica serovar Typhimurium DT104 to antibiotics. Foodborne Pathog Dis 2010; 7: 1165-70.

[95] Langeveld WT, Veldhuizen EJA, Burt SA. Synergy between essential oil components and antibiotics: a review. Crit Rev Microbiol 2014; 40(1): 76-94.
[http://dx.doi.org/10.3109/1040841X.2013.763219] [PMID: 23445470]

[96] Ribeiro DA, Damasceno SS, Boligon AA, *et al.* Chemical profile and antimicrobial activity of Secondatia floribunda A. DC (Apocynaceae). Asian Pac J Trop Biomed 2017; 7(8): 739-49.
[http://dx.doi.org/10.1016/j.apjtb.2017.07.009]

[97] Ballard E, Coote PJ. Enhancement of antibiotic efficacy against multi-drug resistant Pseudomonas aeruginosa infections via combination with curcumin and 1-(1-naphthylmethyl)-piperazine. J Antimicrob 2016; 2(2): 1000116. [6p].

[98] Negi N, Prakash P, Gupta ML, Mohapatra TM. Possible role of curcumin as an efflux pump inhibitor in multi drug resistant clinical isolates of Pseudomonas aeruginosa. J Clin Diagn Res 2014; 8(10): DC04-7.
[PMID: 25478340]

[99] Rasamiravaka T, Labtani Q, Duez P, El Jaziri M. The formation of biofilms by Pseudomonas aeruginosa: a review of the natural and synthetic compounds interfering with control mechanisms. BioMed Res Int 2015; 2015: 759348. [17p].
[http://dx.doi.org/10.1155/2015/759348] [PMID: 25866808]

[100] Mukanganyama S, Chirisa E, Hazra B. Antimycobacterial activity of diospyrin and its derivatives against Mycobacteium aurum. Res Pharm 2012; 2(1): 1-13.

[101] Knezevic P, Aleksic V, Simin N, Svircev E, Petrovic A, Mimica-Dukic N. Antimicrobial activity of Eucalyptus camaldulensis essential oils and their interactions with conventional antimicrobial agents against multi-drug resistant *Acinetobacter baumannii*. J Ethnopharmacol 2016; 178: 125-36.
[http://dx.doi.org/10.1016/j.jep.2015.12.008] [PMID: 26671210]

[102] Chovanová R, Mikulášová M, Vaverková S. *In vitro* antibacterial and antibiotic resistance modifying effect of bioactive plant extracts on methicillin-resistant Staphylococcus epidermidis. Int J Microbiol

2013; 2013: 760969. [7p].
[http://dx.doi.org/10.1155/2013/760969] [PMID: 24222768]

[103] Horiuchi K, Shiota S, Kuroda T, Hatano T, Yoshida T, Tsuchiya T. Potentiation of antimicrobial activity of aminoglycosides by carnosol from Salvia officinalis. Biol Pharm Bull 2007; 30(2): 287-90.
[http://dx.doi.org/10.1248/bpb.30.287] [PMID: 17268067]

[104] Boonyanugomol W, Kraisriwattana K, Rukseree K, Boonsam K, Narachai P. *In vitro* synergistic antibacterial activity of the essential oil from Zingiber cassumunar Roxb against extensively drug-resistant Acinetobacter baumannii strains. J Infect Public Health 2017; 10(5): 586-92.
[http://dx.doi.org/10.1016/j.jiph.2017.01.008] [PMID: 28162962]

[105] Abreu AC, Serra SC, Borges A, *et al*. Combinatorial activity of flavonoids with antibiotics against drug-resistant Staphylococcus aureus. Microb Drug Resist 2015; 21(6): 600-9.
[http://dx.doi.org/10.1089/mdr.2014.0252] [PMID: 25734256]

[106] Jeong D, Joo SW, Shinde VV, Cho E, Jung S. Carbohydrate-based host-guest complexation of hydrophobic antibiotics for the enhancement of antibacterial activity. Molecules 2017; 22(8): 1311. [15p].
[http://dx.doi.org/10.3390/molecules22081311] [PMID: 28786953]

[107] Wang SY, Sun ZL, Liu T, Gibbons S, Zhang WJ, Qing M. Flavonoids from *Sophora moorcroftiana* and their synergistic antibacterial effects on MRSA. Phytother Res 2014; 28(7): 1071-6.
[http://dx.doi.org/10.1002/ptr.5098] [PMID: 24338874]

[108] Sagdic O, Ozturk I, Kisi O. Modeling antimicrobial effect of different grape pomace and extracts on *S. aureus* and *E. coli* in vegetable soup using artificial neural network and fuzzy logic system. Expert Syst Appl 2012; 39(8): 6792-8.
[http://dx.doi.org/10.1016/j.eswa.2011.12.047]

[109] Chan BC, Han XQ, Lui SL, *et al*. Combating against methicillin-resistant *Staphylococcus aureus* - two fatty acids from Purslane (Portulaca oleracea L.) exhibit synergistic effects with erythromycin. J Pharm Pharmacol 2015; 67(1): 107-16.
[http://dx.doi.org/10.1111/jphp.12315] [PMID: 25212982]

[110] Eumkeb G, Siriwong S, Thumanu K. Synergistic activity of luteolin and amoxicillin combination against amoxicillin-resistant *Escherichia coli* and mode of action. J Photochem Photobiol B 2012; 117: 247-53.
[http://dx.doi.org/10.1016/j.jphotobiol.2012.10.006] [PMID: 23159507]

[111] Siriwong S, Thumanu K, Hengpratom T, Eumkeb G. Synergy and mode of action of ceftazidime plus quercetin or luteolin on Streptococcus pyogenes. Evidence-Based Complem Altern Med 2015; p. 759459. [12p]

[112] Liu H, Mou Y, Zhao J, *et al*. Flavonoids from *Halostachys caspica* and their antimicrobial and antioxidant activities. Molecules 2010; 15(11): 7933-45.
[http://dx.doi.org/10.3390/molecules15117933] [PMID: 21060300]

[113] Maisuria VB, Hosseinidoust Z, Tufenkji N. Polyphenolic extract from maple syrup potentiates antibiotic susceptibility and reduces biofilm formation of pathogenic bacteria. Appl Environ Microbiol 2015; 81(11): 3782-92.
[http://dx.doi.org/10.1128/AEM.00239-15] [PMID: 25819960]

[114] Wang S, Wang C, Gao L, *et al*. Rutin inhibits Streptococcus suis biofilm formation by affecting cps biosynthesis. Front Pharmacol 2017; 8: 379. [12p].
[http://dx.doi.org/10.3389/fphar.2017.00379] [PMID: 28670278]

[115] Chan WK, Tan LT, Chan KG, Lee LH, Goh BH. Nerolidol: A sesquiterpene alcohol with multi-faceted pharmacological and biological activities. Molecules 2016; 21(5): 529. [40p].
[http://dx.doi.org/10.3390/molecules21050529] [PMID: 27136520]

[116] Varela MF, Andersen JL, Ranjana KC, *et al*. Bacterial resistance mechanisms and inhibitors of

multidrug efflux pumps belonging to the major facilitator superfamily of solute transport systems 2017.
[http://dx.doi.org/10.2174/9781681082912117050006]

[117]   Kalia NP, Mahajan P, Mehra R, *et al.* Capsaicin, a novel inhibitor of the NorA efflux pump, reduces the intracellular invasion of Staphylococcus aureus. J Antimicrob Chemother 2012; 67(10): 2401-8.
[http://dx.doi.org/10.1093/jac/dks232] [PMID: 22807321]

[118]   Wang Z, Fan G, Hryc CF, *et al.* An allosteric transport mechanism for the AcrAB-TolC multidrug efflux pump. eLife 2017; 6: e24905. [19p].
[PMID: 28355133]

[119]   Floyd JL, Smith KP, Kumar SH, Floyd JT, Varela MF. LmrS is a multidrug efflux pump of the major facilitator superfamily from *Staphylococcus aureus*. Antimicrob Agents Chemother 2010; 54(12): 5406-12.
[http://dx.doi.org/10.1128/AAC.00580-10] [PMID: 20855745]

[120]   Kumar S, Mukherjee MM, Varela MF. Modulation of bacterial multidrug resistance efflux pumps of the major facilitator superfamily. Int J Bacteriol 2013; 2013(15p): 204141.
[PMID: 25750934]

[121]   Lekshmi M, Ammini P, Adkei J, *et al.* Modulation of antimicrobial efflux pumps of the major facilitator superfamily in *Staphyloccus aureus*. AIMS Microbiol 2018; 4(1): 1-18.
[http://dx.doi.org/10.3934/microbiol.2018.1.1]

[122]   Blanco P, Hernando-Amado S, Reales-Calderon JA, *et al.* Bacterial multidrug efflux pumps: Much more than antibiotic resistance determinants. Microorganisms 2016; 4(1): 14. [19p].
[http://dx.doi.org/10.3390/microorganisms4010014] [PMID: 27681908]

[123]   Sun J, Deng Z, Yan A. Bacterial multidrug efflux pumps: mechanisms, physiology and pharmacological exploitations. Biochem Biophys Res Commun 2014; 453(2): 254-67.
[http://dx.doi.org/10.1016/j.bbrc.2014.05.090] [PMID: 24878531]

[124]   Paulsen IT, Park JH, Choi PS, Saier MH Jr. A family of Gram-negative bacterial outer membrane factors that function in the export of proteins, carbohydrates, drugs and heavy metals from Gram-negative bacteria. FEMS Microbiol Lett 1997; 156(1): 1-8.
[http://dx.doi.org/10.1016/S0378-1097(97)00379-0] [PMID: 9368353]

[125]   Quistgaard EM, Löw C, Guettou F, Nordlund P. Understanding transport by the major facilitator superfamily (MFS): structures pave the way. Nat Rev Mol Cell Biol 2016; 17(2): 123-32. [10p].
[http://dx.doi.org/10.1038/nrm.2015.25] [PMID: 26758938]

[126]   Swick MC, Morgan-Linnell SK, Carlson KM, Zechiedrich L. Expression of multidrug efflux pump genes acrAB-tolC, mdfA, and norE in *Escherichia coli* clinical isolates as a function of fluoroquinolone and multidrug resistance. Antimicrob Agents Chemother 2011; 55(2): 921-4.
[http://dx.doi.org/10.1128/AAC.00996-10] [PMID: 21098250]

[127]   Aly SA, Debavalya N, Suh SJ, Oryazabal OA, Boothe DM. Molecular mechanisms of antimicrobial resistance in fecal Escherichia coli of healthy dogs after enrofloxacin or amoxicillin administration. Can J Microbiol 2012; 58(11): 1288-94.
[http://dx.doi.org/10.1139/w2012-105] [PMID: 23145826]

[128]   Liu M, Heng J, Gao Y, Wang X. Crystal structures of MdfA complexed with acetylcholine and inhibitor reserpine. Biophys Rep 2016; 2(2): 78-85.
[http://dx.doi.org/10.1007/s41048-016-0028-1] [PMID: 28018966]

[129]   Vila J, Sáez-López E, Johnson JR, *et al.* Escherichia coli: an old friend with new tidings. FEMS Microbiol Rev 2016; 40(4): 437-63.
[http://dx.doi.org/10.1093/femsre/fuw005] [PMID: 28201713]

[130]   Hooper DC, Jacoby GA. Mechanisms of drug resistance: quinolone resistance. Ann N Y Acad Sci 2015; 1354: 12-31.

[http://dx.doi.org/10.1111/nyas.12830] [PMID: 26190223]

[131] Rampioni G, Pillai CR, Longo F, *et al.* Effect of efflux pump inhibition on *Pseudomonas aeruginosa* transcriptome and virulence. Sci Rep 2017; 7(1): 11392. [14p].
[http://dx.doi.org/10.1038/s41598-017-11892-9] [PMID: 28900249]

[132] Klančnik A, Možina SS, Zhang Q. Anti-Campylobacter activities and resistance mechanisms of natural phenolic compounds in Campylobacter. PLoS One 2012; 7(12): e51800. [10p].
[http://dx.doi.org/10.1371/journal.pone.0051800] [PMID: 23284770]

[133] Oh E, Jeon B. Contribution of surface polysaccharides to the resistance of *Campylobacter jejuni* to antimicrobial phenolic compounds. J Antibiot (Tokyo) 2015; 68(9): 591-3.
[http://dx.doi.org/10.1038/ja.2015.26] [PMID: 25757605]

[134] Li X-Z, Plésiat P, Nikaido H. The challenge of efflux-mediated antibiotic resistance in Gram-negative bacteria. Clin Microbiol Rev 2015; 28(2): 337-418.
[http://dx.doi.org/10.1128/CMR.00117-14] [PMID: 25788514]

[135] Woronowicz K, Olubanjo OB, Sha D, Kay JM, Niederman RA. Effects of the protonophore carbonyl-cyanide m-chlorophenylhydrazone on intracytoplasmic membrane assembly in Rhodobacter sphaeroides. Biochim Biophys Acta 2015; 1847(10): 1119-28.
[http://dx.doi.org/10.1016/j.bbabio.2015.06.002] [PMID: 26055662]

[136] Tanaka M, Zhang YX, Ishida H, Akasaka T, Sato K, Hayakawa I. Mechanisms of 4-quinolone resistance in quinolone-resistant and methicillin-resistant *Staphylococcus aureus* isolates from Japan and China. J Med Microbiol 1995; 42(3): 214-9.
[http://dx.doi.org/10.1099/00222615-42-3-214] [PMID: 7884804]

[137] Kraatz M, Whitehead TR, Cotta MA, *et al.* Effects of chlorophyll-derived efflux pump inhibitor pheophorbide a and pyropheophorbide a on growth and macrolide antibiotic resistance of indicator and anaerobic swine manure bacteria. Int J Antibiot 2014; p. 185068. [14 p]

[138] Balganesh M, Dinesh N, Sharma S, Kuruppath S, Nair AV, Sharma U. Efflux pumps of *Mycobacterium tuberculosis* play a significant role in antituberculosis activity of potential drug candidates. Antimicrob Agents Chemother 2012; 56(5): 2643-51.
[http://dx.doi.org/10.1128/AAC.06003-11] [PMID: 22314527]

[139] Szumowski JD, Adams KN, Edelstein PH, Ramakrishnan L. Antimicrobial efflux pumps and Mycobacterium tuberculosis drug tolerance: evolutionary considerations. Curr Top Microbiol Immunol 2013; 374: 81-108.
[http://dx.doi.org/10.1007/82_2012_300] [PMID: 23242857]

[140] Pule CM, Sampson SL, Warren RM, *et al.* Efflux pump inhibitors: targeting mycobacterial efflux systems to enhance TB therapy. J Antimicrob Chemother 2016; 71(1): 17-26.
[http://dx.doi.org/10.1093/jac/dkv316] [PMID: 26472768]

[141] Veziris N, Bernard C, Guglielmetti L, *et al.* Rapid emergence of *Mycobacterium tuberculosis* bedaquiline resistance: lessons to avoid repeating past errors. Eur Respir J 2017; 49(3): 1601719.
[http://dx.doi.org/10.1183/13993003.01719-2016] [PMID: 28182568]

[142] Rodrigues L, Ramos J, Couto I, Amaral L, Viveiros M. Ethidium bromide transport across Mycobacterium smegmatis cell-wall: correlation with antibiotic resistance. BMC Microbiol 2011; 11: 35. [10p].
[http://dx.doi.org/10.1186/1471-2180-11-35] [PMID: 21332993]

[143] Li XZ, Zhang L, Nikaido H. Efflux pump-mediated intrinsic drug resistance in Mycobacterium smegmatis. Antimicrob Agents Chemother 2004; 48(7): 2415-23.
[http://dx.doi.org/10.1128/AAC.48.7.2415-2423.2004] [PMID: 15215089]

[144] Roy SK, Pahwa S, Nandanwar H, Jachak SM. Phenylpropanoids of *Alpinia galanga* as efflux pump inhibitors in *Mycobacterium smegmatis* mc^2 155. Fitoterapia 2012; 83(7): 1248-55.
[http://dx.doi.org/10.1016/j.fitote.2012.06.008] [PMID: 22735598]

[145] Gomes RA, Ramirez RRA, Maciel KS, *et al.* Phenolic compounds from Sidastrum micranthum (A. St.-Hil.) fryxell and evaluation of acacetin and 7,4′-di-O-methylisoscutellarein as modulator of bacterial drug resistance. Quim Nova 2011; 34(8): 1385-8.
[http://dx.doi.org/10.1590/S0100-40422011000800016]

[146] Salaheen S, Peng M, Joo J, Teramoto H, Biswas D. Eradication and sensitization of methicillin resistant *Staphylococcus aureus* to methicillin with bioactive extracts of berry pomace. Front Microbiol 2017; 8: 253.
[http://dx.doi.org/10.3389/fmicb.2017.00253] [PMID: 28270804]

[147] Gupta VK, Tiwari N, Gupta P, *et al.* A clerodane diterpene from *Polyalthia longifolia* as a modifying agent of the resistance of methicillin resistant Staphylococcus aureus. Phytomedicine 2016; 23(6): 654-61.
[http://dx.doi.org/10.1016/j.phymed.2016.03.001] [PMID: 27161406]

[148] Chan BC, Ip M, Gong H, *et al.* Synergistic effects of diosmetin with erythromycin against ABC transporter over-expressed methicillin-resistant *Staphylococcus aureus* (MRSA) RN4220/pUL5054 and inhibition of MRSA pyruvate kinase. Phytomedicine 2013; 20(7): 611-4.
[http://dx.doi.org/10.1016/j.phymed.2013.02.007] [PMID: 23541215]

[149] Kuete V, Omosa LK, Tala VR, *et al.* Cytotoxicity of Plumbagin, Rapanone and 12 other naturally occurring Quinones from Kenyan Flora towards human carcinoma cells. BMC Pharmacol Toxicol 2016; 17(1): 60. [10p].
[http://dx.doi.org/10.1186/s40360-016-0104-7] [PMID: 27998305]

[150] Omosa LK, Midiwo JO, Mbaveng AT, *et al.* Antibacterial activities and structure-activity relationships of a panel of 48 compounds from Kenyan plants against multidrug resistant phenotypes. Springerplus 2016; 5(1): 901. [15p].
[http://dx.doi.org/10.1186/s40064-016-2599-1] [PMID: 27386347]

[151] Limaverde PW, Campina FF, da Cunha FAB, *et al.* Inhibition of the TetK efflux-pump by the essential oil of Chenopodium ambrosioides L. and α-terpinene against *Staphylococcus aureus* IS-58. Food Chem Toxicol 2017; 109(Pt 2): 957-61.
[http://dx.doi.org/10.1016/j.fct.2017.02.031] [PMID: 28238773]

[152] Cirino ICS, Menezes-Silva SMP, Silva HT, de Souza EL, Siqueira-Júnior JP. The essential oil from Origanum vulgare L. and its individual constituents carvacrol and thymol enhance the effect of tetracycline against *Staphylococcus aureus*. Chemotherapy 2014; 60(5-6): 290-3.
[http://dx.doi.org/10.1159/000381175] [PMID: 25999020]

[153] Hyldgaard M, Mygind T, Meyer RL. Essential oils in food preservation: mode of action, synergies, and interactions with food matrix components. Front Microbiol 2012; 3: 12. [12p].
[http://dx.doi.org/10.3389/fmicb.2012.00012] [PMID: 22291693]

[154] Zhang J, Sun Y, Wang Y, *et al.* Non-antibiotic agent ginsenoside 20(S)-Rh2 enhanced the antibacterial effects of ciprofloxacin *in vitro* and *in vivo* as a potential NorA inhibitor. Eur J Pharmacol 2014; 740: 277-84.
[http://dx.doi.org/10.1016/j.ejphar.2014.07.020] [PMID: 25054686]

[155] Diniz-Silva HT, Magnani M, de Siqueira S, de Souza EL, de Siqueira-Júnior JP. Fruit flavonoids as modulators of norfloxacin resistance in Staphylococcus aureus that overexpresses norA. Lebensm Wiss Technol 2016; 85B: 324-6.
[http://dx.doi.org/10.1016/j.lwt.2016.04.003]

[156] Fiamegos YC, Kastritis PL, Exarchou V, *et al.* Antimicrobial and efflux pump inhibitory activity of caffeoylquinic acids from Artemisia absinthium against gram-positive pathogenic bacteria. PLoS One 2011; 6(4): e18127. [12p].
[http://dx.doi.org/10.1371/journal.pone.0018127] [PMID: 21483731]

[157] Cabral V, Luo X, Junqueira E, *et al.* Enhancing activity of antibiotics against Staphylococcus aureus: Zanthoxylum capense constituents and derivatives. Phytomedicine 2015; 22(4): 469-76.

[http://dx.doi.org/10.1016/j.phymed.2015.02.003] [PMID: 25925969]

[158] Goncalves de Brito-Filho S, Macial J, Teles YC, *et al.* Phytochemical study of Pilosocereus pachycladus and antibiotic-resistance modifying activity of syringaldehyde. Braz J Pharmacognosy 2017; 27: 453-8.
[http://dx.doi.org/10.1016/j.bjp.2017.06.001]

[159] Diniz-Silva HT, Cirino IC, Falcão-Silva VdosS, Magnani M, de Souza EL, Siqueira-Júnior JP. Tannic acid as a potential modulator of norfloxacin resistance in *Staphylococcus aureus* overexpressing NorA. Chemotherapy 2016; 61(6): 319-22.
[http://dx.doi.org/10.1159/000443495] [PMID: 27144278]

[160] Maia GLA, Falcão-Silva VdosS, Aquino PGV, *et al.* Flavonoids from *Praxelis clematidea* R.M. King and Robinson modulate bacterial drug resistance. Molecules 2011; 16(6): 4828-35.
[http://dx.doi.org/10.3390/molecules16064828] [PMID: 21666549]

[161] Roy SK, Kumari N, Gupta S, Pahwa S, Nandanwar H, Jachak SM. 7-Hydroxy-(E--3-phenylmethylene-chroman-4-one analogues as efflux pump inhibitors against *Mycobacterium smegmatis* mc^2 155. Eur J Med Chem 2013; 66: 499-507.
[http://dx.doi.org/10.1016/j.ejmech.2013.06.024] [PMID: 23832254]

[162] Gröblacher B, Kunert O, Bucar F. Compounds of *Alpinia katsumadai* as potential efflux inhibitors in *Mycobacterium smegmatis*. Bioorg Med Chem 2012; 20(8): 2701-6.
[http://dx.doi.org/10.1016/j.bmc.2012.02.039] [PMID: 22459211]

[163] Gröblacher B, Maier V, Kunert O, Bucar F. Putative mycobacterial efflux inhibitors from the seeds of *Aframomum melegueta*. J Nat Prod 2012; 75(7): 1393-9.
[http://dx.doi.org/10.1021/np300375t] [PMID: 22789014]

[164] Bame JR, Graf TN, Junio HA, *et al.* Sarothrin from Alkanna orientalis is an antimicrobial agent and efflux pump inhibitor. Planta Med 2013; 79(5): 327-9.
[http://dx.doi.org/10.1055/s-0032-1328259] [PMID: 23468310]

[165] Mabhiza D, Chitemerere T, Mukanganyama S. Antibacterial Properties of Alkaloid Extracts from Callistemon citrinus and Vernonia adoensis against *Staphylococcus aureus* and *Pseudomonas aeruginosa*. Int J Med Chem 2016; 2016: 6304163. [7p].
[http://dx.doi.org/10.1155/2016/6304163] [PMID: 26904285]

[166] Aghayan SS, Kalalian Mogadam H, Fazli M, *et al.* The effects of berberine and palmatine on efflux pumps inhibition with different gene patterns in *Pseudomonas aeruginosa* isolated from burn infections. Avicenna J Med Biotechnol 2017; 9(1): 2-7.
[PMID: 28090273]

[167] Bag A, Chattopadhyay RR. Efflux-pump inhibitory activity of a gallotannin from Terminalia chebula fruit against multidrug-resistant uropathogenic *Escherichia coli*. Nat Prod Res 2014; 28(16): 1280-3.
[http://dx.doi.org/10.1080/14786419.2014.895729] [PMID: 24620744]

[168] Ebrahimi A, Eshraghi A, Mahzoonieh MR, Lotfalian S. Antibacterial and antibiotic-potentiation activities of Levisticum officinale L. extracts on pathogenic bacteria. Int J Infect 2017; 4(2): e38768. [4p].

[169] Pourahmad Jaktaji R, Mohammadi P. Effect of total alkaloid extract of local Sophora alopecuroides on minimum inhibitory concentration and intracellular accumulation of ciprofloxacin, and acrA expression in highly resistant *Escherichia coli* clones. J Glob Antimicrob Resist 2018; 12: 55-60.
[http://dx.doi.org/10.1016/j.jgar.2017.09.005] [PMID: 28939469]

[170] Zhou XY, Ye XG, He LT, *et al.* In vitro characterization and inhibition of the interaction between ciprofloxacin and berberine against multidrug-resistant *Klebsiella pneumoniae*. J Antibiot (Tokyo) 2016; 69(10): 741-6.
[http://dx.doi.org/10.1038/ja.2016.15] [PMID: 26932407]

[171] Tankeo SB, Lacmata ST, Noumedem JA, Dzoyem JP, Kuiate JR, Kuete V. Antibacterial and

antibiotic-potentiation activities of some Cameroonian food plants against multi-drug resistant Gram-negative bacteria. Chin J Integr Med 2014; 20(7): 546-54.
[http://dx.doi.org/10.1007/s11655-014-1866-7] [PMID: 24972582]

[172] Dzotam JK, Kuete V. Antibacterial and antibiotic-modifying activity of methanol extracts from six Cameroonian food plants against multidrug-resistant enteric bacteria. BioMed Res Int 2017; 2017: 1583510. [19p].
[http://dx.doi.org/10.1155/2017/1583510] [PMID: 28904944]

[173] Rafiq Z, Narasimhan S, Vennila R, Vaidyanathan R. Punigratane, a novel pyrrolidine alkaloid from *Punica granatum* rind with putative efflux inhibition activity. Nat Prod Res 2016; 30(23): 1-6.
[http://dx.doi.org/10.1080/14786419.2016.1146883] [PMID: 26912266]

[174] Miller SI. Antibiotic resistance and regulation of the Gram-negative bacterial outer membrane barrier by host innate immune molecules. mbio 2016 ; 7(5)e01541-16 [3p].

[175] Krishnamoorthy G, Leus IV, Weeks JW, Wolloscheck D, Rybenkov VV, Zgurskaya HI. Synergy between active efflux and outer membrane diffusion defines rules of antibiotic permeation into gram-negative bacteria. MBio 2017; 8(5): e01172-17. [16p].
[http://dx.doi.org/10.1128/mBio.01172-17] [PMID: 29089426]

[176] Chaves TP, Fernandes FHA, Santana CP, *et al.* Evaluation of the interaction between the Poincianella pyramidalis (Tul.) LP Queiroz extract and antimicrobials using biological and analytical models. PLoS One 2016; 11(5): e0155532. [23p].
[http://dx.doi.org/10.1371/journal.pone.0155532] [PMID: 27192209]

[177] Menezes IR, Santana TI, Varela VJ, *et al.* Chemical composition and evaluation of acute toxicological, antimicrobial and modulatory resistance of the extract of *Murraya paniculata*. Pharm Biol 2015; 53(2): 185-91.
[http://dx.doi.org/10.3109/13880209.2014.913068] [PMID: 25255929]

[178] Llarrull LI, Fisher JF, Mobashery S. Molecular basis and phenotype of methicillin resistance in *Staphylococcus aureus* and insights into new beta-lactams that meet the challenge. Antimicrob Agents Chemother 2009; 53(10): 4051-63.
[http://dx.doi.org/10.1128/AAC.00084-09] [PMID: 19470504]

[179] Lim D, Strynadka NC. Structural basis for the beta lactam resistance of PBP2a from methicillin-resistant *Staphylococcus aureus*. Nat Struct Biol 2002; 9(11): 870-6.
[PMID: 12389036]

[180] Fishovitz J, Hermoso JA, Chang M, Mobashery S. Penicillin-binding protein 2a of methicillin-resistant Staphylococcus aureus. IUBMB Life 2014; 66(8): 572-7.
[http://dx.doi.org/10.1002/iub.1289] [PMID: 25044998]

[181] Peacock SJ, Paterson GK. Mechanisms of methicillin resistance in Staphylococcus aureus. Annu Rev Biochem 2015; 84: 577-601.
[http://dx.doi.org/10.1146/annurev-biochem-060614-034516] [PMID: 26034890]

[182] Lee JW, Ji YJ, Lee SO, Lee IS. Effect of Saliva miltiorrhiza bunge on antimicrobial activity and resistant gene regulation against methicillin-resistant Staphylococcus aureus (MRSA). J Microbiol 2007; 45(4): 350-7.
[PMID: 17846590]

[183] Santiago C, Lim KH, Loh HS, Ting KN. Prevention of cell-surface attachment and reduction of penicillin-binding protein 2a (PBP2a) level in methicillin-resistant *Staphylococcus aureus* biofilms by Acalypha wilkesiana. BMC Complement Altern Med 2015; 15: 79. [7p].
[http://dx.doi.org/10.1186/s12906-015-0615-6] [PMID: 25880167]

[184] Santiago C, Pang EL, Lim KH, Loh HS, Ting KN. Inhibition of penicillin-binding protein 2a (PBP2a) in methicillin resistant *Staphylococcus aureus* (MRSA) by combination of ampicillin and a bioactive fraction from *Duabanga grandiflora*. BMC Complement Altern Med 2015; 15: 178. [7p].
[http://dx.doi.org/10.1186/s12906-015-0699-z] [PMID: 26060128]

[185] Catteau L, Olson J, Bambeke F, *et al.* Ursolic acid from shea butter tree (*Vitellaria paradoxa*) leaf extract synergizes with β-lactams against methicillin-resistant *Staphylococcus aureus* [Abstract]. FASEB J; 31(1 Suppl 1000.5).

[186] Bessa LJ, Palmeira A, Gomes AS, *et al.* Synergistic effects between thioxanthones and oxacillin against methicillin-resistant *Staphylococcus aureus*. Microb Drug Resist 2015; 21(4): 404-15. [http://dx.doi.org/10.1089/mdr.2014.0162] [PMID: 25789724]

[187] Jiménez-Arellanes A, Luna-Herrera J, Cornejo-Garrido J, *et al.* Ursolic and oleanolic acids as antimicrobial and immunomodulatory compounds for tuberculosis treatment. BMC Complement Altern Med 2013; 13: 258. [11p]. [http://dx.doi.org/10.1186/1472-6882-13-258] [PMID: 24098949]

[188] van Duijkeren E, Schink AK, Roberts MC, Wang Y, Schwarz S. Mechanisms of bacterial resistance to antimicrobial agents. Microbiol Spectr 2018; 6(1) [http://dx.doi.org/10.1128/microbiolspec.ARBA-0019-2017] [PMID: 29327680]

[189] Ruppé É, Woerther PL, Barbier F. Mechanisms of antimicrobial resistance in Gram-negative bacilli. Ann Intensive Care 2015; 5(1): 61. [15p]. [http://dx.doi.org/10.1186/s13613-015-0061-0] [PMID: 26261001]

[190] Andersen JL, He GX, Kakarla P, *et al.* Multidrug efflux pumps from Enterobacteriaceae, *Vibrio cholerae* and *Staphylococcus aureus* bacterial food pathogens. Int J Environ Res Public Health 2015; 12(2): 1487-547. [http://dx.doi.org/10.3390/ijerph120201487] [PMID: 25635914]

[191] Wang CM, Chen HT, Wu ZY, Jhan YL, Shyu CL, Chou CH. Antibacterial and synergistic activity of pentacyclic triterpenoids isolated from *Alstonia scholaris*. Molecules 2016; 21(2): 139. [11p]. [http://dx.doi.org/10.3390/molecules21020139] [PMID: 26821000]

[192] Wilson TJ, Blackledge MS, Vigueira PA. Resensitization of methicillin-resistant *Staphylococcus aureus* by amoxapine, an FDA-approved antidepressant. Heliyon 2018; 4(1): e00501. [http://dx.doi.org/10.1016/j.heliyon.2017.e00501] [PMID: 29349359]

[193] Quave CL, Estévez-Carmona M, Compadre CM, *et al.* Ellagic acid derivatives from Rubus ulmifolius inhibit *Staphylococcus aureus* biofilm formation and improve response to antibiotics. PLoS One 2012; 7(1): e28737. [16p]. [http://dx.doi.org/10.1371/journal.pone.0028737] [PMID: 22242149]

[194] Green AE, Rowlands RS, Cooper RA, Maddocks SE. The effect of the flavonol morin on adhesion and aggregation of *Streptococcus pyogenes*. FEMS Microbiol Lett 2012; 333(1): 54-8. [http://dx.doi.org/10.1111/j.1574-6968.2012.02598.x] [PMID: 22591139]

[195] Sharma G, Raturi K, Dang S, Gupta S, Gabrani R. Combinatorial antimicrobial effect of curcumin with selected phytochemicals on *Staphylococcus epidermidis*. J Asian Nat Prod Res 2014; 16(5): 535-41. [Abstract]. [http://dx.doi.org/10.1080/10286020.2014.911289] [PMID: 24773066]

[196] Rathinam P, Vijay Kumar HS, Pragasam Viswanathan P. Eugenol exhibits anti-virulence properties by competitively binding to quorum sensing receptors. Biofouling The Journal of Bioadhesion and Biofilm Research 2017; 33 (8).

[197] Kim HS, Lee SH, Byun Y, Park HD. 6-Gingerol reduces *Pseudomonas aeruginosa* biofilm formation and virulence *via* quorum sensing inhibition. Sci Rep 2015; 5: 8656. [11p]. [http://dx.doi.org/10.1038/srep08656] [PMID: 25728862]

[198] Hobby GH, Quave CL, Nelson K, Compadre CM, Beenken KE, Smeltzer MS. *Quercus cerris* extracts limit *Staphylococcus aureus* biofilm formation. J Ethnopharmacol 2012; 144(3): 812-5. [http://dx.doi.org/10.1016/j.jep.2012.10.042] [PMID: 23127649]

[199] Das MC, Sandhu P, Gupta P, *et al.* Attenuation of *Pseudomonas aeruginosa* biofilm formation by Vitexin: A combinatorial study with azithromycin and gentamicin. Sci Rep 2016; 6: 23347. [13p].

[http://dx.doi.org/10.1038/srep23347] [PMID: 27000525]

[200]   Kumar L, Chhibber S, Harjai K. Zingerone inhibit biofilm formation and improve antibiofilm efficacy of ciprofloxacin against *Pseudomonas aeruginosa* PAO1. Fitoterapia 2013; 90: 73-8.
[http://dx.doi.org/10.1016/j.fitote.2013.06.017] [PMID: 23831483]

[201]   Kumar L, Chhibber S, Harjai K. Structural alterations in *Pseudomonas aeruginosa* by zingerone contribute to enhanced susceptibility to antibiotics, serum and phagocytes. Life Sci 2014; 117(1): 24-32.
[http://dx.doi.org/10.1016/j.lfs.2014.09.017] [PMID: 25277943]

[202]   Santajit S, Indrawattana N. Mechanisms of antimicrobial resistance in ESKAPE pathogens. BioMed Res Int 2016; vol. Article ID 2016; 2475067(8p)
[http://dx.doi.org/10.1155/2016/2475067]

[203]   Chandra H, Bishnoi P, Yadav A, *et al.* Antimicrobial resistance and the alternative resources with special emphasis on plant-based antimicrobials—A review. Plants 2017; 6:16 [11p].

[204]   Tsai CJY, Loh JMS, Proft T. Galleria mellonella infection models for the study of bacterial diseases and for antimicrobial drug testing. Virulence 2016; 7(3): 214-29.
[http://dx.doi.org/10.1080/21505594.2015.1135289] [PMID: 26730990]

[205]   Mooyottu S, Flock G, Upadhyay A, Upadhyaya I, Maas K, Venkitanarayanan K. Protective effect of carvacrol against gut dysbiosis and Clostridium difficile associated disease in a mouse model. Front Microbiol 2017; 8: 625. [10p].
[http://dx.doi.org/10.3389/fmicb.2017.00625] [PMID: 28484429]

[206]   Quave CL, Lyles JT, Kavanaugh JS, *et al. Castanea sativa* (European Chestnut) leaf extracts rich in ursene and oleanene derivatives block *Staphylococcus aureus* virulence and pathogenesis without detectable resistance. PLoS One 2015; 10(8): e0136486. [32p].
[http://dx.doi.org/10.1371/journal.pone.0136486] [PMID: 26295163]

[207]   Cech NB, Junio HA, Ackermann LW, Kavanaugh JS, Horswill AR. Quorum quenching and antimicrobial activity of goldenseal (*Hydrastis canadensis*) against methicillin-resistant *Staphylococcus aureus* (MRSA). Planta Med 2012; 78(14): 1556-61.
[http://dx.doi.org/10.1055/s-0032-1315042] [PMID: 22814821]

[208]   Qi Z, Kelley E. The WHO traditional medicine strategy 2014–2023. Perspect Sci 2014; 346(6216) (Suppl.): S5-6.

[209]   Schmidt BM, Ribnicky DM, Lipsky PE, Raskin I. Revisiting the ancient concept of botanical therapeutics. Nat Chem Biol 2007; 3(7): 360-6.
[http://dx.doi.org/10.1038/nchembio0707-360] [PMID: 17576417]

[210]   Nichols D, Cahoon N, Trakhtenberg EM, *et al.* Use of ichip for high-throughput in situ cultivation of "uncultivable" microbial species. Appl Environ Microbiol 2010; 76(8): 2445-50.
[http://dx.doi.org/10.1128/AEM.01754-09] [PMID: 20173072]

[211]   Arias CA, Murray BE. A new antibiotic and the evolution of resistance. N Engl J Med 2015; 372(12): 1168-70.
[http://dx.doi.org/10.1056/NEJMcibr1500292] [PMID: 25785976]

[212]   Hunter P. Antibiotic discovery goes underground: The discovery of teixobactin could revitalise the search for new antibiotics based on the novel method the researchers used to identify the compound. EMBO Rep 2015; 16(5): 563-5.
[http://dx.doi.org/10.15252/embr.201540385] [PMID: 25832105]

[213]   Cooper MA, Shlaes D. Fix the antibiotics pipeline. Nature 2011; 472(7341): 32.
[http://dx.doi.org/10.1038/472032a] [PMID: 21475175]

[214]   Hu Y, Coates AR. Enhancement by novel anti-methicillin-resistant *Staphylococcus aureus* compound HT61 of the activity of neomycin, gentamicin, mupirocin and chlorhexidine: in vitro and in vivo studies. J Antimicrob Chemother 2013; 68(2): 374-84.
[http://dx.doi.org/10.1093/jac/dks384] [PMID: 23042813]

CHAPTER 4

Molecular Modelling Approaches to Antibacterial Drug Design and Discovery

Agnieszka A. Kaczor[1,2,*], **Prasanthi Medarametla**[2], **Damian Bartuzi**[1], **Magdalena Kondej**[1], **Dariusz Matosiuk**[1] and **Antti Poso**[2]

[1] *Department of Synthesis and Chemical Technology of Pharmaceutical Substances with Computer Modelling Lab, Faculty of Pharmacy with Division for Medical Analytics, 4A Chodzki St., PL-20059 Lublin, Poland*

[2] *School of Pharmacy, University of Eastern Finland, Yliopistonranta 1, P.O. Box 1627, FI-70211 Kuopio, Finland*

Abstract: Projects on design and discovery of antibacterial compounds are at present one of the main research lines in academia and to the lesser extent in pharmaceutical industry. Application of computer-aided drug design (CADD) techniques to drug discovery approaches may lead to a reduction of up to 50% in the cost of drug design. Effective drug design is facilitated when the 3D structure of a drug target is known from experimental or molecular modeling studies (*e.g.* from homology modelling). Nowadays, diverse techniques of molecular docking and molecular dynamics (MD) constitute important computational tools to study drug-protein interactions at the molecular level. Ligand-based and receptor-based methods of virtual screening are becoming more and more powerful for identification of potential hits. It should be stressed, however, that the main issue with target-based automated HTS approaches as well as virtual screening methods is the fact that identified substances although active on the target, are frequently ineffective in the host. In this chapter we present successes and challenges of molecular modelling techniques as applied to antibacterial drugs. The covered techniques are: homology modeling, molecular docking (including virtual screening), molecular dynamics, quantitative structure-activity relationship (QSAR), pharmacophore models. In spite of the successes, there are specific problems and challenges connected with application of CADD to antibacterial drug discovery. CADD techniques enable to design the compound active on a given target, often without considerations if a molecule is able to reach the target. It is thus needed to develop rules for effective bacterial penetration to be used for filtering compound libraries instead of Lipinski's filters. Next, CADD methods are capable to address only partially the problem of antibiotic resistance. However, progress in *in silico* pharmacology and toxicology allows to design safer molecules which is important for antibacterial drugs used in relatively high concentrations.

---

* **Corresponding authors Agnieszka A. Kaczor:** Department of Synthesis and Chemical Technology of Pharmaceutical Substances with Computer Modelling Lab, Faculty of Pharmacy with Division for Medical Analytics, 4A Chodzki St., PL-20059 Lublin, Poland; Tel: +48814487272; Fax: +48814487272; E-mail: agnieszka.kaczor@umlub.pl

In summary, the importance of CADD techniques in academia and industry for discovery of novel antibacterial compounds cannot be overestimated. Although experimental verification of computational results is still required, these methods limit significantly the number of necessary experiments.

Keywords: Antibacterial drugs, Homology modelling, Molecular docking, Molecular dynamics, Pharmacophore models, QSAR, Virtual screening.

INTRODUCTION

The availability of antibiotics in clinical practice revolutionized the therapy of infectious illnesses. Without antibacterial drugs, infectious diseases would be the top reason of morbidity and mortality in human populations [1]. The World Health Organization (WHO) reports that infectious and parasitic illnesses are nowadays a reason of about 16% of all deaths worldwide and over 40% of deaths in Africa. The majority of antibiotics currently used were discovered in the 'golden age' of the antibiotic development which lasted from 1930's to 1960's [2]. However, the over-prescription and misuse of antibacterial drugs [3] led to the development of resistant strains of many microorganisms [4]. The spread of resistant microbes results in a human health crisis and we are witnessing the emergence of pathogens resistant to all available antibiotics [5]. Drug-resistant bacterial infections more often lead to hospitalizations, treatment failures and the persistence of drug-resistant pathogens [6]. In particular, organisms such as methicillin-resistant *Staphylococcus aureus*, *Clostridium difficile*, multi-drug-resistant *Mycobacterium tuberculosis*, *Neisseria gonorrhoeae*, carbapenem-resistant *Enterobacteriaceae* and bacteria that produce extended spectrum β-lactamases, such as *Escherichia coli* are the major concern [6]. Design and discovery of antibacterial drugs are thus still one of the main challenges in current pharmaceutical industry. Unfortunately, most pharmaceutical companies have stopped or have significantly limited investments to antibiotic discovery programs, as the return on investment has been mostly negative for recently launched antibiotics [7]. Nowadays only a few small companies continue their projects on antibacterial drugs. At present, 43 small molecules are in the antibiotic development pipeline from late preclinical stage (7 compounds) through Phase 1 (11 molecules), Phase 2 (13 molecules) to Phase 3 (12 molecules) [8]. Most of these molecules belong to known antibiotic classes which have been modified to address the problems of resistance [8].

It is clear that new antibacterial drugs belonging to structurally new classes with possibly new mechanisms of action are urgently needed. Progress in genomic, transcriptomic and proteomic technologies as well as in bioinformatics [9] and synthetic biology [10, 11] enables better characterization of bacteria, including bacterial processes such as bacterial survival, persistence in the host and infection [12]. It can thus help to identify bacterial components as potential targets for the discovery of new antibacterial drugs. Molecular modelling techniques are of high importance for this purpose because application of computer-aided drug design (CADD) techniques to drug discovery approaches may lead to a reduction of up to 50% in the cost of drug design [13], although this estimation might be a bit too optimistic (authors honest opinion). CADD methods can be divided into two classes, namely structure-based (SB) and ligand-based (LB) drug discovery [14]. In general, computational techniques have been developed and commonly used for pharmacology hypothesis development and testing in drug discovery projects [15].

Application of structure-based techniques to drug design and discovery requires the availability of protein 3D structure. If such a structure is not known from experimental studies, homology modelling should be utilized, if possible. Homology models may be used for molecular docking to study ligand-protein interactions at the molecular level and for subsequent molecular dynamics of ligand-protein complexes. Molecular dynamics is currently widely used to study the dynamic nature of proteins, the effect of solvents and ions as well as such phenomena as ligand selectivity, ligand binding reversibility (in particular QM/MM techniques) and allosterism. High-throughput docking is also a commonly applied method of virtual screening, an approach that enables to search large databases of compounds and to limit the number of chemical compounds subjected to experimental (usually *in vitro*) tests. Moreover, ligand-based or fragment-based virtual screening techniques are also in use. Finally, quantitative structure-activity relationship (QSAR) studies and ligand or structure-based pharmacophore models can be a helpful guide for lead compound optimization.

In this chapter, we discuss challenges in the design and discovery of antibacterial drugs, review shortly the currently important antibacterial drug targets and focus on molecular modeling techniques (homology modelling, molecular docking, molecular dynamics, QSAR, pharmacophore models, virtual screening), their basis and case studies of their application for antibacterial drug design.

CHALLENGES IN DESIGN AND DISCOVERY OF ANTIBACTERIAL DRUGS

The discovery of new small-molecule antibiotics has been stalled for many years [16]. An ideal, non-existing antibiotic kills or inhibits the growth of all harmful bacteria in a host without affecting beneficial gut microbes or causing undue toxicity to the host [17]. Instead, antibacterial agents against Gram-negative or Gram-positive bacteria but not against the holistic bacteria spectrum are available.

The main challenge in the discovery of new (and ideal) antibiotics is related to drug resistance [18]. However, other difficulties and challenges can be attributed to (i) human factors (irresponsible applications of antibiotics and underestimating of microbes), (ii) scientific failure and (iii) unfavourable legal and economic factors such as increased costs, licensing, as well as strict regulations [2, 19].

Antibiotic resistance is based on the microorganisms response to antibiotics *via* bacterial adaptation and evolution [20]. Antibiotic resistance is thus an adaptive trait acquired after challenge with therapeutic antibiotics [21]. As a consequence of genetic plasticity "survival of the fittest" occurs [20] due to mutational adaptations, acquisition of genetic material and/or alteration of gene expression. The molecular mechanisms of antibiotics resistance involve decreased drug permeability, active efflux, alteration or bypass of the drug target, production of antibiotic-modifying enzymes, and physiological states such as biofilms that are less susceptible to antibiotic activity [22]. In order to inhibit bacterial growth, antibacterial drugs have to cross the cell envelopes, which may require activation and reaching the target at a concentration high enough to exert an effect [21]. These steps are connected with the classic resistance mechanisms. Based on the biochemical classification, the resistance mechanisms can be divided into mechanisms which modify the antibiotic target or antibiotic concentration itself [21]. Target modification may be caused by target mutation (*e.g.* quinolone resistance by mutations in pathogen topoisomerases), target replacement (beta-lactam resistance due to the acquisition of chimeric penicillin-binding proteins, PBPs), target enzymatic modification (*e.g.* resistance to vancomycin through the re-organization of the cell wall), or target protection (*e.g.* protection of bacterial topoisomerases from the inhibitory activity of quinolones by the QnrA protein) [21]. Lowering of antibiotic concentrations occurs by impeding the entry of the antibiotic or by extruding the antibiotic through efflux pumps [21]. Recently some other resistance mechanisms revealed by the search for elements that contribute towards the characteristic phenotype of susceptibility to antibiotics in a given species (the intrinsic resistome) have been described. Moreover, the community level resistance resulting from biofilms is different from cellular level resistance mechanisms and creates new challenges to combat bacterial infections. Thus, inhibitors of bacterial biofilm formation are a promising strategy to combat antibiotic resistance. Due to the significance of the efflux-related multi-drug resistance, novel compounds which inhibit bacterial efflux pumps are also potentially able to kill bacteria having over-expressed multi-drug resistance efflux systems [23]. Another important strategy is to use antibiotic adjuvants, *i.e.* non-antibiotic molecules that increase the activity of an antibiotic [22]. Antibiotic resistance is accelerated by the misuse and overuse of antibiotics (*e.g.* inappropriate prescribing [24]), as well as poor infection prevention and control. It is also accompanied by uncontrolled and excessive use of antibiotics in agriculture [24], contributing to the fast spread of antibiotic resistance [2].

The problem of antibiotic resistance is differentiated for Gram-positive and Gram-negative bacteria [25] as they show different antibiotic susceptibility patterns. Gram positive bacteria have no outer (LPS) membrane but possess a thick layer of peptidoglycan. This makes them sensitive to cell-wall active antibiotics (*e.g.* penicillin/beta-lactam or vancomycin-type antibiotics). These organisms are able to escape antibiotic activity through several mechanisms including β-lactamase production, altered penicillin-binding proteins, aminoglycoside-modifying enzymes, modification of the target site of the antibiotic, and active efflux [26]. Development of multiple resistances to antibiotics in Gram-positive pathogens (*e.g.* staphylococci, enterococci and pneumococci) became a health threat during the past 30 years [27]. This resistance is based on acquisition of resistance genes by predominant epidemic subpopulations (clonal complexes) [27], *e.g.* emergence and spread of methicillin-resistant *Staphylococcus aureus*. In order to kill Gram-negative bacteria, the antibiotics need to traverse the LPS layer *via* porin proteins. Depending on antibiotic molecule shape and other properties (*e.g.* charge), some antibiotics, like benzylpenicillin cannot cross whereas ampicillin can, leading to intrinsic antibiotic resistance to the former drug. Porins may be subjected to mutations changing the resistance character of the pathogen. Moreover, efflux proteins may also be present in Gram negative cell walls which is important for antibiotics that act intracellularly (by lowering the intracellular antibiotic concentration to a level where the antibiotic becomes inactive). In addition to efflux pumps and porin mutations mechanisms of antibiotic resistance in Gram-negative bacteria include production of β-lactamases, target site mutations, over production of enzymes and drug modification [28].

Recent advances in antibacterial drug design and discovery, including structure-based drug design (SBDD), the genomic approach, anti-virulence strategy, targeting non-multiplying bacteria and the use of bacteriophages can be useful in overcoming antibiotic resistance [29]. In particular, SBDD include the successful design of new compounds that target resistant mutant proteins, as well as the development of drugs that target multiple proteins involved in specific biochemical pathways [30]. With the emergence of genomic information, a number of antibacterial targets have been pursued over the last 25 years often using SBDD [31]. Moreover, drug resistance can also be considered in the early stages of drug discovery, through the use of strategies to delay the development of resistance [30].

One of the main scientific problems regarding discovery of new antibacterial drugs is a proper target selection [16]. In this regard, the most convenient antibacterial targets are characterized by their low propensity for rapid resistance selection [16]. There are, however, other important issues that should be considered: (i) crucial function of a target in bacteria so that its inhibition or blockade leads to inhibition of bacterial growth or death; (ii) conservation of target structure among bacterial species; (iii) considerable structural differences in comparison to possible homologous human targets to avoid toxicity; and (iv) "druggability" of the chosen target [16]. In the light of these facts multi-target drugs could overcome at least a part of these difficulties [16].

The success of antibacterial screening depends on the quality of the chemicals assayed [16]. In the 'golden era' of antibiotics discovery the search for antibacterial drugs among natural products was very successful [16]. Chemical libraries, however, are less useful for antibacterial screening. Both HTS methods and computer-assisted drug discovery methods are often connected with too high expectations. Both methods are capable to identify active hits on the target but frequently ineffective in the host. This can be mainly attributed to permeability and efflux, which frequently prevent them from crossing cell wall of bacteria [2, 23]. Next, the hit-to-lead ratios (0.001%), both with synthetic and natural products libraries are equal [2, 23].

A specific scientific problem is connected with Gram-negative bacteria, which are particularly efficient in keeping out drugs [2, 32] as their outer membrane constitutes a barrier for amphipathic molecules. All antibiotics have to be amphipathic as they need to be water-soluble on one hand and possess ability to cross the cytoplasmic membrane on the other hand. The multidrug-resistant pumps eject all drugs leaking in through the outer membrane [2]. They mainly recognize molecules on the basis of polarity and the more favourable ones are amphipathic molecules [32]. Hydrophilic compounds penetration of the inner membrane is limited, assisting the outer membrane in being a perfect barrier.

The number of molecules that are able to break into the bacterial cell is limited, and this can be partially attributed to the tailoring of compound libraries using Lipinski's rules filters in order to increase the probability of oral bioavailability after administration [2, 32]. It is however rather unlikely that random libraries without any filters applied can perform better [2]. Probably, there are still parts of chemical space with more matching properties for antibacterial drug discovery if scientists manage to elaborate rules for effective bacterial penetration [2, 32]. Due to poor penetration, antibacterial drugs are effective at micromolar concentrations which is two to three times greater than for drugs applied for eukaryotic targets. Indeed, this high antibiotic concentration significantly increases toxicity, and decrease the possibility of finding of good lead compounds [32].

The above limitations are accompanied by legal and economic problems [32]. Clinical trials for novel antibiotics can last only a couple of days during the infection. It is difficult to indicate a clear-cut end points of a new molecules during clinical trials as most of treated patients are infected by drug-susceptible bacteria [2]. Moreover, because of ethical aspects, administration of placebos is avoided in patients [32]. Treatment of bacterial infection is short time and takes usually no longer than a week. Furthermore, the problem of antibiotic resistance limits the usefulness of a drug on the market. In contrast, patients suffering from chronic diseases require even a life-lasting treatment. This can be visualised by the comparison of annual sales of the top cholesterol-lowering drug atorvastatin - $12 billion during the duration of patent protection and only $2.5 billion for bringing the highest profit antibiotic - levofloxacin [32]. It should be emphasized, however, that an antibiotic market is still large enough to be attractive for the discovery of new antibiotics [2].

DRUG TARGETS FOR ANTIBIOTICS

Only a small fraction from about two hundred bacteria conserved essential proteins, is currently considered a possible drug target [2]. Antibiotics target key elements of microbial metabolism (Fig. **1**). β-lactams, in particular cephalosporins or penicillin, stop synthesis of bacterial cell wall. Antibiotics also target DNA gyrase (quinolones), DNA-directed RNA polymerase (rifampicin), protein synthesis (chloramphenicol, macrolides, aminoglycosides, clindamycin, oxazolidinones and tetracyclines) and enzymes (trimethoprim and sulphonamides) [33]. The most potent antibacterial drugs hit only three pathways or targets: cell wall synthesis, the ribosome, as well as DNA topoisomerase and gyrase [32]. The currently important drug targets for antibacterial drug discovery have been recently reviewed [2] and involve, among others, MurA-MurF enzymes targeted by inhibitors of cell wall biosynthesis, peptide deformylase (PDF), DNA gyrase and type IV topoisomerase (TPIV), fatty acid biosynthesis (FAB), FtsZ and ribosomes. Below a short description of antibacterial drug targets is provided. The detailed discussion, in particular description of structural aspects of these targets is available in our earlier review [2].

The cell wall is key for bacterial survival, and proteins that participate in its biosynthesis are important antibiotic targets [34]. The main constituent of the cell envelope of most bacteria is peptidoglycan [35], of which synthesis is one of the most important biogenesis pathways in bacteria and most of the steps of peptidoglycan synthesis have been studied as potential drug targets [36]. In this regard, a number of inhibitors of Mur enzymes, MurA-F (in particular for the amide ligases MurC, MurD, MurE and MurF [37]), which are engaged in the bio-synthesis of UDP-N-acetylmuramyl-pentapeptide [38] have been developed [2].

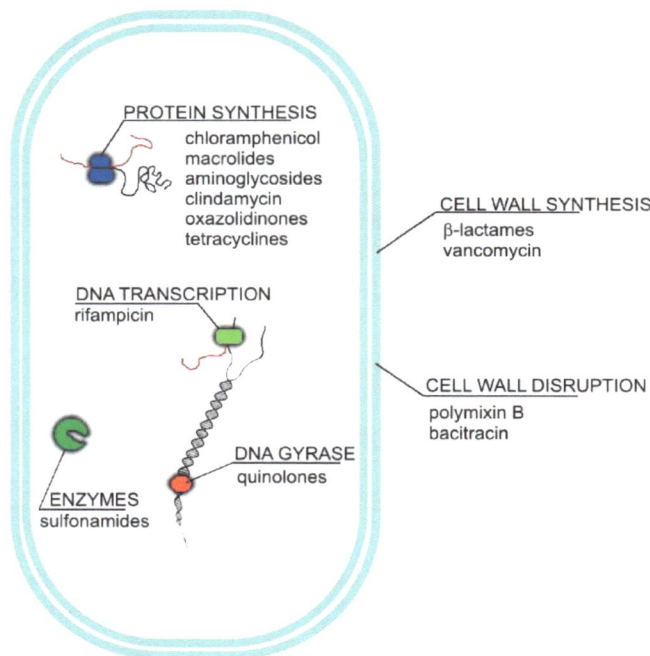

Fig. (1). Drug targets for antibiotics.

Peptide deformylase (PDF) is a class of metalloenzyme involved in catalyzing the removal of the N-formyl group from N-terminal methionine following translation [39]. In this reaction methionyl peptide and formate are produced which are crucial for bacteria survival. Peptide deformylase is thus considered a new target in antibacterial, antimalarial and anticancer drug discovery. By application of structure-based techniques assisted with high throughput screening, a number of chemical classes of PDF inhibitors with improved efficacy and specificity have been developed [2, 39].

DNA gyrase and topoisomerase IV are type IIA bacterial enzymes which are targeted by highly potent antibiotics [2, 40]. These drugs operate by inhibiting the topoisomerase molecule from relegating DNA strands after cleavage and convert the topoisomerase molecules into a DNA damaging agent [41]. Availability of high resolution crystal structures of both enzymes enabled the design of numerous classes of inhibitors with dual mechanism of action, including benzimidazoles, benzothiazoles, thiazolopyridines, imidiazopyridazoles, pyridines, indazoles, pyrazoles, imidazopyridines, triazolopyridines, pyrrolopyrimidines and pyrimidoindoles [42].

Fatty acids biosynthesis (FAB) is a metabolic pathway, essential for both eukaryotic and prokaryotic cells [2]. The differences in this process between bacteria and humans makes FAB an ideal target in antibacterial drug discovery. Recently, β-ketoacyl-acyl carrier protein synthase III (FabH), which catalyzes the first step of fatty acid biosynthesis, has been studied as a drug target [43], and FabH inhibitors [2] can be antibacterial drug candidates.

FtsZ (named after filamenting temperature-sensitive mutant Z) is a microbial protein which is involved in cytokinesis and may be targeted by antibacterial drugs [2]. This is a prokaryotic homologue to the eukaryotic protein tubulin. FtsZ is highly conserved among bacteria, and may be targeted by broad-spectrum antibiotics, while it is structurally different from eukaryotic tubulin which allows to avoid toxicity [44]. Many FtsZ-interacting molecules have been published and some of them are potent antibacterial agents [2, 45].

Ribosomes are major targets for antibacterial drugs *e.g.* oxazolidinones [2]. Antibiotics inhibit ribosome function by interfering in messenger RNA translation or by blocking the formation of peptide bonds at the peptidyl transferase centre *via* binding of drugs to the ribosomal subunits [46]. The new high-resolution structures (typically by electron microscopy) of the bacterial ribosomes and their complexes with antibiotics have greatly improved our understanding of ribosomal function and opened the possibilities for structure-based drug design [47].

MOLECULAR MODELLING TECHNIQUES FOR DESIGN AND DISCOVERY OF ANTIBACTERIAL DRUGS

Protein 3D Structure Prediction

Bacterial genome has been solved for many bacterial species through the advancement of sequencing technology. There is still a large gap between the available sequence data and available structural data. *Escherichia coli* has 1 810 184 sequences for various strains reported in RefSeq and whereas PDB has only 6876 *Escherichia coli* protein structures. The reported structures of established targets include those involved in cell wall synthesis and general protein synthesis of bacteria. However, increased antimicrobial resistance to existing antibiotics and therapies insists on the search for new targets. Thus, many research groups are working towards identifying new targets for antibacterial drug discovery using bioinformatic approaches [48 - 50]. Experimental techniques such as TraDis (Transposon Directed Insertion Sequencing) are reported to identify candidate genes for bacterial functionality [51]. Since protein structure determines its function the structural information is vital for identifying protein functionality, understanding the substrate specificity and to study binding interactions between protein and ligand. Experimental structure determination techniques include

X-Ray crystallography, nuclear magnetic resonance (NMR) and electron microscopy (EM). Despite advancements of EM, NMR and X-ray, three dimensional structure determination is expensive, tedious and challenging. Hence, the gap between the solved structural data and available sequence data underlines the importance of alternative methods for structure determination. Theoretical structure prediction methods are providing a helping hand to bridge the gap between target identification methods and experimental structure determination methods. These theoretical methods are especially useful in structure based drug design for targets whose three-dimensional structure is not known.

There are various methods available for the structure prediction: (i) homology modelling (or comparative modelling), (ii) fold recognition (or threading) and (iii) *ab initio* modelling (or first principle methods). Homology modelling and fold recognition methods mainly depend on the availability of identical or homologous protein structures (template) whereas *ab initio* modelling depends on physical chemistry principles. Fold recognition method also predicts the structure based on the homologous protein folds available in structural databases such as PDB. *Ab initio* methods predict the native fold based on scoring functions and conformational search methods. Even though a lot of efforts have been made towards the *ab initio* and fold recognition methods, homology modelling is preferred based on its reliability and accuracy [52]. Automation of algorithms also made homology modelling an easy tool for structure prediction of new targets. There are several online resources available for structure prediction implementing these approaches for model building. Protein structure prediction methods and their basic methodology are presented in Fig. (**2**). Some of structure prediction tools are listed in Table **1**.

Table 1. Protein structure prediction tools.

Method	Tools	References or Links
Homology Modelling	MODELLER	Standalone (free for academic users) [53]
	ModWeb	https://modbase.compbio.ucsf.edu/modweb/
	SWISS-MODEL	https://swissmodel.expasy.org
	ESyPred3D	http://www.unamur.be/sciences/biologie/urbm/bioinfo/esypred/
	ROBETTA	http://robetta.bakerlab.org
	Phyre	http://www.sbg.bio.ic.ac.uk/phyre2/html/page.cgi?id=index
	Prime	Standalone (GUI) Commercial application [54]

(Table 1) contd.....

Method	Tools	References or Links
Threading/ Fold recognition	I-TASSER	http://zhanglab.ccmb.med.umich.edu/I-TASSER/
	Raptor-X	http://raptorx.uchicago.edu/StructurePrediction/predict/
	HHpred	https://toolkit.tuebingen.mpg.de/hhpred
	GenTHREADER	http://bioinf.cs.ucl.ac.uk/psipred/?genthreader=1
	IntFOLD	http://www.reading.ac.uk/bioinf/IntFOLD/IntFOLD3_form.html
	TM-Fold	https://zhanglab.ccmb.med.umich.edu/TM-fold/
	DescFold	http://protein.cau.edu.cn/DescFold/prhps.html
	MUSTER	https://zhanglab.ccmb.med.umich.edu/MUSTER/
	SPARKS X	http://sparks-lab.org/yueyang/server/SPARKS-X/
	3D- PSSM	http://www.sbg.bio.ic.ac.uk/~3dpssm/index2.html
Ab initio Modelling	NovaFold	Commercial application
	QUARK	Webserver [http://zhanglab.ccmb.med.umich.edu/QUARK/]
	ROBETTA	http://robetta.bakerlab.org/submit.jsp

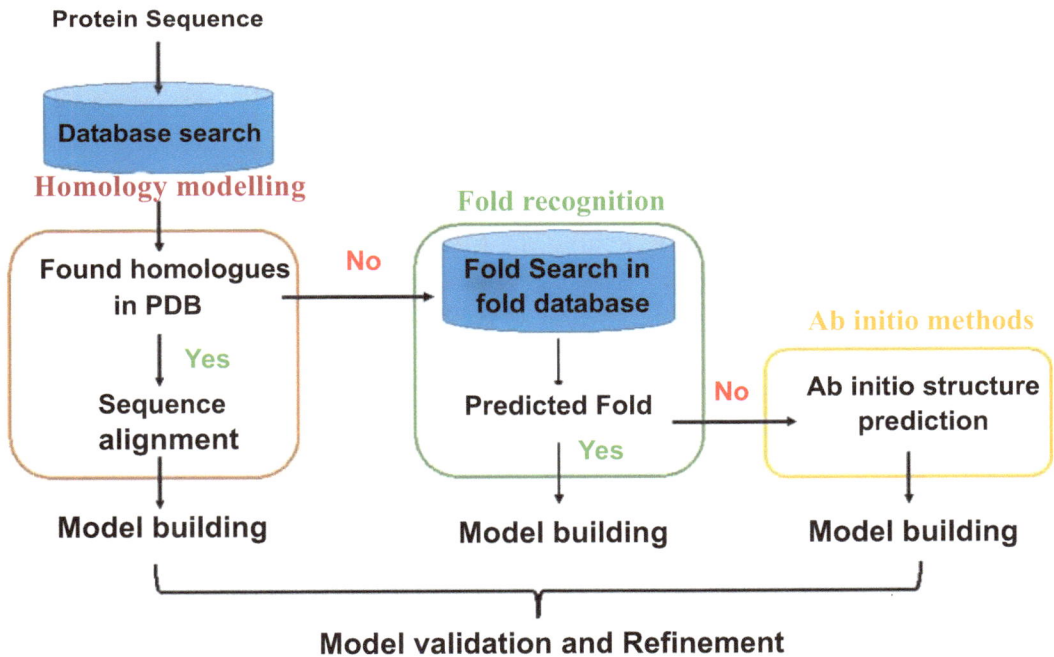

Fig. (2). Protein structure prediction methods.

Comparative/Homology Modelling

The major hypothesis involved here is that structural features are highly preserved during the evolution compared with sequential and functional changes [55]. General steps followed during homology modelling: (i) database search and template selection: the sequence of the protein of interest (query) will be searched for its homologous protein crystal structure (template); (ii) sequence structure alignment: alignment of the query sequence to the template structure, (iii) model building and (iv) model validation and refinement.

Database Search and Template Selection

Initially, the query sequence will be searched against protein sequences present in RCSB PDB to identify homologues. It provides the information about potential templates, based on % identity and % homology. % Identity refers to the same residues present in the query and the template while % Homology refers to similar type of residues present in the query and the template. Homology search is carried out using various methods such as sequence-sequence alignment (BLAST [56]), profile-sequence alignments (PSI-BLAST [57]) or profile-profile alignments (HMM-HMM). BLAST [58], PSI-BLAST, SSEARCH, FASTA [59] and HMMER [60] are some of the widely used similarity searching programs. From the search results, the template with highest % identity and % homology is typically selected to be a template. Accuracy of the homology model depends on the degree of homology of the query sequence to the template and its alignment so the template selection influences the model structure. While selecting the template, one should consider important parameters such as %identity, % homology, protein family and structural quality of the template structure. Usually, the template with highest sequence identity is selected. If the query has sequence identity more than 80%, we can expect the model of high accuracy. If the query has low sequence identity with the template (less than 30%), then much care is needed while alignment and model building. Generally, PSI-BLAST is preferred in case of low sequence identity as it constructs a position specific scoring matrix (PSSM) based on multiple sequence alignment of initial top scoring results of BLAST search [61]. It considers this PSSM for the next iteration rather than standard matrices during the alignment. This gives the opportunity to expand the search also to distant related sequences. Multi template modelling is also an option for low sequence identity where you build the model using multiple templates instead of a single template. If templates have similar identity and homology, the same family or subfamily templates are preferred during template selection. Multiple sequence alignment or construction of the phylogenetic tree is helpful for identifying similar family of proteins. Template resolution is also an important parameter to consider while modelling because errors in the template structure lead to poor quality models. Best resolution templates give typically better models if the alignment is done properly. One should consider the purpose of modelling also during the template selection. If our aim is to understand the protein-ligand interactions, it is better to select the template with similar co-crystallized ligand and in general similarity over the ligand-binding domain is more important than the overall identity. If we are at the initial step of wrong template selection, the entire process will go wrong and will end up with wrong models. Thus, one should consider all these aspects during the template selection.

Sequence-Structure Alignment

The alignment produced during the template search method is usually far from optimal. Thus, once the homologue structural template is found, the query sequence should be aligned again to the template structure using sequence-structure alignment methods such as pairwise sequence alignment and profile based alignment. Alignment reliability cannot be estimated exactly always as one of the structure is unavailable. Mostly, pairwise alignment from the BLAST or PSI-BLAST is reliable and manual intervention may be beneficial in case of insertions/deletions for targets having high sequence homologue templates. For the targets with low sequence homologue templates alignment quality is assessed based on region specific stability. Multiple sequence alignment [62] (MSA) is helpful in identifying conserved regions among evolutionary sequences and in improving model quality especially where the sequence identity is low. MUSCLE, CLUSTAL-W and T-coffee are some of the popular online tools available for MSA [63]. If the conserved region residues are misaligned among the family, manual curation is needed for improving the alignment. Alignment confidence can also be checked based on the comparison of structure based multiple sequence alignments. Tong *et al.* reported that shift based on secondary structural elements improves alignment accuracy [64]. Deriving the consensus alignment based on different methods is also useful for alignment improvement, in case of low sequence identity. If it is required, multi-template modelling is also an option to achieve the reliable alignment to cover the entire query sequence length. Alignment is the most critical step in the entire process of model development and it is the determinant for the model quality. Misalignment of one residue during the alignment can distort the entire structure and lead to a poor quality model. Alignment should be checked thoroughly at this step to reduce errors in the final model. Especially it is important to check that possible gaps do not occur along the secondary structural elements. As discussed above, method of alignment also influences the quality of homology models. For water-soluble proteins methods such as pairwise alignment and multiple sequence alignments will produce reliable quality models. In case of membrane proteins modelling accuracy is improved using profile-profile alignments or HMM-HMM (Hidden

Markov Models) methods [65].

Model Building

Model development is the next step after the optimal alignment is achieved. In the first step of the model building, backbone residue coordinates are copied to the model. If the aligned residues are identical, also side chain atom coordinates can be copied to the model. Loops are modelled after the construction of backbone and side chain residues. The probability of predicting the exact conformation of loop residues is a challenge in modelling. There are several online tools available for loop modelling, such as ModLoop, SuperLooper, FREAD, RCD+, SA-Mot, LoopIng [66]. After the loop modelling, side chain prediction is done using existing rotamer libraries or other conformational search methods. If the % identity or homology is high between the query and template, side chain coordinates will also be copied along with backbone residues as discussed above. If not, side chain placement is carried out with the help of rotamers extracted from high resolution crystal structures. Backbone structure and neighboring residues conformation is taken into account during rotamer search, which favors particular rotamer conformation to the backbone. Further, global model optimization is carried out using molecular mechanics and sometimes with subsequent molecular dynamics to remove steric clashes. However, molecular dynamics simulations may sometimes worsen the model compared to its native (non-MD) state [67]. There are also tools available online for model refinement such as 3D Refine (http://sysbio.rnet.missouri.edu/3Drefine/), ModRefiner (https://zhanglab.ccmb. med.umich.edu/ModRefiner/).

Model Validation

The developed model should be evaluated for its quality and possible errors. Most errors arise from the alignment and the selected template structure. If the errors are localized at a certain region of the model such as regions far from the binding site, they are less problematic for modelling. If the sequence identity is more than 50%, model can be compared with the template structure and model is expected to be close enough to the template structure. If it is less than 30%, there is possibility for large errors than expected [68]. Generally, models are checked for their stereo-chemical quality based on the defined bond lengths, bond angles, dihedral angles and contacts. Servers like SAVES (The Structure Analysis and Verification Server), JCSG and STAN provides quality check for protein models. These servers include validation tools such as Ramachandran plot, PROCHECK, WHATCHECK, ProSA-II, Verify-3D and ERRAT [69]. Ramachandran plot provides the information of protein residues in the allowed region and disallowed region based on dihedral angles. PROCHECK and WHATCHECK gives the stereochemical quality plots of each residues. PROCHECK also includes G-factor, which represents protein residues with unusual geometry. G factor below -0.5 indicates "unusual" geometry and less than -1.0 means "very unusual" geometry. ProSA-II calculates the energy using statistical potential mean forces and provides a parameter *i.e.* Z-score [70]. Verify-3D [71] determines the compatibility of the model with its sequence based on the information retrieved from existing structures. ERRAT factor is a statistical measure of non-bonded interactions between different atom types in the protein model. Factor above 90 indicates high quality of the model resembling crystal structures of 1Å to 2.0Å. Factor value near to 90 indicates quality resembling the crystal structures of 2.5Å to 3Å. All these parameters provide the information whether the model is of reliable quality or not. If the model quality is poor, one or all these steps can be iterated until we get a model of reliable quality. The developed model quality can also be determined using experiments like site-directed mutagenesis based on relative locations of the residues.

Fold Recognition/Threading

Fold recognition/threading methods are useful when there is no clear homologous known protein structure available (beyond twilight zone). In this method, query sequence is searched in structural database (template fold database) to identify the similar structural fold. The hypothesis is that proteins adopt similar structural fold even without detectable sequence similarity. This differs from homology modelling in search method and scoring.

Initially query target sequence is searched in fold databases rather than sequence or structural database. These fold databases contain native protein folds derived from the structural repositories like PDB. The template fold which fits the query sequence is identified and then build the model. This search is carried out using prediction based methods (PBM) or distance based methods (DBM) (knowledge based potentials). In PBM, fold information is deposited in the form of 1D profiles (such as α−helices, left handed helix, β−sheets, coil and strands) [72, 73]. The secondary structure of query sequence is predicted and then searched against these profiles of fold database. Alignment of the query structural elements and fold database is done using dynamic programming or heuristic approaches [74]. The fold which fits with the query fold with high score is selected to build the model. In DBM, initially 3D model of the query protein is generated and then searched against the fold database. Here, fit of query to fold is inspected based on statistically derived knowledge-based potentials [75]. Usually, backbone information is only traced during the search ignoring the side chain conformations for efficiency. Once the perfect fold is found, model building follows by combining all folds together into a single model. Thus, it is common to observe gaps during process as the entire target sequence is fitted to different template folds.

To inspect the sequence-fold alignment and the fit of each fold to the entire target sequence, each fold recognition algorithm uses its own alignment methods and scoring functions. Good scoring functions should identify the similar to native fold of target sequence. These scoring functions are derived through statistical analysis of various parameters such as pair potentials, correlation of predicted secondary structure and observed secondary structure and accessibility. Initial scoring functions were based on pairwise residue-residue contact potentials (*e.g.*: PROSPECT II). Then, residue environment such as hydrophobicity was included to predict the native fold and proved to be effective with 85% success rate [76, 77]. Machine learning techniques such as random forest (RF), neural networks (NN), support vector machines (SVM) were also implemented in various fold recognition algorithms [78]. DescFold, DN-Fold, RF-Fold are some of the fold recognition programs derived scoring functions based on classification methods. Recently, Meta servers overtook the traditional servers, which includes various scoring functions and methods and build a consensus model. Some of the servers are listed in Table **1**.

Ab initio Modelling

Ab initio modelling (also referred as *de novo* modelling) is a complex structure prediction method when compared with homology modelling and fold recognition methods. If a target protein has no homologous protein present in the structural database (which is occasional), this method is usually helpful. The method predicts the native structure of target protein only from the sequence based on physical principles [79]. This prediction is mainly based on the fact that native state or functional state of the protein structure corresponds to its global minimum energy conformation. *Ab initio* method generates a number of possible conformations based on physics based energy functions such as AMBER, CHARMM, OPLS and UNRES [80] and knowledge based methods used in ROSETTA and I-TASSER [81, 82]. The knowledge based functions are empirical functions derived from the existing PDB structures. After the conformational search, lowest energy structure will be selected as a final model. Conformational space is explored using methods such as Monte Carlo simulations and molecular dynamics. This search is computationally expensive and demanding because of the high number of degrees of freedom of polypeptide chain. Previous *ab initio* methods did not use the knowledge of existing protein structures. Recent methods improved the *ab initio* prediction by including existing structural information and profile-based fragments (ROSETTA and I-TASSER). These algorithms also include the conformational clustering process. Here, the generated conformations are clustered and centroid of the system is selected as final model. Refer to Table (**1**) for *ab initio* servers and programs.

Protein Structure Prediction in Anti-Bacterial Drug Design

Homology modelling is helpful to understand the binding environment of target proteins and enzymes. It also helps to inspect the binding mode of ligands and their mechanism of action. Some case studies illustrating the use of homology modelling are discussed below.

Quinolones are used to treat various infections caused by microorganisms such as *Streptococcus pneumoniae, Escherichia coli, Haemophilus influenzae, Neisseria gonorrhoeaea, Salmonella typhi* and *Staphylococcus aureus.* The molecular target of broad spectrum quinolone antibiotics is DNA gyrase/topoisomerases. DNA gyrase consists of two subunits encoded by genes gyrA and gyrB; GyrA introduces the negative supercoiling and GyrB provides ATP required for the process. Quinolone resistance is majorly due to the chromosomal mutations localized in Quinolone Resistance Determining Region (QRDR), between amino acids 67 and 106 of subunit A. Mutations of Ser83Phe/Tyr and Asp87Tyr/Gly in QRDR are reported in *Salmonella typhi* clinical isolates [83]. To understand the binding characteristics of fluoroquinolones, Kumar *et al.* built homology models of *Salmonella typhi* topoisomerase complexes. They built the protein complex using *Escherichia coli* GyrA subunit and *Staphylococcus aureus* GyrB subunit. Final complex was modelled using the crystal structure of *Staphylococcus aureus* topoisomerase complex co-crystallized with ciprofloxacin. The model was validated using PROCHECK for its stereochemical quality and Verify-3D for sequence-structure relationship. Mutant complexes were also generated likewise and then subjected to dynamic simulations to check the stability of complexes. Docking of fluoroquinolones into both wild type and mutant complexes of *Salmonella typhi* revealed the role of mutations in drug resistance. Further, molecular dynamics simulations on wild type and mutant complexes provided insights into binding interactions. These simulations also revealed the importance of hydrogen bonding between Ser 83 of GyrA and fluoroquionolones, and this residue is absent in mutant complex. Gyrase and topoisomerases are similar in their mode of action with similar catalytic sites such as ATP binding site and DNA cleavage site. Thus, the dual targeting of gyrase and topoisomerases can be helpful to find novel inhibitors which are capable of evading these resistance mechanisms. Even though several compounds like closthiomide [84], haloemodin [85], pyrrolopyrimidines [86], pyridylureas [87], quercetin analogues [88], pyrazolopyridones [89], naphthoquinones [90] and pyridine-carboxamide ureas [91] are reported acting on both these targets, there is an urge for potent antibacterial compounds targeting them.

DNA gyrase is an important target in anti-tubercular drug discovery [92]. Napthoquinone derivatives are reported as DNA gyrase inhibitors particularly in *Mycobacterium tuberculosis*. Diosypirin is one of the napthoquinione derivatives and it has shown potential as gyrase B inhibitor. Chetty and Soliman [93] proposed a new allosteric binding site for diosyprin, distant from conventional ATP binding and catalytic binding sites, by using homology modelling. They constructed the homology model of *Mycobacterium tuberculosis* DNA gyrase based on the templates of *Escherichia coli* and *Thermus thermophilus*. The model was used to study possible binding pockets and putative binding mode of diosyprin by docking. These studies revealed an allosteric binding pocket near to the ATP binding site. This predicted novel binding site that can be explored in future to target gyrase B for the identification of novel antibacterial compounds.

Serine/threonine protein kinases (STPK) play an important role in the pathogenesis of tuberculosis and other bacterial infections [94]. The importance of protein kinases in regulating key processes responsible for *Mycobacterium tuberculosis*, viability and virulence makes them good targets for tuberculosis treatment. *Mycobacterium tuberculosis* has eleven functional STPKs, nine transmembrane proteins (PknA, PknB, PknD, PknE, PknF, PknH, PknI, PknJ and PknL) and two cytosolic proteins (PknG and PknK). PknI is involved in cell division and growth regulation of *Mycobacterium tuberculosis*. Kandaswamy's group used homology modelling to understand the binding characteristics of serine/threonine protein kinase PknI of *Mycobacterium tuberculosis* [95]. They built a homology model of PknI based on its nearest homolog protein (having 30% sequence identity), namely PknB of *Mycobacterium tuberculosis*. They also predicted the active site using pharmacophore model, based on other kinases, and then used this for further docking studies. Based on pharmacophore model analysis, Lys41, Asp90, Val92 and Asp96 residues were predicted to be important for PknI function. Further, the site-directed mutagenesis studies on PknI confirmed the importance of Lys41 as mutation of this residue to methionine hindered the binding of ATP.

Aminoacyl-tRNA synthetases (aaRSs) are one of validated targets in antimicrobial drug discovery. aaRSs are involved in protein synthesis by transferring the related amino acid to its cognate tRNA. They are present in all bacterial pathogens and are structurally distinct from their respective eukaryotic aaRSs. aaRSs are widely studied as drug targets in different organisms such as *Staphylococcus aureus*, *Clostridium difficile* [96] and *Mycobacterium tuberculosis*. Inhibition of these aaRSs leads to the depletion of tRNAs, protein synthesis inhibition, cell growth arrest and finally result in cell death. Isloleucyl-tRNA synthetase (IleRS), Methionyl-tRNA synthetase (MetRS), Threonyl- tRNA synthetase (ThrRS), Phenylalanyl- tRNA synthetase (PheRS) and AspartynyltRNA synthetase (AspRS) are some of aaRSs studied for the identification of novel antibacterial agents [97]. Muciprocin is fine. The only FDA approved drug for the treatment of skin infections such as impetigo, traumatic lesions and for nasal carriage caused by methicillin resistant *Staphylococcus aureus* (MRSA) targeting IleRS [98]. MetRS is also explored to design new inhibitors against *Staphylococcus aureus*, affecting the bacterial growth [99 - 102]. Liu *et al.* used hybrid virtual screening methodology to identify new MetRS inhibitors based on the *Staphylococcus aureus* MetRS homology model [103]. Initially, they screened Specs molecular database using structure based pharmacophore model and selected 1000 hits. Due to the lack of 3D structure of *Staphylococcu aureus* MetRS, a protein model was developed based on its nearest available homologous *Escherichia coli* MetRS (of 32% sequence identity). MODELLER [104] was used to build the model. The model was validated using Ramachandran plot and RMSD with the template. The developed homology model of *Staphylococcu aureus* MetRS was used for the docking of initial 1000 hits, of which 15 hits were selected for experimental screening. Most compounds exhibited good MIC values *in vitro* ranging from 4 to 64 µg/ml against *Staphylococcu aureus* and four other strains (MRSA, *Escherichia coli*, *Pseudomonas aeruginosa* and *Klebsiella pneumonia*). This is an example how theoretical structure prediction methods can be used to identify new inhibitors. The PheRS, a tetrameric protein, also plays a major role in MRSA infections. Unfortunately, there are no crystal structure of *Staphylococcus aureus* PheRS. Elbaramawi *et al.* reported a homology model of *Staphylococcus aureus* PheRS and they used the homology model to identify new inhibitors against PheRS [105]. The model was built by MOE [106] using AMBER force field and based on the structure of *Staphylococcus haemolyticus* PheRS (PDB ID: 2RHQ). The *Staphylococcus haemolyticus* PheRS has 93% sequence identity with *Staphylococcus aureus* PheRS and thus, it was selected as the template for the model building. The model was validated using different methods such as Ramachandran plot, Verify-3D and ProSA. Reported PheRS inhibitors (phenylthiazolylurea sulfonamides and ethanolamine derivatives) were docked in the model. It revealed important binding sites for aminoacylation and also the role of magnesium in binding of subunits. Other docking studies related to aaRS are described in the docking section below.

Molecular Docking

Molecular Docking as an Approach to Study Ligand-Protein Interactions

Structure-based drug design strategies were critical for the successful discovery of some drugs present in the market, like HIV protease inhibitors [107]. Prediction of protein-ligand interactions is the main principle involved in structure-based drug design and docking is the most commonly used method for predicting these interactions. Docking proved helpful from hit identification to lead identification. Use of these methods in drug discovery has been raised through the years. In the docking procedure, ligands are placed in the target binding site to identify the possible binding conformation and its orientation. Once the conformation fitting into the binding site is found, it is scored using scoring functions. Typically, the scoring is in terms of binding free energy. This methodology is automated in many programs like DOCK [108], AutoDock [109], FlexX [110], Glide [111], GOLD [112], MOE-Dock [106] and CDOCKER [113], implementing various search algorithms and scoring functions [114]. Automation of docking algorithms has made screening of large databases simple and (if enough CPU power is available) fast. The availability of three dimensional structure of the protein is essential for any docking. Small molecule databases such as ZINC [115] and ASINEX [116] are available online for virtual screening. Docking procedure consists of three key components (i) representation; (ii) conformational search and (iii) scoring and ranking. Basic docking procedures and algorithms are shown in Fig. (3).

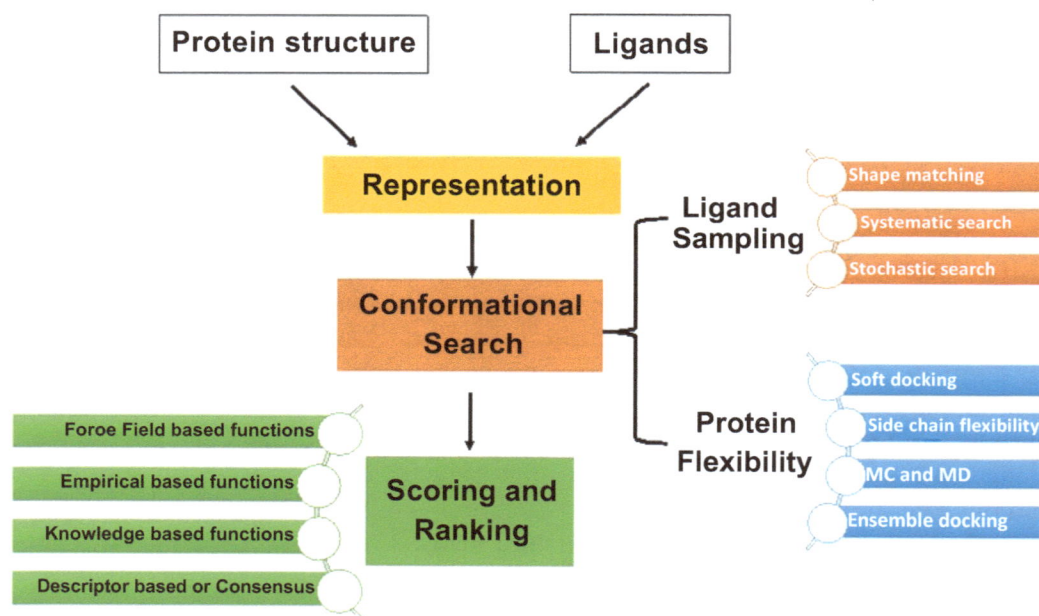

Fig. (3). Docking methodology and algorithm.

Representation

Protein and ligand in docking are represented by atoms, grid or the surface. Initial docking programs represent the exposed protein residues with atoms. However, usage of all atom-pair interactions increased the complexity of predictions. Thus, this method is typically used for final ranking *via* potential energy functions as implemented in DARWIN program [117]. Another popular representation is so called solvent accessible protein surfaces calculated using solvent probe *i.e.* Connolly surfaces [118]. Here, the probe molecule will be rolled over the protein's van der Waals surface to see the accessible surface for interaction. This is implemented in DOCK program to predict protein-ligand binding. Still another method is grid representation. In this method, protein will be represented by potential energy grid points, usually by electrostatic and van der Waals potentials [119]. The final interaction potential is predicted using probe molecules. Unlike surface representation method, here probes are atoms (C, N, O and H) or molecular fragments (C=O, COO⁻, N-H and O-H *etc.*) found in various drug molecules. Grid representation also takes more time as it needs to consider each fragment separately. However, it is a single time procedure for a protein and can be stored and used for further calculations. This is implemented in many programs such as AutoDock, revised version of DOCK and Glide.

Conformational Search

Ligand flexibility is explored using conformational search algorithms: systematic search and stochastic or random search. In systematic methods, search is done by altering the degrees of freedom systematically. These methods include matching algorithm and incremental construction algorithm. In matching algorithms, ligand atoms will be matched to the protein binding space pseudoatoms based on the shape complementarity. If a suitable ligand match is found, it is considered as one of the binding conformations. The method does not consider any binding interactions except the shape matching/complementarity. This is implemented in earlier versions of DOCK. As it only considers the matching of ligand atoms to the shape, there is a possibility to generate binding modes that may occupy existing protein atoms and resulting false positives. The DirectedDock algorithm overcame this drawback by considering binding groups and their interactions along with shape complementarity. Some programs like FLOG generate ligand conformations based on rotatable bonds and then the generated conformational database is matched into the target binding site [120]. The other systematic method is incremental construction method, where ligands will be fragmented based on flexible rotatable bonds. Among generated fragments, the rigid fragment is identified and matched to the binding site points based on its shape and binding groups available for interactions. Once possible anchor conformation is found, flexible fragments are added to the anchor sequentially, based on interacting groups. Dock 4.0 implemented this method considering only shape complementarity while FlexX used chemical complementarity. Unlike FlexX and

DOCK 4.0, Hammerhead (Glide) program uses this method with automatic anchor selection to avoid bias at initial stage [121].

Stochastic methods are computationally expensive because of their exhaustive search algorithms. Although, no method is 100% accurate enough finding the exact biological active conformation, the probability of finding global minimum energy conformation is high through the stochastic methods. These methods modify ligand conformations randomly. Genetic Algorithm (GA) and MonteCarlo (MC) methods are popular methods under this category. In MC method, ligand conformations are generated by random bond rotations. The generated conformation is minimized and its binding energy is calculated in the binding site. If it is below the threshold of certain energy criteria, it is discarded and then generates a new conformation by bond rotation. This process is repeated until a minimum binding energy conformation is generated. Thus, this method increases the possibility of predicting the accurate binding mode. Programs like Glide, AutoDock, ICM, MCDOCK and Prodock use this method for docking. GA method generates the conformation randomly using principle of evolution and natural selection. Ligand conformations are generated randomly based on the rotation and translation of dihedral angles. Dihedral angles of ligand are stored as chromosomes and then they are changed randomly (like mutations or crossover in biology). Binding energy is calculated for each conformation considering its position and orientation in the binding site. If it has less energy than the parent conformation, this is taken to the next generation for further mutations and crossovers. Several mutations and cross overs take place until it generates a minimum energy conformation. Best docking modes are taken based on the interaction energy. GOLD, AutoDock and DARWIN implemented this method. Even though, most of the programs try to predict the global minimum energy conformation of the ligand, the global minima conformation may not always be the biological active conformation.

Most of the docking programs consider protein as a rigid body. Previously, protein flexibility is overlooked in docking methodology based on the hypothesis that protein side chain conformational flexibility during ligand binding is negligible in comparison with ligand flexibility. Recent advancements in induced-fit docking [122], molecular dynamics [123] and QM/MM methods [124], prove the importance of protein flexibility in binding affinity prediction [125]. A small change in protein flexibility can totally erase the binding affinity of a molecule. Thus, now many sampling algorithms consider the protein flexibility in docking with different approaches such as soft docking, ensemble docking and induced-fit docking. Initially, soft docking methods were implemented in many programs, to simulate protein flexibility, by softening van der Waals potentials of protein residues to accommodate ligands [126]. Even though, this method is computationally economic, it increased the threat of false positives where diverse ligands fit into the binding pocket. The side chain flexibility of protein residues during ligand binding is further explored by rotamer libraries [127, 128]. These rotamer libraries are extracted from existing experimental protein side chain conformations. Another method is to dock ligands into an ensemble of protein conformations such as apo proteins and proteins with co-crystallized ligands. This is implemented in various programs like DOCK, FlexE and Glide. DOCK uses different structural conformations *via* combined grids to generate the ensemble of potentials to predict the binding free energies. FlexE uses each protein structure individually and then combines all protein conformations to generate a new ensemble protein conformation for docking. Glide also uses the same approach, initially considering individual rigid grid conformations and then combining all grids to give an ensemble scoring. Induced-fit docking is an approach where certain residues will be defined as flexible to allow ligand flexibility within the binding site region. Programs, such as Glide, initially generate ligand poses by softening the potentials (likewise in soft docking) and then explore rotamer conformational flexibility by mutating defined residues. It gives opportunity to find the ligand that can induce conformational changes in the protein. After the identification of proper ligand conformation with possible rotamers, minimization follows. These methods help to identify ligands that induce conformational changes in the protein.

Scoring and Ranking

Scoring is the determination of strength of the interactions (or binding affinity) between binding groups of ligand and protein. Scoring function should reliably recognize the correct binding pose of ligand with low RMSD to the co-crystallized complex within reasonable computational time. Even though many scoring functions are available, most of them are failing to rank the correct poses in the top list and there is large variation between targets and scoring algorithms, as some methods work well with one type of targets while giving basically useless results with other targets.

Scoring functions can be incorporated into the docking algorithms at different stages. Some programs integrated scoring functions during the conformational search and other programs at the end of the search stage. Usually, docking algorithms like genetic algorithms need to integrate the scoring function for conformational search, as it needs to check the fitness score of each conformation. There are three main classes of scoring methods: force field based functions, empirical scoring functions and knowledge based functions. Recently, Liu and Wang included descriptor based scoring function in this classification along with traditional three scoring functions [128].

Force field scoring functions are mainly based on different force field originating individual non bonded interaction energy components, such as bond stretching/bending, torsional energies, van der Waals interactions and electrostatic interactions. The first docking scoring functions were derived from force fields such as AMBER or CHARMM (implemented in DOCK and AutoDock). Generally, force field (FF) based methods measure the potential energy of the system. Equation 1 is the example of FF scoring function implemented in DOCK.

$$E = \sum_{i=1}^{lig} \sum_{j=1}^{rec} \left[\frac{A_{ij}}{r_{ij}^{12}} - \frac{B_{ij}}{r_{ij}^{6}} + 332 \frac{q_i q_j}{D r_{ij}} \right] \tag{1}$$

Here, r_{ij} – distance between ligand atom i and protein atom j, A_{ij} and B_{ij} – VDW repulsion and attraction parameters, q_i and q_j - atomic charges and D - dielectric constant. These functions mostly depend on electrostatic terms and often electrostatic interaction contributions are overestimated in the case of charged ligands, leading to false positives. These methods are also problematic in the light of solvent and entropy effects. Even though, FF based methods such as Free Energy Perturbations (FEP) and Thermodynamic Integrations (TI) consider solvent effects explicitly, these methods are computationally expensive which limit their usage in the virtual screening of large libraries. Poisson-Boltzmann/surface area (PB/SA) model and Generalized-Born/surface area (GB/SA) models consider the solvent implicitly. Usually, these methods are used after the general scoring methods in docking.

Empirical scoring functions are regression-based scoring functions derived from a dataset of known protein-ligand complexes. Here, protein-ligand complexes with known experimental binding affinity are used for the derivation of equations. These scoring functions are summation of various weighted energy terms such as hydrogen bonding, electrostatic potential, VDW energy, hydrophobicity, entropy and desolvation energy. For example, ChemScore estimates the total binding free energy based on empirical terms such as hydrogen bonding and lipophilicity (equation 2).

$$\Delta G_{binding} = \Delta G_0 + \Delta G_{hbond} v_0 + \Delta G_{metal} v_1 + \Delta G_{lipo} v_2 + \Delta G_{rot} v_3 \tag{2}$$

In the above equation, each component is the product of physical contributions of each energy term and its weighted coefficient determined by regression. v_0, v_1, v_2 and v_3 are weighted coefficients determined from the training dataset of known complexes correlating with their binding affinity. These scoring functions are fast and efficient, if compared with FF scoring functions, due to their individual energy terms. However, their applicability always depends on the structural range of the dataset used for training. To be noted, as these are derived from certain protein-ligand complexes, unfavorable conformations are typically not penalized enough. Many docking programs are using their own empirical scoring functions due to increased availability of protein-ligand complexes. GlideScore, ChemScore, Xscore, PLP, MedusaScore [129] are some of these empirical functions implemented in various programs.

Knowledge based scoring functions are also referred to as potential mean force (PMF) functions. These functions are derived by statistical means based on the experimentally determined protein-ligand complexes in the knowledge base. Protein and ligand atom types are classified based on their molecular environment. Then, distance dependent atom pair potentials are derived from their occurrence of frequency of particular atom pair using inverse Boltzmann constant (equation 3). Here, the occurrence of frequency of atom pair is assumed to be a measure of its energetic contribution to the binding.

$$\omega(r) = -k_B T \ln \left[\frac{\rho(r)}{\rho * (r)} \right] \tag{3}$$

Here, $\omega(r)$ – distance dependent pair-wise potential, k_B is the Boltzmann constant, T – absolute temperature of the system, $\rho(r)$ – numerical density of the protein-ligand atom pair at a distance r, $\rho*(r)$ – numeric density of atom pair in a reference state where interatomic distance is zero. Due to their implicit treatment of atom pair potentials, this method includes all energetic factors information. These scoring functions are computationally efficient in their speed and accuracy due to their pairwise atom treatment. These functions do not fit the experimental binding affinity data, thus these are thought to be more robust and general. Even though, knowledge based scoring functions are as fast as empirical, finding the initial reference state is challenging. This problem is more prominent during virtual screening to find the accurate ligand binding mode. As these functions are derived from complexes, these are not sensitive in predicting different ligand positions. To circumvent this problem, some scoring functions included the iterative mode where they calculate the potentials till they reproduce the experimental pair distributions (ITScore). Extension to many-body interactions to account for hydrogen bonding and other directional interaction terms is also a problem with these scoring functions. DrugScore, SMoG2001 [130], ITScore, MScore, KECSA and DSX are some of the scoring functions derived based on this principle.

Descriptor-based or machine learning scoring functions have recently gained popularity in the docking algorithms. These methods are similar to empirical scoring functions in their method of derivation as they are also derived from existing protein-ligand complexes. Like quantitative structure activity relationship (QSAR) methods, these functions are actually based on descriptors. These descriptors, such as occurrence of atomic pairs within a cutoff distance, physicochemical descriptors (van der Waals interactions, electrostatic interactions, aromatic interactions, metal atom interactions), geometrical descriptors (surface property and shape matching) and energy effects (entropic effects and desolvation), are considered for the development of these functions. Scoring functions are derived using various regression based methods such as multi linear regression (MLR), kernel-based regression (K-PLS) and machine learning methods such as random forest (RF), neural networks (NN) and bayes classification. Despite the progress of these methods in docking and screening, one should consider respective applicability domain while using them. Recently, Ain *et al.* have reviewed machine learning scoring functions with the detailed classification and their application in protein-ligand binding affinity prediction [131]. NNScore, RF-Score, SFCscore, ID-score and GemAffinity are some scoring functions developed in this category [132]. For example, RF-score is used in the virtual screening of DHQase2 protein, of *Mycobacterium tuberculosis* and *Streptomyces coelicolor,* resulting in 100 new inhibitors containing 48 new core scaffolds [133]. In addition to these functions, consensus scoring is another approach which combines various scoring functions to improve the performance of protein-ligand binding prediction. Here, various individual scores are combined to give a final scoring eliminating errors in individual scoring functions to predict true binders. X-Cscore [134], MulitScore [135], SeleX-CS [136], GFscore are such scoring functions derived in this process of predicting true protein-ligand complexes. Some of the popular docking programs and algorithms are tabulated in Table **2**.

Table 2. Docking programs and associated scoring functions.

	Software	Search algorithm	Scoring functions
1	AutoDock	Stochastic method (GA)	$\Delta G = \left(\Delta V_{bound}^{L-L} - \Delta V_{unbound}^{L-L} \right) + \left(\Delta V_{bound}^{P-P} - \Delta V_{unbound}^{P-P} \right) + \left(\Delta V_{bound}^{P-L} - \Delta V_{unbound}^{P-L} + \Delta S_{conf} \right)$
2	GOLD	Stochastic method (GA)	$\text{GOLD score} = E_{H-bond,ext} + E_{vdW,ext} + E_{vdW,int} + E_{torsion,int} + \left(E_{H-bond,int} + S_{con} + S_{cov} \right)$

(Table 2) contd.....

	Software	Search algorithm	Scoring functions
3	Glide	Systematic search	$$\text{XP Glide score} = E_{coul} + E_{vdW} + E_{bind} + E_{penalty}$$ $$E_{bind} = E_{hyd\_enclosure} + E_{hb\_nn\_motif} + E_{hb\_cc\_motif} + E_{PI} + E_{hb\_pair} + E_{phobic\_pair}$$
4	FlexX	Shape matching (Incremental construction	$$\Delta G_{bind} = \Delta G_0 + \Delta G_{rot} NROT + \Delta G_{hb} \sum_{h-bonds} f(\Delta R, \Delta a) + \Delta G_{ionic} \sum_{\substack{ionic\\interactions}} f(\Delta R, \Delta a) + \Delta G_{aromatic} \sum_{aromatic} f(\Delta R, \Delta a) + \Delta G_{lipo} \sum_{lipo} f(\Delta R, \Delta a)$$
5	MOE	Systematic and Stochastic	London-dG $\Delta G = c + E_{flex} + \sum_{h-bonds} c_{HB} f_{HB} + \sum_{m-lig} c_M f_M + \sum_{atom i} \Delta D_i$ Affinity-dG $\Delta G = C_{hb} f_{hb} + C_{ion} f_{ion} + C_{mlig} f_{mlig} + C_{hh} f_{hh} + C_{hp} f_{hp} + C_{aa} f_{aa}$

Docking is a huge subject including various methods such as protein-ligand docking, protein-protein docking, ensemble docking, inverse docking, flexible docking and dynamic docking. Docking algorithms are still in the process of active development. Despite advancements and development of various methods for scoring and ranking, there is no perfect scoring function till date, to predict the accurate binding mode of ligands. Even though docking has its own limitations it has been a good support for the drug discovery.

Application of Molecular Docking in Anti-Bacterial Drug Discovery

Docking is useful from initial virtual screening, hit identification, hit optimization to lead identification and optimization. It not only predicts protein-ligand interactions but also protein-protein interactions. The method has been useful for the identification of inhibitors against various bacterial targets. Here, we highlighted some of such case studies.

MscL is a mechanosensitive channel of large conductance, an attractive target for antibacterial drug discovery, conserved in bacterial species [137]. MscL protects the bacteria from acute hypoosmotic shock by converting mechanical tension to electrochemical response. This channel acts as an entry point for ions, drugs and small molecules. MscL channel opens up to 30Å diameter in *Escherichia coli* [138]. Many groups explored this MscL channel to design new antibacterial compounds. Propyl parabens, which are used as preservatives in food, pharmaceutical and cosmetic industry, are reported acting on MscL based on docking studies [139]. Iscla *et al.* reported MscL influence on the potency of widely used antibiotic Streptomycin [140]. In this study, *in vivo* liquid culture growth experiments revealed the MscL-dependent growth inhibition of streptomycin. They also showed dihydrostreptomycin effecting MscL activity by using patch clamp assays. Ramiz *et al.* reported the discovery of a new antimicrobial agent targeting MscL based on docking. The homology model based studies led to this discovery. They developed *Escherichia coli* MscL homology model from *Mycobacterium tuberculosis* MscL. MscL of *Escherichia coli* is of 136 amino acids in length and homopentamer in structure. Initial *denovo* design of ligands based on the pharmacophore model followed by docking resulted in an active compound *i.e.* 1,2,4-tris(2'-(4''-phenol)ethyl)benzene (Fig. **4**). Further, functional group modification and iterative docking studies in Autodock, led to a novel class of antibacterial preclinical agent, 1,3,5-tris((1E)-2'-(4''-benzoic acid)vinyl)benzene (referred to as Ramizol) [141, 142].

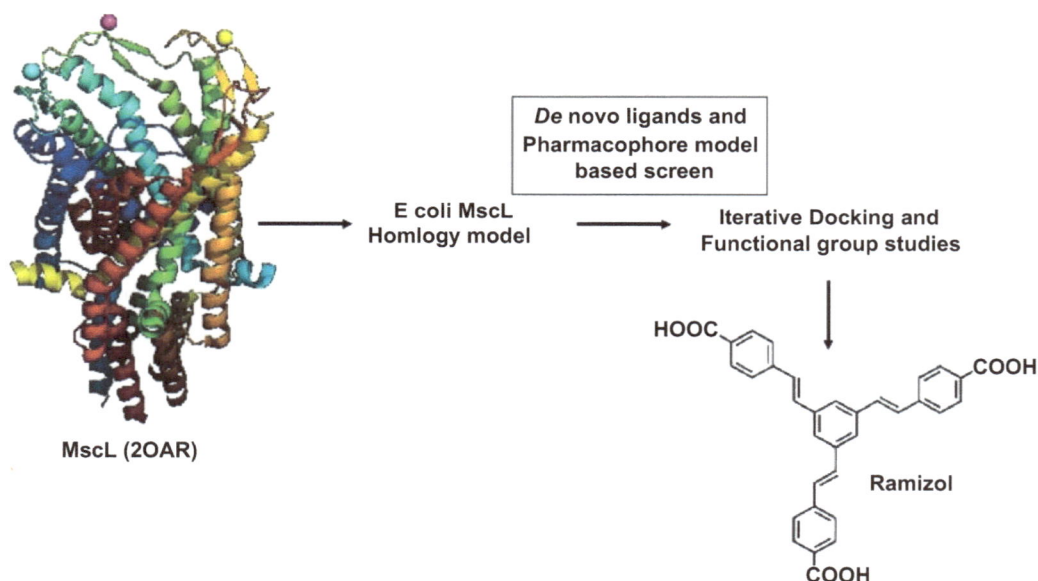

Fig. (4). Case study: MscL homology based docking studies led to a preclincial agent.

As discussed in homology modelling section, aaRSs are important targets in antibiotic drug discovery. The FDA approved drug, muciprocin, is used in the treatment of skin infections. Muciprocin activity is due to its selective binding affinity to the IleRS [143]. Shortly after the use of muciprocin, resistance is observed in clinical isolates of *S. aureus* due to V588F or V631F mutations in IleRS. Hurdle *et al.* used the modelling techniques to understand the binding characteristics of muciprocin with IleRS mutants [144]. They generated mutated protein models of IleRS using SwissPDB and then minimized. Muciprocin is docked into these mutated models along with the wild type IleRS to estimate the binding energy of muciprocin. Binding free energies calculated by docking are correlated to the degree of resistance observed in *in vitro* binding data. They modelled the intermediate Ile-AMP in the active site of IleRS to mimic the reaction of amino acyl transfer and conducted docking studies. These studies support the lack of fitness in muciprocin resistant strains is due to the decreased affinity of the Ile-AMP reactive intermediate. There are also studies reported the benefit of targeting of more than one aaRS to overcome the resistance [145].

Thioredoxin reductases (TrxR) are flavoproteins belong to pyridine nucleotide-disulfide oxidoreductase family [146]. They catalyze the reduction of thioredoxin protein by NADPH and plays a critical role in DNA synthesis. Even though, TrxR is present in both mammalian and bacterial cells, they differ in their structure and mechanism of action. This makes TrxR an interesting target to treat bacterial infections caused by organisms such as *Mycobacterium tuberculosis* and *Staphylococcus aureus* [147]. These organisms are causative agents for various infectious diseases such as tuberculosis, skin and soft tissues infections, pneumonia and endocarditis. TrxR is a homodimer with an NADPH binding site, a FAD prosthetic group, and an active site containing a redox-active disulfide. Bacterial TrxR has high substrate specificity compared with mammalian cells. Mammalian TrxR also differs from bacterial TrxR due to the presence of a selenocysteine residue at the C-terminal tail of its active site. Sweeney *et al.* screened CSD database compounds against *Mycobacterium tuberculosis* TrxR using docking [148]. Based on docking results, they tested nine compounds for their activity in *Mycobacterium tuberculosis* assays. Unfortunately, none of them supported the docking results. They also tested the same compounds in four other species *Staphylococcus aureus, Escherichia coli, Enterococcus faecalis* and *Pseudomonas aeruginosa.* Interestingly, one compound (CSD5376) showed MIC of 8 μg/ml in *Staphylococcus aureus*. Further, testing of this compound (CSD5376) and its analogs on various *Staphylococcus aureus* strains and clinical isolates of *Staphylococcus aureus,* revealed the consistent activity of CSD 5376. But the other analogs of CSD 5376 are inactive. The CSD 5376 showed activity in drug resistant *Staphylococcus aureus* strains. Lack of activity of CSD5376 in *Mycobacterium tuberculosis* can be attributed to thick mycobacterial cell wall of mycolic acids. In antibacterial drug design, permeability is one major problem especially in case of gram negative organisms. Enzyme potency of some compounds and inhibitors may not give rise to antibacterial activity because of the efflux and permeability barriers [149]. Hence it is important to achieve balance between compounds physical properties and the bacterial membrane permeability during the design of antibacterial compounds. Thio redox systems are reported as viable targets in antibacterial drug design based on various studies where the Trx system inhibition showed bactericidal activity. HTS screening of pharmacologically active compounds on various gram positive species such as *Bacillus subtilis, Enterococcus faecalis, Staphylococcus aureus* led to the identification of bactericidal properties of an approved anti-rheumatic drug aurafinon. Further biochemical assays revealed aurafinon's bactericidal properties are because of TrxR inhibition [150]. Ebselen is a new class of inhibitor showed effective inhibition on Trx system in *Escherichia coli* mutants lacking glutathione reductase or glutathione [151]. Ebselen and its analogs are also effective for inhibition of Trx system in various bacterial species such as *Staphylococcus aureus, Mycobacterium tuberculosis, Bacillus antracis* [151]. Epigallocatechin 3-gallate [EGCG] a component of Green TEA extract is also reported to be involved in Trx/TrxR inactivation in *Staphylococcus aureus* [152].

Bacteria use various mechanisms to protect from antibiotics and become resistant to current treatments [153]. Besides the evolution of bacteria using chromosomal mutations, enzymatic degradation of antibiotics and efflux pumps, bacterial persistence is another mechanism adopted by bacteria to escape the drugs and other antibiotics [154]. Bacterial persistence and dormancy, with respect to antibiotics, nutrient depletion and environmental stress conditions, is affected by Toxin-Antitoxin (TA) genes [155]. Toxins are responsible for the bacterial cell growth arrest during stress conditions. During normal growth conditions, antitoxins neutralizes toxins activity. Targeting toxins can be helpful to prevent the bacterial persistence stage during the treatment which eliminates the reoccurrence of infection [156]. These TA systems are divided into six types based on their mechanism of action. These are further divided into subfamilies [157]. Among these, Type II TA systems are widely studied and are established for their role in virulence in organisms like *Escherichia coli* and *Streptococcus pneumoniae*. Specificity is a general problem while designing drugs for homologous proteins because of the cross-talk between proteins. Polom *et al.* studied two homolog TA systems (YefM-YoeB and Axe-Txe) to understand the cross talk and specificity between these homologous complexes [158]. YefM–YoeB is one of the Type II TA system (endoribonuclease) dependent on ribosomes [159]. Axe-Txe is a broad spectrum TA system reported in gram positive organisms and homologous to YefM-YoeB [160]. They built Axe-Txe complex based on the crystal structure of YefM-YoeB in swissmodel. They followed Frankensteins's monster approach of fold recognition method to build the model. Models are evaluated using ProQ and MetaMQAP server. Protein-protein docking is carried out between toxin (Txe) and antitoxin (Axe) using HADDOCK. The three dimensional structural analysis and protein-protein docking provide the information of major residues involved in toxin-antitoxin complex formation. Further, site directed mutagenesis studies are carried out on

Txe toxin. YoeB functional residues are mutated onto Txe system to inspect the specificity between different toxin-antitoxin systems. These mutational studies revealed the specificity role of residue 83 (Asp in Txe and Tyr in YoeB) in YoeB-YefM and Txe-Axe systems. These structural insights may provide information to focus on TA systems for antibacterial drug discovery.

Molecular Dynamics

Molecular Dynamics as an Approach to Study Dynamic Aspects of Ligand-Protein Interactions

Antibacterial compounds usually interact with either bacterial cell walls, disrupting their integrity and destroying their homeostasis, or with enzymes involved in cell wall construction or cell division. All these structures are flexible and constantly undergo conformational changes, so both their full understanding and design of compounds affecting them requires insight into their dynamics. Molecular dynamics simulations provide a unique possibility to observe events in temporal and spatial scale inaccessible for most other methods. Principle behind MD simulations is the calculation of discrete atomic motions. Once a three-dimensional representation of a structure is created, all atoms are assigned with values and directions of forces acting on them, according to the chosen set of pre-defined properties corresponding to particular atom types, called 'force field'. After the initial assignment, atoms are moved - new coordinates and, consequently, new forces are calculated. After several steps an *in silico* simulation of the structure behaviour is prepared. The resulting atom trajectories are a rich source of information about the investigated system, under some conditions. The first one is the proper preparation of the system, the second – careful and thought out data analysis. Compared to these first and last steps, the middle one – simulation itself – might be the shortest one, even if computationally demanding and quite time-consuming.

Preparation of the System

The initial stages of a molecular dynamics study are crucial. Only if the *in silico* model of investigated structure is well-prepared and satisfyingly corresponds to the actual, native material, results may be conclusive. As long as there are no critical errors like missing atoms or overlapping molecules, neither the simulation engines nor trajectory analysis tools will report an error if conditions are improper or the protein model is of low quality – they will simply proceed with their algorithms. Obviously, calculations performed on incorrect starting structure, or with inappropriate force field will not yield conclusive results. If the problem remains unnoticed even at the simulation analysis step, some revolutionary discoveries might be postulated, which most probably do not match any experimental results. Little oversights at the beginning of a computational study may lead to regrettable waste of time and resources.

The first issue in design of an MD study is to define the scale of investigated events (Fig. **5**). Depending on one's expectations, different modifications of MD should be used. For instance, simulations of large membrane (or cell wall) patches may require coarse-grained simulation approach to reach reasonable timescales [161]. On the other hand, if more specific interactions between small molecule and cell wall or protein are to be investigated, all-atom approach would be more appropriate [162]. When both atomistic resolution and long timescale are needed, accelerated MD may be a good choice [163].

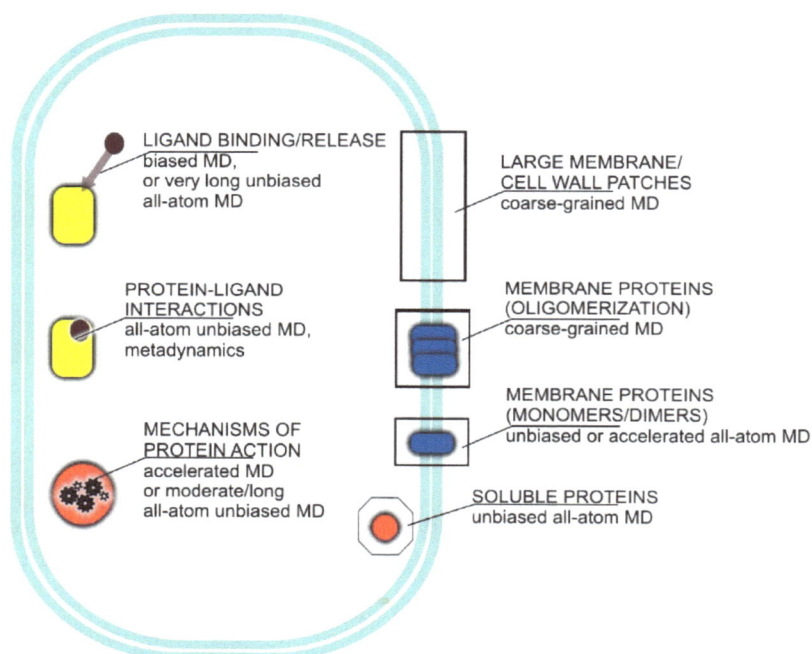

Fig. (5). Molecular dynamics approaches to antibacterial drug design and discovery.

Depending on the nature of the most important component of the simulation, various force fields can be chosen. For instance, all-atom simulations of proteins can be performed using force fields designed for proteins, *e.g.* Amber [164], CHARMM [165] or OPLS [166]. On the other hand, all-atom lipid simulations would require force fields adjusted for lipids. For example, Stockholm lipids is a force field prepared exclusively for lipids (although it uses the same atom names as Amber, and can be used together with that protein force wield in one simulation) [167]. Unfortunately, this well performing force field does not include numerous parameters for lipids essential in bacterial membranes. In contrary, CHARMM force field, originally developed for proteins, was recently extended with large number of lipid parameters, enabling construction of complicated membrane systems [168]. Also a Lipid14 force field, being an extension of Amber, offers a wide choice of lipid residues [169]. Notably, a useful comparison of the mentioned force fields was published recently [170]. It is worth mentioning, that when a force field of one's choice does not offer a particular topology, it can be easily created with automated tools [171]. However, one has to be aware that accurate parametrization of a molecule is much more challenging task, and automatic generation of parameters won't guarantee obtaining relevant results.

Except of the above-mentioned all-atom force fields, numerous coarse-grained force fields are available. They allow for construction of larger systems and reaching longer timescales thanks to joining atoms, functional groups, entire residues or molecules into grains. They are usually, however, less versatile than all-atom ones. This is due to the fact, that investigation of various phenomena requires various graining patterns. Coarse-grained force fields were recently described in more detail by Barnoud and Minticelli [161]. Notably, coarse-grained simulations may be used for initial equilibration of the system, that can be further processed as all-atom representation, which was recently applied by Berglund *et al.* [172].

Once the force field is chosen, the decision on the simulation program should be made. While force fields describe interactions between atoms and molecules and their choice may significantly affect results, the simulation engine utilizes them for calculations, and the code quality affects calculation speed. It is also responsible for interface quality. There are commercial MD packages, which frequently have intuitive user interface, with user support ensured by the developer. For instance, YASARA is a very user-friendly molecular modelling package which allows for quick simulation setup and real-time view of a simulated box [173]. Other popular packages include Scigress [174], MOE [113], Discovery Studio [175], Desmond [176], CHARMM [177] or AMBER [164]. User support and comfortable graphical user interface provided by commercial packages are of course an advantage, yet it is worth notice that *e.g.* NAMD [178], which is freely available for academic use, can be used together with VMD [179] as a graphic interface. On the other hand, Gromacs [180], which is a broadly used open-source molecular dynamics program, despite absence of GUI is a very attractive due to its speed, versatility and rich support from community.

Simulation

Despite the significant computational resources needed to perform an MD simulation, this is the shortest step of the study. The resources needed depend on the complexity of a simulated system – small water-soluble protein can be simulated in a small truncated octahedron simulation box which, together with GPU support, can be performed even on a reasonable quality personal computer [181], especially if only a docking refinement is needed. On the other hand, simulation of large membrane patches with lipopolysaccharides will force the use of a cuboid box with large amounts of water, which involves calculation of a large number of nonbonding interactions (Fig. **6**). Moreover, one should keep in mind that in most cases simulations should be repeated at least three times to prove reliability of results. Such simulations would take significant amount of time on a regular PC, and should rather be performed on larger clusters. In absence of such possibility, one can consider establishing a Beowulf cluster in a lab.

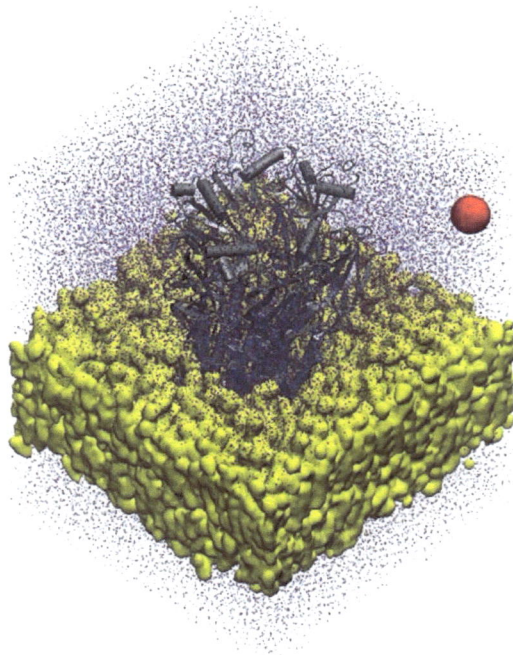

Fig. (6). Membrane-immersed protein simulation box. Increase of the membrane size causes enormous increase in the number of water molecules which involves the necessity of calculation of additional non-bonding interactions. The diameter of the red sphere presents the area of typical cut-off distance (1.2 nm).

Trajectory Analysis

Molecular dynamics simulations provide a wealth of data. Analysis of all variables is not always necessary or purposeful, however. In contrast to drug design studies on human proteins, where exact mechanism of action is important and subtle differences between conformational changes induced by drugs play crucial role, antibacterial drugs do not have to be that precise, since bacterial proteins usually do not have human counterparts. Therefore, in many drug design studies aiming at bacterial proteins MD is used just as a docking refinement and validation, or as a source of conformations further processed by virtual screening. Simulations performed in such works reach approximately 30 ns, which is too short to observe *e.g.* mechanisms of protein action. In these cases, analysis of protein-ligand contacts together with RMSD and RMSF is usually enough to fulfil the purpose of this part. On the other hand, when more detailed insight into protein function is needed, information theory-based methods like MutInf [182] or NbIT [183] may be useful. Analysis of ligand-membrane complex trajectories may in turn benefit *e.g.* from comparing solvent accessible area radial distribution functions or water penetration of the membrane core, measuring membrane thickness or lipid surface areas. Also in this case, however, ligand – lipid interactions are frequently among the most informative properties.

Application of Molecular Dynamics for Antibacterial Drug Discovery

A great part of studies on bacteria as infective agents focuses on bacterial barriers and their components. Bacterial cell walls, surrounding single cells, as well as components of biofilm, which is a form of collective bacterial life, are a potential target for antibacterial drugs. Moreover, these structures play an important role in protecting cell interior from undesired chemicals like antibiotics. Biofilm structure allows also for more efficient quorum sensing and easier sustaining sufficient concentrations of extracellular enzymes in the area. Therefore, deeper understanding of these structures and their properties would facilitate design of drugs that can permeate through them or destroy them.

A number of recent MD studies focus particularly on biofilms (Fig. **7**). For instance, Kuttel *et al.* investigated exopolysaccharide from *Burkholderia* biofilm with three methods: NMR, fluorescence microscopy and all-atom molecular dynamics [184]. The computational part of the study involved simulations of the polysaccharide together with hexane molecules or amphiphilic compounds, performed in CHARMM36 force field with NAMD. The saccharide topologies were modified to include O-methyl groups. Their simulations demonstrated, that the investigated exopolysaccharide is highly flexible in water environment. They also show that it can develop extensive interactions with hydrophobic ligand –

hexane, but these interactions were mostly nonspecific. Interestingly, a situation when polysaccharide form a pocket and surrounds the ligand was observed. Such interaction was quite stable, and it was able to persist for nanoseconds. Similar observation was made for the amphiphilic signalling molecule, which lasted inside the pocket formed by the chain for several nanoseconds. Another interesting observation for the signalling molecule was that it could 'walk' through the polysaccharide chain, which may be relevant mechanism in bacterial communication within a biofilm.

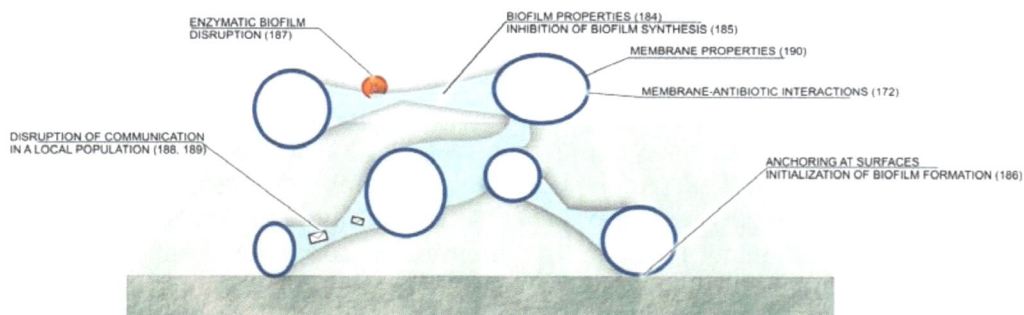

Fig. (7). Summary of recent applications of MD to antibacterial drug design.

Synthesis of biofilm is frequently addressed in studies of antibacterial compounds. Inhibition of the extracellular polymer formation would help to prevent biofilm formation on implants, which is a frequent problem. Gupta *et al.* address this issue with molecular modelling, virtual screening and molecular dynamics study [185]. They constructed a model of IcaA protein, responsible for biofilm formation in *Staphylococcus aureus*, a bacterium responsible for large part of iatrogenic infections. Authors suggest, that ligands such as clindamycin, linezolid, teicoplanin and CCG may affect the biofilm formation. In their study, they use Desmond to perform MD simulation that aims to refine a protein-ligand complex, which can be a basis for structure-based design of new derivatives. Unfortunately, authors decided to perform only one 20 ns simulation, which is too short timescale to draw any deeper conclusions. However, the study quite well presents a workflow of *in silico* antibacterial drug design.

A more complete, state-of-the-art *in silico* drug design study targeting biofilm formation was recently reported by Luo *et al.* The authors focus on the sortase A protein, utilized by *Streptococcus mutans* to anchor to solid surfaces and consequently initialize the biofilm formation [186]. As a result, *Streptococcus mutans* is able to cause dental caries. In order to find novel, effective inhibitors of the enzyme, they screened two libraries of compounds against its structure, and nine best hits were subjected to MD simulation, free energy calculations and ADMET analysis. First, the X-ray structure of protein was used for molecular docking performed with DOCK6. Then, MD simulations were performed in Gromacs, with Amber ff99SB force field. Notably, authors used dodecahedron box, which greatly decreases a number of water molecules to calculate. On the other hand, they used slightly old version of Gromacs (4.5.5), which did not support the Verlet scheme, that could give additional boost to simulations. Standard RMSD and RMSF analyses were performed, with known inhibitors – curcumin and kaempferol-3-rutinoside – as a reference.

If a biofilm is already built, there are some ways to destroy it. For instance, application of alginate lyase is suggested to be a promising approach in treatment of Pseudomonas aeruginosa infections. Cho *et al.* has recently undertaken an effort to model a complex of the enzyme with biofilm components, in order to design a more efficient mutant [187]. Specifically, they prepared a homology model of the enzyme in complex with alginate, which was subsequently simulated in AMBER with Amber ff03 force field. The simulation served as a relaxation and refinement step of modelling. On the basis of the final structure, Authors selected the residues crucial for the enzymatic activity. This was the starting point for site-directed mutagenesis, which confirmed conclusions drawn from simulations. The next step involved preparation of more active mutants, which eventually turned out to be successful.

Formation of the biofilm which is, as mentioned, a form of collective bacterial settlement, requires communication between participants. Disruption of this communication could be an interesting strategy in drug design. Recently, Rajamanikandan *et al.* focused on inhibition of LuxP protein, responsible for synthesis of bacterial autoinducers [188, 189]. Theirs *in silico* efforts resulted in discovery of potent inhibitors of the protein. The work of Rajamanikandan *et al.* is an example of MD application as a docking refinement tool. The virtual screening and subsequent fine docking performed with Schrödinger software were followed by short molecular dynamics simulations of the obtained complexes. Authors use Desmond in the first of described works, while in the second they employ Gromacs. These simulations were rather short and simple, but they surely contributed to successful identification of potent inhibitors with activity confirmed *in vitro*.

Some antibacterial compounds may interact with bacterial membranes, disturbing their structure. Such interactions also can be investigated with MD. Berglund *et al.* performed simulations of polymyxin B1 with inner and outer membranes of *Escherichia coli* [172]. Polymyxin B1 is a potent antibacterial lipopeptide.

Unfortunately, it presents severe side effects, which limit its use. Therefore, more detailed insights into its action would facilitate design of safer derivatives. Berglund *et al*. prepared several microseconds-long simulations to analyse the mechanism of polymyxin action. They prepared appropriate membrane patches with composition mimicking outer and inner membranes, *i.e.* asymmetric outer membrane with outer leaflet composed of lipopolysaccharide and inner membrane containing 75% phosphatidylethanolamine, 20% phosphatidylglycerol and 5% cardiolipin. An original approach was used for membrane preparation – bilayers were initially simulated as coarse-grained structures in MARTINI force field, and such equilibrated coarse-grained membranes were transcribed into all-atom representation with SUGAR-PIE methodology. Such initially equilibrated simulation boxes were supplemented with several copies of ligand and further simulated as all-atom system with GROMOS 53A6 and GROMOS-CKP parameters. Interestingly, no spontaneous penetration of LPS layer was observed, even when an additional pulling force was applied. However, an additional simulation of a simplified outer membrane composed exclusively of lipid A molecules resulted in an event of spontaneous penetration of the bilayer by a lipid tail of polymyxin. Analysis of this event indicated that interaction of alpha-gamma-diaminobutyric acid residues from polymyxin with phospholipid phosphate groups at the membrane surface, which facilitated insertion of the membrane tail. On the other hand, simulations of the inner membrane with polymyxin resulted in rapid spontaneous penetration of membrane, which deepened over the rest of simulation time. As the lipoprotein molecules dove deeper, the diaminobutyric acid residues dragged some water molecules into the membrane core.

Results of the above-mentioned study generally stay in line with experimental results. They clearly show, that the lipopolysaccharide – containing outer layer of the outer membrane of Gram-negative bacteria is a barrier difficult to cross by some drugs. Therefore, LPS properties are important from drug design point of view. Molecular dynamics may serve as a useful supplementary tool in studies on LPS. In their recent work, Blasco *et al*. investigated LPS with both NMR and MD [190]. They used CHARMM-GUI service for construction of simulation boxes, which were subsequently simulated in CHARMM and NAMD software with CHARMM force field. Results of MD were in agreement with NMR, proving reliability of the data. The experiment revealed, that polysaccharide chains of the antigen attached to lipid A are extended due to space limitations resulting from dense packing, and that calcium ions play important role in maintaining membrane structure.

QSAR

QSAR as a Method Applied in Drug Design

Growing worldwide incidence rate and the advent of multi-drug resistant bacteria raise the need for novel antibiotics. QSAR-based rational approaches are useful to meet the requirement of rational drug design as they render rapid and cost-efficient design and optimization of new drug candidates [191]. These techniques are based on statistics which correlate activities of ligand-protein interactions with molecular descriptors [14]. QSAR relies on the assumption that structurally related molecules tend to display similar pattern of interactions with molecular targets and similar biological activity. As a results it gives a mathematical description how these interactions and resulting pharmacological profile vary with the structural properties of the ligand. These models result from calculation of a correlation between experimentally determined biological activities and various molecular descriptors of small molecules and can be used for prediction of biological activity of an unknown compound. QSAR concept has been step-by-step developed from 0D to 2D [192]. In classical or 2D QSAR approaches, the biological activity is correlated to physical and chemical descriptors such as electronic, hydrophobic and steric features of molecules [14]. Due to limitations of these 2D models, 3D-QSAR has been developed with different advancements like CoMFA or CoMSiA. In 3D QSAR methods, in addition to physical and geometric features of ligands, quantum chemical features are also applied [14]. Some reports are highlighting also the limitations of 3D-QSAR. In order to overcome the limitations of 3D-QSAR, more advanced QSAR approaches like 4D, 5D and 6D-QSAR have been evolved [192]. A clear systematic multidimensional QSAR classification involves the static ligand representation (3D), multiple ligand representation (4D), ligand-based virtual or pseudo receptor models (5D), multiple solvation scenarios (6D) and real receptor or target-based receptor model data (7D) [193].Widely used QSAR methods involve recent fragment-based QSAR methods such as fragment-similarity-based QSAR (FS-QSAR), fragment-based QSAR (FB-QSAR), Hologram QSAR (HQSAR), and top priority fragment QSAR in addition to 3D- and nD-QSAR methods such as comparative molecular field analysis (CoMFA), comparative molecular similarity analysis (CoMSIA), Topomer CoMFA, self-organizing molecular field analysis (SOMFA), comparative molecular moment analysis (COMMA), autocorrelation of molecular surfaces properties (AMSP), weighted holistic invariant molecular (WHIM) descriptor-based QSAR (WHIM), grid-independent descriptors (GRIND)-based QSAR, 4D-QSAR, 5D-QSAR and 6D-QSAR methods [194].

The main steps of QSAR can be summarized as presented in Fig. (**8**) [14]. Cherkasov *et al.* [195] list possible reason of errors in QSAR modelling: failure to take account of data heterogeneity, use of inappropriate endpoint units, use of confounded descriptors, use of non-interpretable descriptors, errors in descriptor values, poor transferability of QSARs, inadequate or undefined applicability domain, unacknowledged omission of data points, use of inadequate data, replication of chemicals in a data set, narrow range of endpoint values, over-fitting of data, use of excessive numbers of descriptors in a QSAR, inadequate or missing statistic measures, incorrect calculation, lack of descriptor auto-scaling, misuse or misrepresentation of statistics, no consideration of distribution of residuals, inadequate training and/or test set selection, inadequate QSAR model validation and lack of mechanistic interpretation.

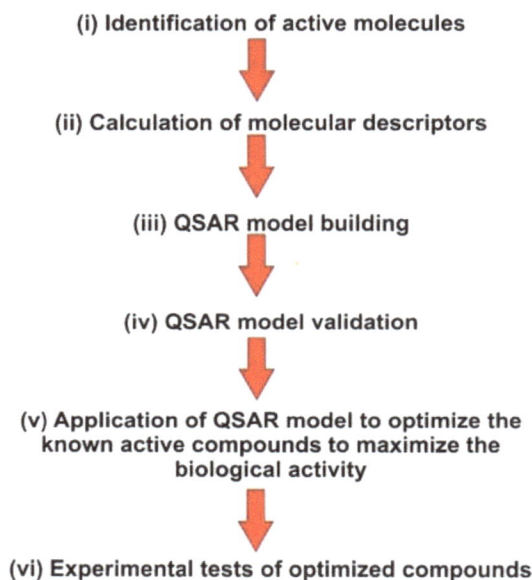

(i) Identification of active molecules

(ii) Calculation of molecular descriptors

(iii) QSAR model building

(iv) QSAR model validation

(v) Application of QSAR model to optimize the known active compounds to maximize the biological activity

(vi) Experimental tests of optimized compounds

Fig. (8). The main steps of QSAR.

Application of QSAR for Antibacterial Drug Discovery

There is a number of reported cases of application of QSAR methods to antibacterial drug discovery. In particular, those related to tuberculosis have been recently reviewed [191, 196 - 198].

Friggeri *et al.* [199] used 71 pyrrole derivatives active against *Mycobacterium tuberculosis* to generate through a recent new 3D QSAR protocol, 3D QSAutogrid/R, a number of predictive 3D QSAR models on compounds aligned by a previously reported pharmacophore model. The pharmacophore model was constructed using 32 imidazole derivatives with antitubercular activity and comprised of a hydrogen bond acceptor feature, two aromatic ring features, and a hydrophobic feature. 3 best monoprobe 3D QSAR models, depicting different interaction modes were selected for further analysis. A final multiprobe 3D QSAR model was then obtained representing the first quantitative pharmacophoric model able to correlate the structural features of pyrrole derivatives with their pharmacological activity. The model was validated by external set of 13 newly synthesized R-4-amino-3-isoxazolidinone derivatives which were found to be active at micromolar level against *Mycobacterium tuberculosis* and the predicted bioactivities were in good agreement with the experimental values. In particular, two derivatives of monocarbamates and dicarbamates displayed best pharmacological activity.

Lee *et al.* [200] modeled inhibitory activities of monocyclic nitroimidazoles against *Mycobacterium tuberculosis* deazaflavin-dependent nitroreductase (DDN) by application of molecular docking, pharmacophore alignment and CoMSIA techniques. First, they docked the compounds to DDN binding site, then constructed a pharmacophore model using GALAHAD and applied it as molecular alignment tool for measuring Mtb inhibitory activity to construct 3D-QSAR model. Pharmacophore model involved one hydrogen bond donor, five hydrogen bond acceptors, and two hydrophobic centers in a monocyclic nitroimidazole. A statistically significant CoMSIA resulted from a training set using pharmacophore-based molecular alignment. The q^2 was 0.681. The CoMSIA model displayed R^2 of 0.611 between the predicted and experimental activities against excluded test sets. The constructed model reveals that electrostatic, hydrophobic and hydrogen bonding interactions are crucial for ligand-enzyme interactions.

Shah *et al.* [201] used ligand-based and structure-based methods to study the physicochemical properties of 2,3-dideoxy hex-2-enopyranosid-4-uloses against *Mycobacterium tuberculosis* H37Rv. Statistically significant 3D-QSAR models with good correlation and predictive power resulted from CoMFA steric and electrostatic fields (R^2 of 0.797, q^2 of 0.589) and CoMSIA with combined steric, electrostatic, hydrophobic and hydrogen bond acceptor fields (R^2 of 0.867, q^2 of 0.570). Analysis of CoMFA and CoMSIA contours revealed that the presence of optimal size and length of steric groups around C-1 are crucial while substitution with electron acceptor group at C-6 position of enones leads to increased activity. Furthermore, molecular docking was applied to study ligand-protein interactions at the molecular level.

Lee *et al.* [202] studied a series of reverse hydroxamate derivatives with antibacterial activity against *E. coli* PDF, using 2D and 3D QSAR methods,

(CoMFA, CoMSIA), and hologram QSAR (HQSAR). Statistically significant models with good predictability were obtained from all three approaches (CoMFA R^2 of 0.957, q^2 of 0.569; CoMSIA R^2 of 0.924, q^2 of 0.520; HQSAR R^2 of 0.860, q^2 of 0.578). The best HQSAR model was constructed applying atoms, bonds, connections, hydrogen atoms and chirality information with a fragment size of 7-10. Among the generated models the CoMFA model displayed the best predictability and was mapped on the PDF binding site obtaining meaningful correlation between receptor binding site and the ligand-based CoMFA contour map.

Huang *et al*. [203] generated 2D-QSAR model based on molecular fingerprints to obtain the bioactive molecular fingerprints from a data set of DNA-gyrase inhibitors with new structure and mechanism. The fingerprints were converted into molecular fragments which were recombined to obtain compound library used subsequently for virtual screening with molecular docking software. 2D QSAR model was based on Learn Molecular Property protocol, as implemented in Pipeline Pilot (SciTegic Inc., USA). The Learn Molecular Property is a technique to derive a regression model which can build a partial least-squares regression of 2D QSAR model based on molecular descriptors. Fang *et al*. [204] used SYBYL X-2.0 to generate CoMFA and CoMSIA models for a series of flavonoids as DNA gyrase inhibitors. The q^2 for CoMFA was 0.743 and for CoMSIA 0.708 supporting high predictive capabilities. Molecular docking revealed that the studied flavonoids inhibited DNA gyrase by interacting with adenosine-triphosphate (ATP) pocket in a same orientation.

Yu *et al*. [205] reported synthesis, evaluation, and CoMFA study of 21 fluoroquinophenoxazine derivatives as bacterial topoisomerase IA inhibitors. As molecules in the set were relatively rigid, they used rigid core alignment. CoMFA analysis was carried out and resulted in reasonable statistics (q^2 of 0.688 and R^2 of 0.806). The predictive power model was investigated applying a test set of 7 compounds, obtaining R^2 of 0.767. Analysis of contour maps revealed that a moderate steric substituent would be favored at the 6 position of the quinophenoxazine moiety which can explain why 6-substituted amino derivatives were more potent than the 6-fluro compounds. Moreover, a bulky substituent is not tolerated at position 9 and electron rich group is required here. Kathiravan *et al*. [206] used series of new 2,4,6-tri-substituted pyridine derivatives which are topoisomerase inhibitors for building QSAR model. First, they obtained a five-point pharmacophore with one hydrophobic group (H4), four aromatic rings (R5, R6, R7 and R8). The pharmacophore model yielded a 3D-QSAR model with good partial least-square (PLS) statistic results. The compounds were also docked to topoisomerase binding site to study their pattern of ligand-protein interactions.

Yamaz *et al.* [207] performed 4D-QSAR studies on a series of 87 penicillin analogues using the electron conformational-genetic algorithm (EC-GA) approach. Hybrid 4D-QSAR approach (EC–GA) was used to explain the pharmacophore and to predict antibacterial activity. In this technique, each conformation of the compound is represented by a matrix (ECMC) with both electron structural parameters and interatomic distances as matrix elements. Multiple comparisons of these matrices made it possible to distinguish a smaller number of matrix elements (ECSA) which represent the pharmacophore groups.

Quorum sensing (QS) is communication between bacterial cells use by microorganisms to coordinate the expression of certain genes applying small signal compounds. This mechanism can regulate bacterial behaviors including bioluminescence, biofilm formation and reproduction. Quorum sensing inhibitors (QSIs) are an attractive alternative to the antibiotics and are not connected with producing drug resistance [208]. Wang *et al.* [208] studied the acute (15 min) and chronic (24 h) toxicity of some potential QSIs on both Gram-negative and Gram-positive bacteria. They generated QSAR models for both the acute and chronic toxicity, applying the interaction energies between QSIs and the relevant proteins, and the frontier orbital energies.

Li *et al.* [209] generated 2D and 3D QSAR models based on the electronic and hydrophobic properties of the quinolones, which were applied to quantify the effect of various structural features of the molecules on their genotoxicity variation. The analysis made it possible to conclude that quinolones with hydrophilic substituents with less H-bond donors and negative charge at the 1-position of the quinolone ring exhibited a positive correlation with genotoxicity increase.

Zanni *et al.* [210] developed *in silico* strategy based on QSAR molecular topology to identify synthetic molecules as antimicrobial agents not susceptible to one or several mechanisms of resistance such as: biofilms formation (BF), ionophore (IA) activity, epimerase (EI) activity or SOS system (RecA inhibition). Molecular topology paradigm studies the positions and interconnections among the atoms of a molecule using graph theory.

A few reports on QSAR for ribosome targeting compounds have been also published [211 - 213]. Setny and Trylska [213] searched for novel aminoglycosides by combining fragment-based virtual screening and 3D-QSAR scoring. The QSAR model, based on CoMFA and CoMSIA was generated for already reported ligands which were selected in order to cover both O5 and O6 substituted neamine derivatives, and to provide biological data that was possible to standardize.

Pharmacophore Models

Importance of Pharmacophore Models in Drug Design

Pharmacological activity of a drug is a consequence of its interactions with a molecular target. The ligand-protein interactions depend on chemical groups, bonds, and their 3D-arrangements towards each other. The 3D-orientations of chemical functionalities responsible for biological activity of a small molecule towards its target can be summarized by pharmacophore models [214] which can be described as molecular framework defining the necessary structural properties for compound pharmacological activity [14]. Pharmacophores are then applied to describe molecules on a 2D or 3D level by identification of the key elements responsible for molecular recognition [215]. In pharmacophore models, chemical functionalities are considered as features which can be derived from a series of active molecules or from protein-ligand interactions obtained from experimental approaches (X-ray, NMR) or molecular docking [214]. As chemical features used in pharmacophore model are well understood by medicinal chemists, these models are intuitive and their usage has been increasingly successful in computer-assisted drug discovery [216]. In spite of that, pharmacophore models have not fulfilled all expectations, in particular in demand to limit the costs of drug design and discovery [217].

If structure of a target is not known, pharmacophore models can be constructed applying the chemical characteristics of ligand set [218]. Such pharmacophore mapping is one of the main techniques in drug design in the absence of structural information of a target protein [219]. Binding site features can be then taken into by investigating the bioactive conformation of the studied compounds [220]. If target structural information is available, a pharmacophore model can be built using binding site characteristics [221]. Pharmacophore models which apply acidic/basic residues and hydrogen bond acceptors and donors as chemical features are considered to be most promising [222]. Pharmacophore models were initially applied to discovery of lead compounds but later the usage was extended to lead optimization [219]. Pharmacophore models can also be applied for virtual screening of large databases [221]. Pharmacophores are also applicable for ADME-tox modeling, side effect, and off-target prediction as well as target identification [215]. Most commonly used software for generating pharmacophore models includes DISCO, GASP and Catalyst with GASP and Catalyst performing better than DISCO in reproducing the pharmacophore models [223].

Pharmacophore model construction steps can be summarized as follows [14]: (i) identification of active compounds sharing the same mode of interactions with the molecular target of interest; (ii) defining atom types and connectivity for 2D pharmacophore models or ligand conformations for 3D models; (iii) ligand alignment; (iv) model building; (v) model selection and (vi) model validation. Construction of a pharmacophore model with balanced sensitivity and specificity is crucial to reduce false negative and false positive results, respectively [220]. Spatial constraints may be used for regions occupied by inactives and refined if the model is too restrictive [220]. The performance and applicability of pharmacophore models depends on the definition and positioning of chemical features and the superposition methods applied to align 3D pharmacophore models and the compounds [216].

Application of Pharmacophore Models for Antibacterial Drug Discovery

Ananthula *et al.* [224] constructed 3D pharmacophore model by using 21 diverse PDF inhibitors and HypoGen of Catalyst. The model was validated using 78 compounds. Pharmacophore model emphasized the significance of two acceptors, one donor and one hydrophobic feature for the pharmacological activity. The pharmacophore model was used for virtual screening of an in-house database and 10 compounds with top scores were selected. However, the virtual screening results have been not experimentally validated. The inhibitors were also docked into the binding site of PDF to gain insight into ligand-enzyme interactions.

Azam and Thathan [225] generated a pharmacophore model for DNA gyrase inhibitors using 49 molecules from a series of pyridine-3-carboxamide-6-yl-urea derivatives. The best fitted model AADDR.13 was constructed with R^2 of 0.918. and validated using test set molecules with R^2 of 0.78. They used XP molecular docking to identify key hydrogen bond interactions with ATP-binding pocket, which are crucial for inhibitor binding. They also calculated free binding energy using the MM-GBSA rescoring approach to validate the binding affinity. Finally, they performed 10 ns molecular dynamics simulations to determine the stability of selected ligand-protein complexes. Radwan and Abdel-Mageed [226] performed molecular modelling studies of quinoxaline-2-carboxamide 1,4-di-n-oxide derivatives as antimycobacterial agents. They used the LigandScout program to develop a pharmacophore model to further optimize the antimycobacterial activity of this series of compounds. Moreover, they used Dock6 to investigate the molecular interactions of the studied compounds with DNA gyrase.

Saha *et al.* [227] generated a 3D pharmacophore model for *Mycobacterium* sulfotransferase. Pharmacophore modelling was carried out using DISCOtech and GASP module of Sybyl-X 2.1. 5 molecules from various chemical classes were selected based on the assumption that the molecules bind with the binding site in a similar manner. 4 models were constructed after GASP (Genetic Algorithm Similarity Program) refinement of seven models (D-1 to D-7) generated by using

DISCOtech. The final GASP model-1 was characterized by two hydrogen bond acceptor, two hydrogen bond donor and four hydrophobic points.

Inhibitors of aryl acid adenylating enzymes (AAAE), involved in siderophore biosynthesis in *Mycobacterium tuberculosis*, are potential antitubercular agents [228]. Tawari and Degani [228] reported a robust pharmacophore model and investigation of structure-activity relationship of several nucleoside bisubstrate analogs as MbtA inhibitors. The constructed pharmacophore model revealed the significance of two hydrogen bond donors and one hydrogen bond acceptor features. Moreover, it was determined that an aromatic ring at the distal part of molecule away from the two aromatic rings of adenyl moiety is a critical feature for inhibitor binding.

Stapylococcus aureus sortase A enzyme participates in adherence of bacteria with the cell wall of host cell and can be an attractive molecular target for potential antibacterial agents against methicillin resistant *Staphylococcus aureus* [229]. Uddin *et al*. [229] identified 3D pharmacophoric features within a series of rhodanine, pyridazinone, and pyrazolethione analogs as *Staphylococcus aureus* Sortase A inhibitors. Pharmacophore model was built applying Genetic Algorithm with Linear Assignment of Hypermolecular Alignment of Database. The found pharmacophoric features were used to create alignment hypothesis for 3D QSAR.

Acinetobacter baumannii is a multi-drug resistant Gram-negative bacterium, which is opportunistic human pathogen. RND family efflux pumps are significant for multi-drug resistance in Gram-negative bacteria [230]. Yilmaz *et al*. [230] generated 3D-common features pharmacophore model by applying the HipHop method. The model revealed that the hydrogen bond acceptor feature of nitrogen in the thiazole ring and the oxygen of the amide substituted at the second position of the benzothiazole ring system were important for binding to the target protein.

Fluoroquinolones possess a broad spectrum of activity against Gram-negative and Gram-positive bacteria as well as mycobacteria and parasites. Fengxian and Reti [231] studied the genotoxicity values of 21 quinolones to establish a quantitative structure-activity relationship model and 3D Pharmacophore model separately to screen dominant substituent positions for the full factorial experimental design, which is used to analyze the main influence and second-order interaction effect of dominant positions and substituents on the genotoxicity of fluoroquinolones.

Ghorab *et al*. [232] reported synthesis, antimicrobial evaluation and molecular modelling of novel sulfonamides carrying a biologically active quinazoline nucleus. A LigandScout was used to obtain pharmacophore model for the *Staphylococcus aureus* growth inhibition. The degree of fitting of the test set compounds to the generated model revealed a qualitative measure of inhibition of

Staphylococcus aureus.

Tawari and Dagani [233] reported pharmacophore modelling and density functional theory analysis for a series of nitroimidazole compounds with antitubercular activity. The generated model involves 5 features: a nitro group, three hydrogen bond acceptor features, and a distal aromatic ring. SAR analysis clarified that hydrophobic substitutions at the para-position of distal aromatic ring could lead to more potent analogs.

Inosine 5'-monophosphate dehydrogenase (IMPDH) is a crucial enzyme for the de novo synthesis of guanosine nucleotides and constitutes an attractive drug target for the immunosuppressive, antiviral, antibacterial and anticancer therapeutic areas [234]. A chemical feature-based pharmacophore model of IMPDH inhibitors was constructed by applying HypoRefine protocol of Discovery Studio 2.5. The best model consisted of one hydrogen-bond donor, one hydrogen-bond acceptor, one aromatic ring and one hydrophobic feature, as well as two excluded volumes.

No pharmacophore models have been reported for ribosome-targeting compounds.

Virtual Screening

Virtual Screening as a Method of Searching Large Databases

In silico methods, such as virtual high throughput screening (VS) and *de novo* structure-based rational drug design are widely used and powerful approaches in drug discovery [235]. In particular, VS methods have been applied to economize on the time and cost of finding active molecules [235] as recent progress in hardware and software enabled quick screening of large databases of small compounds against a given target. Virtual screening is nowadays a method of choice to search large databases of compounds and to select compounds for *in vitro* testing (Fig. **9**) [236].

There are two main approaches for computational screening: structure-based virtual screening and ligand-based virtual screening. If a target 3D structure is available from experimental of molecular modelling studies, high-throughput docking is a method of choice. In virtual screening, the docking hit rates for water-soluble protein are approximately 5–10% of the molecules tested, resulting in hits with micromolar to mid-micromolar affinity [237]. These hit rates for soluble proteins are better than average HTS hit rates. High-throughput docking identifies compounds predicted to interact with a considered binding site as opposed to classical HTS which evaluates general capability of a ligand to bind, inhibit, or allosterically alter the target's function [238]. This method often applies limited conformational sampling of protein and ligand and a simplified approximation of binding energy in order to screen large libraries in a reasonably short time [238].

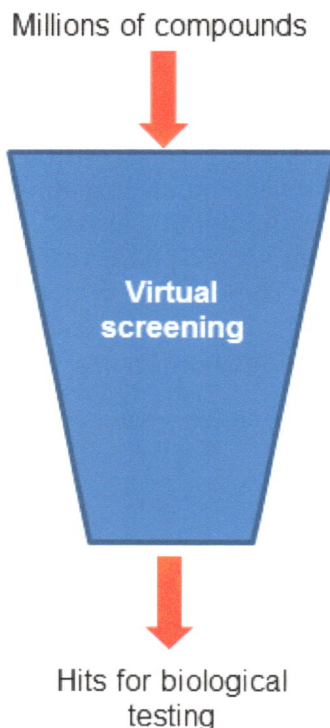

Fig. (9). The general idea of virtual screening.

Ligand-based approaches include similarity searching, QSAR models, and fingerprint and pharmacophore searching [235]. In particular, pharmacophore searches are nowadays a common tool for virtual screening of databases to find new active molecules which could be developed into drugs [239]. Pharmacophore screening is capable of finding molecules with different scaffolds, but with a similar 3D arrangement of most important interacting chemical functionalities [220]. The choice of a technique depends on the availability of information on ligands or a target. It can be recommended that a range of approaches is used in parallel to maximize the chance of identification a suitable hit for further optimization [235]. It should be emphasized that both ligand- and structure-based approaches have been successfully applied in many research projects [235]. Although structure-based methods are more frequently applied, ligand-based methods have resulted in discovery of a great number of potent drugs [14].

A very popular approach to identification of active compounds for a given target when structural data on target is available is to screen fragments. Fragment-based drug discovery (FBDD) has brought a revolution in drug design and discovery [240] with many FBDD leads being developed into clinical trials or approved in the past few years [241]. Fragment-based virtual screening aims to identify small chemical fragments, which may bind only weakly to the subpockets of a given target, and then growing them or combining them to obtain a lead with a higher affinity [242].

Application of Virtual Screening for Antibacterial Drug Discovery

Tomašić *et al.* [243] carried out virtual screening for potential ATP-competitive inhibitors targeting MurC and MurD ligases, using a protocol of consecutive hierarchical filters. Experimental validation of selected compounds confirmed that they found weak inhibitors possessing dual inhibitory activity which require further optimization. Samal *et al.* [244] constructed a homology model of MurD from *Salmonella typhimurium* using MODELLER software and refined the model in molecular dynamics simulations using GROMACS. The refined model was applied for virtual screening of Zinc Database using Dockblaster software. The best inhibitor, 3-(amino methyl)-n-(4-methoxyphenyl)aniline, was efficient in inhibition of peptidoglycan biosynthesis.

Howard *et al.* [245] identified a structurally novel class of PDF inhibitors containing a 2-thioxo-thiazolidin-4-one heterocycle substituted by an arylidene group at the 5-position and a hexanoic acid side chain at the 3-position using independently high-throughput screening and virtual ligand screening. Data mining and analogue made it possible to derive a structure-activity relationship for the side chain region which is in accordance with the docked structure. Gao *et al.* [246] reported ligand and structure-based approaches for the identification of PDF inhibitors. They built a pharmacophore model for PDF inhibitors and used it to screen Zinc database. The best compounds were docked to PDF binding site and their pharmacokinetics and toxicity were evaluated using OSIRIS software. However, this study lacks experimental validation.

Bacterial DNA gyrase is often subjected to virtual screening. Ghosh and Bagchi [247] searched for novel compounds with anti-tubercular activity and constructed QSAR models for subsequent usage in virtual screening. QSAR models were built based on structurally related fluoroquinolone derivatives which are DNA gyrase inhibitors. The models were used to screen a library of 5280 compounds based on fluoroquinolone template and the best compounds were docked to DNA gyrase active site. The authors concluded that hydrophobic characteristics of the compounds accompanied by few hydrogen bond interactions are necessary for antimicrobial activity for the fluoroquinolone derivatives. This study also lacks experimental validation. Kolaric and Minovski [248] used a similar approach for this purpose. Maharaj and Soliman [249] proposed 10 compounds as DNA gyrase inhibitors by combination of homology modelling, pharmacophore/structure-based virtual screening, molecular dynamics simulations and per-residue energy contribution. The compounds displayed better computed binding energy with DNA gyrase than novobiocin. No experimental validation is provided. Islam and Pillay [250] used pharmacophore model for virtual screening to search for DNA gyrase inhibitors. The best compounds were subjected to molecular docking and subsequent molecular dynamics, however no experimental validation is provided. Saxena *et al.* [251] used a similar approach and constructed a pharmacophore model for DNA gyrase inhibitors which consists of HBA, HY, and RA features and used this model to screen their in-house database. *In vitro* enzymatic inhibition studies for 15 most promising candidates revealed that the compounds exhibit inhibition at 30 µM. The same research group used structure-based virtual screening to screen a commercial Asinex database [252]. They found 15 compounds with IC_{50} values in the range of 1.5-45.5 µM against *Mycobacterium smegmatics* GyrB and 1.16-25 µM in MTB supercoiling assay. Lead 11 was the most promising compound with inhibition of MTB DNA gyrase supercoiling with an IC50 of 1.16±0.25 µM, and *Mycobacterium smegmatics* GyrB IC50 of 1.5±0.12 µM. Werner *et al.* [253] reported computer-aided identification of novel 3,5-substituted rhodanine derivatives with activity against *Staphylococcus aureus* DNA gyrase. They used the virtual screening tool Shape Signatures to screen for molecules with shape similar to novobiocin, a known gyrase B inhibitor. The best compounds were validated in molecular docking. In order to experimentally confirm these results MIC were determined as well as inhibition of DNA gyrase was evaluated.

Sirdevi *et al.* [254] used structure-based virtual screening against *Mycobacterium tuberculosis* topoisomerase I (Topo I). The found hit, hydroxycamptothecin, was active at 6.25 µM and was optimized to obtain its 15 derivatives. The most promising compound was screened for *in vivo* using zebrafish model and was found to be more potent than first line anti-tubercular drugs, isoniazid and rifampicin. Other reported case of virtual screening against various topoisomerases concern compounds with anticancer activity.

Chan *et al.* [255] identified a new class of FtsZ inhibitors bearing the pyrimidine-quinuclidine scaffold by structure-based virtual screening and *in vitro* screening of natural products library. Similar approach but without experimental validation was used by Vijayalakshmi *et al.* [256]. They also performed molecular dynamics of selected ligand-protein complexes.

Pérez-Castillo *et al.* [257] derived QSAR models for FabH inhibitors and used them for virtual screening. QSAR models were constructed for a diverse dataset of 296 FabH inhibitors applying an in-house modeling workflow. The models showed high fitting, robustness, and generalization capabilities. They concluded that at least for FabH inhibitors, virtual screening performance is not guaranteed by predictive QSAR models.

There is no reported virtual screening experiment for ribosomes, however the availability of high-resolution ribosome structures makes such experiments possible. The only ribosome-associated case of virtual screening concerns ribosomal phosphoprotein P1 (RPP1) which is acidic phosphoprotein that in association with neutral phosphoprotein P0 and acidic phosphoprotein P2 forms ribosomal P protein complex as (P1)2-P0-(P2)2 [258]. It should be stressed that popular software for virtual screening, such as virtual screening workflow in Schrödinger software are tailored for proteins and may not perform optimally for nucleic acids.

Prediction of Drug-Likeness and ADMET Properties

The term drug-likeness is usually understood as a set of functional groups and/or physicochemical properties which are common for most registered drugs. The basic and simplest method to estimate drug-likeness is Lipinski's rule of five. According to this rule, most drugs possess molecular mass lower or equal 500, lipophilicity (log P) lower or equal 5, the number of hydrogen bond donors lower or equal 5 and the number of hydrogen bon acceptors lower or equal 10. Although Lipinski's rule is a very useful guideline for orally bioavailable small-molecule drug design, it has to some extent been overemphasized. Firstly, only a half of all FDA-approved small-molecule drugs are both used orally and comply with the 'rule-of-five' [259]. Secondly, it does not cover natural product and semisynthetic natural product drugs, which constitute over one-third of all marketed small-molecule drugs. Drug-likeness may be also estimated by application of functional group filters, by examination of building blocks of common drugs or by defining with structural descriptors the chemical space occupied by common drugs and referring it to the investigated compounds.

The applicability of drug-likeness filters for antibacterial drug discovery is, however, limited [260]. At first, these filters assume that the drug is administered orally which is not the case for many antibiotics administered by injection. The properties of these compounds may lie outside the designated range as they can be more polar and possess more ionizable groups for better water solubility. Second, drug-likeness rules are uniform through drug and target classes while it has been observed that many antibiotics are outliers of Lipinski's rule and possess unique physicochemical properties (*e.g.* oral and parenteral cephalosporins, the glycopeptide antibiotics, the ansamycin antibiotics).

The term ADMET describes the disposition of a pharmaceutical compound within an organism. In the case of orally administered drugs, their pharmaceutical effect depends on several factors: absorption in a digestive tract, the first-pass effect (phenomenon of drug metabolism whereby the concentration of a drug is greatly reduced before it reaches the systemic circulation), the active level of the drug in the bloodstream and time within it is reached, the ability of a drug to reach its site of action and the way and efficiency of its excretion. Some of these processes are additionally affected by specific interactions of a drug with various proteins (*e.g.* transport proteins or deactivating enzymes). Usually, preliminary screening aimed to exclude compounds with unfavorable pharmacokinetic profile from experimental studies are performed with usage of computational methods.

The applicability of models such as model of human passive intestinal absorption for discovery of antibiotics is also limited [260]. In such models, it is assumed that orally administered drug would undergo passive absorption from gastrointestinal (GI) tract. Although a number of antibiotics, such as sparfloxacin and chloramphenicol are absorbed passively through the GI epithelium, a large fraction of antibacterials (*e.g.* most oral cephalosporins) are a substrate for biological transporters which leads to different structure-activity relationship, in particular different effect of physicochemical properties on biological activity.

SUMMARY AND PERSPECTIVE

Development of a new drug starting from an idea till reaching the market requires significant time (10-15 years) and money (about 100 mln euro). At the beginning of medicinal chemistry, discovery of new medicinal substances was mostly accidental and became more rational with the development of chemistry and pharmacology. However, only the progress in structural biology and bioinformatics enabled fully rational drug target-oriented design which made it possible to limit both time and cost involved in drug discovery. Indeed, it is estimated that computer-assisted techniques allow to reduce the cost of drug discovery by 50%.

In the light of above, in recent years the importance of computer-aided drug design techniques has increased to become an established and powerful approach for discovery of new potent molecules. Computer-aided drug design applies the structural information of either the target (structure-based) or known ligands with bioactivity (ligand-based) to enable identification of promising drug molecules. Structure-based and ligand-based techniques to develop new inhibitors of bacterial targets have made a valuable contribution to antibacterial drug discovery in recent years, participating in the discovery of a number of molecules that have either reached the market or entered clinical trials. It can be expected that further progress will be achieved in this area with the development of computer hardware and software and availability of computational resources. In particular, capabilities of molecular dynamics might be greatly increased due to the possibility to reach new timescale levels.

In spite of these successes, there are specific problems and challenges connected with application of CADD to antibacterial drug discovery. One of the remaining challenges of structural biology is to address integral membrane proteins, which include many key drug targets. Moreover, CADD techniques enable to design the compound active on a given target, often without considerations if a molecule is able to reach the target. It is thus necessary to develop rules for effective bacterial penetration to be used for filtering compound libraries instead of Lipinski's filters. Moreover, CADD methods are only partially capable to address the problem of antibiotic resistance. However, progress in *in silico* pharmacology and toxicology allows to design safer molecules which is important for antibacterial drugs used in relatively high concentrations.

In this review, we covered recent progress in application of molecular modeling techniques for antibacterial drug design and discovery to facilitate progress in the field. The provided examples of successful antibacterial drug discovery may help to deliver twenty-first century antibiotics capable to control infections in the resistance era.

CONSENT FOR PUBLICATION

Not applicable.

CONFLICT OF INTEREST

The authors declare no conflict of interest, financial or otherwise.

ACKNOWLEDGEMENTS

The paper was developed using the equipment purchased within the project "The equipment of innovative laboratories doing research on new medicines used in the therapy of civilization and neoplastic diseases" within the Operational Program Development of Eastern Poland 2007-2013, Priority Axis I Modern Economy, operations I.3 Innovation promotion. P.M and A.P have received funding from the European Union's Horizon 2020 research and innovation programme under the Marie Sklodowska Curie grant agreement No. 642620.

REFERENCES

[1]   Aminov R. History of antimicrobial drug discovery: Major classes and health impact. Biochem Pharmacol 2017; 133: 4-19.
        [http://dx.doi.org/10.1016/j.bcp.2016.10.001] [PMID: 27720719]

[2]   Kaczor AA, Polski A, Sobótka-Polska K, Pachuta-Stec A, Makarska-Bialokoz M, Pitucha M. Novel antibacterial compounds and their drug targets - successes and challenges. Curr Med Chem 2017; 24(18): 1948-82.
        [http://dx.doi.org/10.2174/0929867323666161213102127] [PMID: 27978802]

[3]   Schmieder R, Edwards R. Insights into antibiotic resistance through metagenomic approaches. Future Microbiol 2012; 7(1): 73-89.
        [http://dx.doi.org/10.2217/fmb.11.135] [PMID: 22191448]

[4]   Mahajan GB, Balachandran L. Sources of antibiotics: Hot springs. Biochem Pharmacol 2017; 134: 35-41.
        [http://dx.doi.org/10.1016/j.bcp.2016.11.021] [PMID: 27890726]

[5]   Lewis K. New approaches to antimicrobial discovery. Biochem Pharmacol 2017; 134: 87-98.
        [http://dx.doi.org/10.1016/j.bcp.2016.11.002] [PMID: 27823963]

[6]   Martens E, Demain AL. The antibiotic resistance crisis, with a focus on the United States. J Antibiot (Tokyo) 2017; 7095: 520-6.

[7]   Fernandes P, Martens E. Antibiotics in late clinical development. Biochem Pharmacol 2017; 133: 152-63.
        [http://dx.doi.org/10.1016/j.bcp.2016.09.025] [PMID: 27687641]

[8]   Bush K, Page MG. What we may expect from novel antibacterial agents in the pipeline with respect to resistance and pharmacodynamic principles. J Pharmacokinet Pharmacodyn 2017; 44(2): 113-32.
        [http://dx.doi.org/10.1007/s10928-017-9506-4] [PMID: 28161807]

[9]   Bansal AK. Role of bioinformatics in the development of new antibacterial therapy. Expert Rev Anti Infect Ther 2008; 6(1): 51-65.
        [http://dx.doi.org/10.1586/14787210.6.1.51] [PMID: 18251664]

[10]   Krishnamurthy M, Moore RT, Rajamani S, Panchal RG. Bacterial genome engineering and synthetic biology: combating pathogens. BMC Microbiol 2016; 16(1): 258.
        [http://dx.doi.org/10.1186/s12866-016-0876-3] [PMID: 27814687]

[11]   Guzmán-Trampe S, Ceapa CD, Manzo-Ruiz M, Sánchez S. Synthetic biology era: Improving antibiotic's world. Biochem Pharmacol 2017; 134: 99-113.
        [http://dx.doi.org/10.1016/j.bcp.2017.01.015] [PMID: 28159623]

[12]   Pulido MR, García-Quintanilla M, Gil-Marqués ML, McConnell MJ. Identifying targets for antibiotic development using omics technologies. Drug Discov Today 2016; 21(3): 465-72.
        [http://dx.doi.org/10.1016/j.drudis.2015.11.014] [PMID: 26691873]

[13]   Taft CA, Da Silva VB, Da Silva CH. Current topics in computer-aided drug design. J Pharm Sci 2008; 97(3): 1089-98.
        [http://dx.doi.org/10.1002/jps.21293] [PMID: 18214973]

[14]   Leelananda SP, Lindert S. Computational methods in drug discovery. Beilstein J Org Chem 2016; 12: 2694-718.
        [http://dx.doi.org/10.3762/bjoc.12.267] [PMID: 28144341]

[15]   Ekins S, Mestres J, Testa B. In silico pharmacology for drug discovery: applications to targets and beyond. Br J Pharmacol 2007; 152(1): 21-37.
        [http://dx.doi.org/10.1038/sj.bjp.0707306] [PMID: 17549046]

[16]   Silver LL. Challenges of antibacterial discovery. Clin Microbiol Rev 2011; 24(1): 71-109.
        [http://dx.doi.org/10.1128/CMR.00030-10] [PMID: 21233508]

[17]   Singh SB, Young K, Silver LL. What is an "ideal" antibiotic? Discovery challenges and path forward. Biochem Pharmacol 2017; 133: 63-73.
[http://dx.doi.org/10.1016/j.bcp.2017.01.003] [PMID: 28087253]

[18]   Dodds DR. Antibiotic resistance: A current epilogue. Biochem Pharmacol 2017; 134: 139-46.
[http://dx.doi.org/10.1016/j.bcp.2016.12.005] [PMID: 27956111]

[19]   Bérdy J. Thoughts and facts about antibiotics: where we are now and where we are heading. J Antibiot 2012; 65(8): 385-95.
[http://dx.doi.org/10.1038/ja.2012.27] [PMID: 22511224]

[20]   Munita JM, Arias CA. Mechanisms of Antibiotic Resistance 2016. http://www.ncbi.nlm.nih.gov/pmc/articles/PMC4888801/
[http://dx.doi.org/10.1128/microbiolspec.VMBF-0016-2015]

[21]   Martinez JL. General principles of antibiotic resistance in bacteria. Drug Discov Today Technol 2014; 11: 33-9.
[http://dx.doi.org/10.1016/j.ddtec.2014.02.001] [PMID: 24847651]

[22]   Wright GD. Antibiotic adjuvants: Rescuing antibiotics from resistance. Trends Microbiol 2016; 24(11): 862-71.
[http://dx.doi.org/10.1016/j.tim.2016.06.009] [PMID: 27430191]

[23]   Spengler G, Kincses A, Gajdács M, Amaral L. New roads leading to old destinations: Efflux pumps as targets to reverse multidrug resistance in bacteria. Mol Basel Switz 2017; 22(3)

[24]   Ventola CL. The antibiotic resistance crisis: part 1: causes and threats. P&T 2015; 40(4): 277-83.
[PMID: 25859123]

[25]   Steinbuch KB, Fridman M. Mechanisms of resistance to membrane-disrupting antibiotics in Gram-positive and Gram-negative bacteria. MedChemComm 2016; 7(1): 86-102.
[http://dx.doi.org/10.1039/C5MD00389J]

[26]   Utili R. (Gram-positive bacterial infections resistant to antibiotic treatment). Ann Ital Med Interna Organo Uff Della Soc Ital. Med Interna 2001; 16(4): 205-19.

[27]   Witte W, Cuny C, Klare I, Nübel U, Strommenger B, Werner G. Emergence and spread of antibiotic-resistant Gram-positive bacterial pathogens. Int J Med Microbiol 2008; 298(5-6): 365-77.
[http://dx.doi.org/10.1016/j.ijmm.2007.10.005] [PMID: 18325835]

[28]   Khoshnood S, Heidary M, Mirnejad R, Bahramian A, Sedighi M, Mirzaei H. Drug-resistant gram-negative uropathogens: A review. Biomed Pharmacother 2017; 94: 982-94.
[http://dx.doi.org/10.1016/j.biopha.2017.08.006] [PMID: 28810536]

[29]   Gadakh B, Van Aerschot A. Renaissance in antibiotic discovery: Some novel approaches for finding drugs to treat bad bugs. Curr Med Chem 2015; 22(18): 2140-58.
[http://dx.doi.org/10.2174/0929867322666150319115828] [PMID: 25787965]

[30]   Ferreira RS, Andricopulo AD. Structure-based drug design to overcome drug resistance: challenges and opportunities. Curr Pharm Des 2014; 20(5): 687-93.
[http://dx.doi.org/10.2174/13816128200514021416 1949] [PMID: 23688077]

[31]   Finn J. Application of SBDD to the discovery of new antibacterial drugs. Methods Mol Biol 2012; 841: 291-319.
[http://dx.doi.org/10.1007/978-1-61779-520-6_13] [PMID: 22222458]

[32]   Lewis K. Platforms for antibiotic discovery. Nat Rev Drug Discov 2013; 12(5): 371-87.
[http://dx.doi.org/10.1038/nrd3975] [PMID: 23629505]

[33]   Coates A, Hu Y, Bax R, Page C. The future challenges facing the development of new antimicrobial drugs. Nat Rev Drug Discov 2002; 1(11): 895-910.
[http://dx.doi.org/10.1038/nrd940] [PMID: 12415249]

[34]   Laddomada F, Miyachiro MM, Dessen A. Structural insights into protein-protein interactions involved in bacterial cell wall biogenesis. Antibiot Basel Switz 2016; 5(2)
[http://dx.doi.org/10.3390/antibiotics5020014]

[35]   Liu Y, Breukink E. The membrane steps of bacterial cell wall synthesis as antibiotic targets. Antibiot Basel Switz 2016; 5(3)
[http://dx.doi.org/10.3390/antibiotics5030028]

[36]   Katz AH, Caufield CE. Structure-based design approaches to cell wall biosynthesis inhibitors. Curr Pharm Des 2003; 9(11): 857-66.
[http://dx.doi.org/10.2174/1381612033455305] [PMID: 12678870]

[37]   Kouidmi I, Levesque RC, Paradis-Bleau C. The biology of Mur ligases as an antibacterial target. Mol Microbiol 2014; 94(2): 242-53.
[http://dx.doi.org/10.1111/mmi.12758] [PMID: 25130693]

[38]   Hrast M, Sosič I, Sink R, Gobec S. Inhibitors of the peptidoglycan biosynthesis enzymes MurA-F. Bioorg Chem 2014; 55: 2-15.
[http://dx.doi.org/10.1016/j.bioorg.2014.03.008] [PMID: 24755374]

[39]   Sangshetti JN, Khan FA, Shinde DB. Peptide deformylase: a new target in antibacterial, antimalarial and anticancer drug discovery. Curr Med Chem 2015; 22(2): 214-36.
[http://dx.doi.org/10.2174/0929867321666140826115734] [PMID: 25174923]

[40]   Tse-Dinh Y-C. Targeting bacterial topoisomerases: how to counter mechanisms of resistance. Future Med Chem 2016; 8(10): 1085-100.
[http://dx.doi.org/10.4155/fmc-2016-0042] [PMID: 27285067]

[41]   Kathiravan MK, Khilare MM, Nikoomanesh K, Chothe AS, Jain KS. Topoisomerase as target for antibacterial and anticancer drug discovery. J Enzyme Inhib Med Chem 2013; 28(3): 419-35.
[http://dx.doi.org/10.3109/14756366.2012.658785] [PMID: 22380774]

[42]   Azam MA, Thathan J, Jubie S. Dual targeting DNA gyrase B (GyrB) and topoisomerse IV (ParE) inhibitors: A review. Bioorg Chem 2015; 62: 41-63.
[http://dx.doi.org/10.1016/j.bioorg.2015.07.004] [PMID: 26232660]

[43]   Song H, Ao G-Z, Li H-Q. Novel FabH inhibitors: an updated article literature review (July 2012 to June 2013). Expert Opin Ther Pat 2013; 24(1): 19-27.

[44]   Panda D, Bhattacharya D, Gao QH, *et al.* Identification of agents targeting FtsZ assembly. Future Med Chem 2016; 8(10): 1111-32.
[http://dx.doi.org/10.4155/fmc-2016-0041] [PMID: 27284850]

[45]   Schaffner-Barbero C, Martín-Fontecha M, Chacón P, Andreu JM. Targeting the assembly of bacterial cell division protein FtsZ with small molecules. ACS Chem Biol 2012; 7(2): 269-77.
[http://dx.doi.org/10.1021/cb2003626] [PMID: 22047077]

[46]   Lambert T. Antibiotics that affect the ribosome. Rev - Off Int Epizoot 2012; 31(1): 57-64.
[http://dx.doi.org/10.20506/rst.31.1.2095] [PMID: 22849268]

[47]   Franceschi F, Duffy EM. Structure-based drug design meets the ribosome. Biochem Pharmacol 2006; 71(7): 1016-25.
[http://dx.doi.org/10.1016/j.bcp.2005.12.026] [PMID: 16443192]

[48]   Chavali AK, D'Auria KM, Hewlett EL, Pearson RD, Papin JA. A metabolic network approach for the identification and prioritization of antimicrobial drug targets. Trends Microbiol 2012; 20(3): 113-23.
[http://dx.doi.org/10.1016/j.tim.2011.12.004] [PMID: 22300758]

[49]   Kim J-H, O'Brien KM, Sharma R, *et al.* A genetic strategy to identify targets for the development of drugs that prevent bacterial persistence. Proc Natl Acad Sci USA 2013; 110(47): 19095-100.
[http://dx.doi.org/10.1073/pnas.1315860110] [PMID: 24191058]

[50]   Singh V, Mizrahi V. Identification and validation of novel drug targets in Mycobacterium tuberculosis.

Drug Discov Today 2017; 22(3): 503-9.
[http://dx.doi.org/10.1016/j.drudis.2016.09.010] [PMID: 27649943]

[51]   Langridge GC, Phan M-D, Turner DJ, *et al.* Simultaneous assay of every *Salmonella Typhi* gene using one million transposon mutants. Genome Res 2009; 19(12): 2308-16.
[http://dx.doi.org/10.1101/gr.097097.109] [PMID: 19826075]

[52]   Xiang Z. Advances in homology protein structure modeling. Curr Protein Pept Sci 2006; 7(3): 217-27.
[http://dx.doi.org/10.2174/138920306777452312] [PMID: 16787261]

[53]   Webb B, Sali A. Comparative protein structure modeling using modeller. Curr Protoc Protein Sci 2016. 86:2.9.1-2.9.37

[54]   Jacobson MP, Pincus DL, Rapp CS, *et al.* A hierarchical approach to all-atom protein loop prediction. Proteins 2004; 55(2): 351-67.
[http://dx.doi.org/10.1002/prot.10613] [PMID: 15048827]

[55]   Andrew JW. 2012. Abagyan. R. (eds.), Homology modeling: Methods and protocols. Humana Press cop. 2012, 857

[56]   Altschul SF, Gish W, Miller W, Myers EW, Lipman DJ. Basic local alignment search tool. J Mol Biol 1990; 215(3): 403-10.
[http://dx.doi.org/10.1016/S0022-2836(05)80360-2] [PMID: 2231712]

[57]   Altschul SF, Madden TL, Schäffer AA, *et al.* Gapped BLAST and PSI-BLAST: a new generation of protein database search programs. Nucleic Acids Res 1997; 25(17): 3389-402.
[http://dx.doi.org/10.1093/nar/25.17.3389] [PMID: 9254694]

[58]   https://blast.ncbi.nlm.nih.gov/Blast.cgi

[59]   http://www.ebi.ac.uk/Tools/sss/fasta/

[60]   http://www.ebi.ac.uk/Tools/hmmer/

[61]   Pearson WR. An introduction to sequence similarity ("homology") searching. Curr Protoc Bioinforma 2013. Chapter 3: Unit3.1

[62]   Sadreyev RI, Grishin NV. Accurate statistical model of comparison between multiple sequence alignments. Nucleic Acids Res 2008; 36(7): 2240-8.
[http://dx.doi.org/10.1093/nar/gkn065] [PMID: 18285364]

[63]   http://www.ebi.ac.uk/Tools/msa/

[64]   Tong J, Pei J, Otwinowski Z, Grishin NV. Refinement by shifting secondary structure elements improves sequence alignments. Proteins 2015; 83(3): 411-27.
[http://dx.doi.org/10.1002/prot.24746] [PMID: 25546158]

[65]   Forrest LR, Tang CL, Honig B. On the accuracy of homology modeling and sequence alignment methods applied to membrane proteins. Biophys J 2006; 91(2): 508-17.
[http://dx.doi.org/10.1529/biophysj.106.082313] [PMID: 16648166]

[66]   http://www.vls3d.com/links/bioinformatics/3d-structure-prediction/modeling-loops

[67]   Raval A, Piana S, Eastwood MP, Dror RO, Shaw DE. Refinement of protein structure homology models *via* long, all-atom molecular dynamics simulations. Proteins 2012; 80(8): 2071-9.
[PMID: 22513870]

[68]   Chothia C, Lesk AM. The relation between the divergence of sequence and structure in proteins. EMBO J 1986; 5(4): 823-6.
[PMID: 3709526]

[69]   https://services.mbi.ucla.edu/SAVES/

[70]   Wiederstein M, Sippl MJ. ProSA-web: interactive web service for the recognition of errors in three-dimensional structures of proteins. Nucleic Acids Res 2007. 35(Web Server issue): W407-410

[http://dx.doi.org/10.1093/nar/gkm290]

[71]   Lüthy R, Bowie JU, Eisenberg D. Assessment of protein models with three-dimensional profiles. Nature 1992; 356(6364): 83-5.
[http://dx.doi.org/10.1038/356083a0] [PMID: 1538787]

[72]   Rost B, Schneider R, Sander C. Protein fold recognition by prediction-based threading. J Mol Biol 1997; 270(3): 471-80.
[http://dx.doi.org/10.1006/jmbi.1997.1101] [PMID: 9237912]

[73]   de la Cruz X, Thornton JM. Factors limiting the performance of prediction-based fold recognition methods. Protein Sci 1999; 8(4): 750-9.
[http://dx.doi.org/10.1110/ps.8.4.750] [PMID: 10211821]

[74]   Dorn M, E Silva MB, Buriol LS, Lamb LC. Three-dimensional protein structure prediction: Methods and computational strategies. Comput Biol Chem 2014; 53PB: 251-76.
[http://dx.doi.org/10.1016/j.compbiolchem.2014.10.001] [PMID: 25462334]

[75]   Kocher JP, Rooman MJ, Wodak SJ. Factors influencing the ability of knowledge-based potentials to identify native sequence-structure matches. J Mol Biol 1994; 235(5): 1598-613.
[http://dx.doi.org/10.1006/jmbi.1994.1109] [PMID: 8107094]

[76]   Huang ES, Subbiah S, Levitt M. Recognizing native folds by the arrangement of hydrophobic and polar residues. J Mol Biol 1995; 252(5): 709-20.
[http://dx.doi.org/10.1006/jmbi.1995.0529] [PMID: 7563083]

[77]   Duan MJ, Zhou YH. A contact energy function considering residue hydrophobic environment and its application in protein fold recognition. Genomics Proteomics Bioinformatics 2005; 3(4): 218-24.
[http://dx.doi.org/10.1016/S1672-0229(05)03030-5] [PMID: 16689689]

[78]   Wei L, Zou Q. Recent progress in machine learning-based methods for protein fold recognition. Int J Mol Sci 2016; 17(12): E2118.
[http://dx.doi.org/10.3390/ijms17122118] [PMID: 27999256]

[79]   Lee J, Wu S, Zhang Y. Ab initio protein structure prediction. From protein structure to function with bioinformatics dordrecht. Springer Netherlands 2009; pp. 3-25.
[http://dx.doi.org/10.1007/978-1-4020-9058-5_1]

[80]   Ołdziej S, Czaplewski C, Liwo A, *et al.* Physics-based protein-structure prediction using a hierarchical protocol based on the UNRES force field: assessment in two blind tests. Proc Natl Acad Sci USA 2005; 102(21): 7547-52.
[http://dx.doi.org/10.1073/pnas.0502655102] [PMID: 15894609]

[81]   Wu S, Skolnick J, Zhang Y. Ab initio modeling of small proteins by iterative TASSER simulations. BMC Biol 2007; 5: 17.
[http://dx.doi.org/10.1186/1741-7007-5-17] [PMID: 17488521]

[82]   Li Z, Yang Y, Zhan J, Dai L, Zhou Y. Energy functions in *de novo* protein design: current challenges and future prospects. Annu Rev Biophys 2013; 42: 315-35.
[http://dx.doi.org/10.1146/annurev-biophys-083012-130315] [PMID: 23451890]

[83]   Kumar M, Dahiya S, Sharma P, *et al.* Structure based *in silico* analysis of quinolone resistance in clinical isolates of Salmonella Typhi from India. PLoS One 2015; 10(5): e0126560.
[http://dx.doi.org/10.1371/journal.pone.0126560] [PMID: 25962113]

[84]   Chiriac AI, Kloss F, Krämer J, Vuong C, Hertweck C, Sahl H-G. Mode of action of closthioamide: the first member of the polythioamide class of bacterial DNA gyrase inhibitors. J Antimicrob Chemother 2015; 70(9): 2576-88.
[http://dx.doi.org/10.1093/jac/dkv161] [PMID: 26174721]

[85]   Duan F, Li X, Cai S, *et al.* Haloemodin as novel antibacterial agent inhibiting DNA gyrase and bacterial topoisomerase I. J Med Chem 2014; 57(9): 3707-14.
[http://dx.doi.org/10.1021/jm401685f] [PMID: 24588790]

[86]   Tari LW, Trzoss M, Bensen DC, *et al.* Pyrrolopyrimidine inhibitors of DNA gyrase B (GyrB) and topoisomerase IV (ParE). Part I: Structure guided discovery and optimization of dual targeting agents with potent, broad-spectrum enzymatic activity. Bioorg Med Chem Lett 2013; 23(5): 1529-36.
[http://dx.doi.org/10.1016/j.bmcl.2012.11.032] [PMID: 23352267]

[87]   Basarab GS, Manchester JI, Bist S, *et al.* Fragment-to-hit-to-lead discovery of a novel pyridylurea scaffold of ATP competitive dual targeting type II topoisomerase inhibiting antibacterial agents. J Med Chem 2013; 56(21): 8712-35.
[http://dx.doi.org/10.1021/jm401208b] [PMID: 24098982]

[88]   Hossion AM, Zamami Y, Kandahary RK, *et al.* Quercetin diacylglycoside analogues showing dual inhibition of DNA gyrase and topoisomerase IV as novel antibacterial agents. J Med Chem 2011; 54(11): 3686-703.
[http://dx.doi.org/10.1021/jm200010x] [PMID: 21534606]

[89]   Cross JB, Zhang J, Yang Q, *et al.* Discovery of pyrazolopyridones as a novel class of gyrase B inhibitors using structure guided design. ACS Med Chem Lett 2016; 7(4): 374-8.
[http://dx.doi.org/10.1021/acsmedchemlett.5b00368] [PMID: 27096044]

[90]   Karkare S, Chung TT, Collin F, *et al.* The naphthoquinone diospyrin is an inhibitor of DNA gyrase with a novel mechanism of action. J Biol Chem 2013; 288(7): 5149-56.
[http://dx.doi.org/10.1074/jbc.M112.419069] [PMID: 23275348]

[91]   Yule IA, Czaplewski LG, Pommier S, Davies DT, Narramore SK, Fishwick CW. Pyridine---carboxamide-6-yl-ureas as novel inhibitors of bacterial DNA gyrase: structure based design, synthesis, SAR and antimicrobial activity. Eur J Med Chem 2014; 86: 31-8.
[http://dx.doi.org/10.1016/j.ejmech.2014.08.025] [PMID: 25137573]

[92]   Blanco D, Perez-Herran E, Cacho M, *et al.* Mycobacterium tuberculosis gyrase inhibitors as a new class of antitubercular drugs. Antimicrob Agents Chemother 2015; 59(4): 1868-75.
[http://dx.doi.org/10.1128/AAC.03913-14] [PMID: 25583730]

[93]   Chetty S, Soliman ME. Possible allosteric binding site on Gyrase B, a key target for novel anti-TB drugs: homology modelling and binding site identification using molecular dynamics simulation and binding free energy calculations. Med Chem Res 2015; 24(5): 2055-74.
[http://dx.doi.org/10.1007/s00044-014-1279-3]

[94]   Prisic S, Husson RN. Mycobacterium tuberculosis Serine/Threonine Protein Kinases. Microbiol Spectr 2014; 2(5)
[http://dx.doi.org/10.1128/microbiolspec.MGM2-0006-2013] [PMID: 25429354]

[95]   Kandasamy S, Hassan S, Gopalaswamy R, Narayanan S. Homology modelling, docking, pharmacophore and site directed mutagenesis analysis to identify the critical amino acid residue of PknI from Mycobacterium tuberculosis. J Mol Graph Model 2014; 52: 11-9.
[http://dx.doi.org/10.1016/j.jmgm.2014.05.011] [PMID: 24955490]

[96]   Eissa AG, Blaxland JA, Williams RO, *et al.* Targeting methionyl tRNA synthetase: design, synthesis and antibacterial activity against Clostridium difficile of novel 3-biaryl-N-benzylpropan-1-amine derivatives. J Enzyme Inhib Med Chem 2016; 31(6): 1694-7.
[http://dx.doi.org/10.3109/14756366.2016.1140754] [PMID: 26899668]

[97]   Zhao Y, Meng Q, Bai L, Zhou H. In silico discovery of aminoacyl-tRNA synthetase inhibitors. Int J Mol Sci 2014; 15(1): 1358-73.
[http://dx.doi.org/10.3390/ijms15011358] [PMID: 24447926]

[98]   Odom RB. Mupirocin (2 percent) ointment in the treatment of primary and secondary skin infections. Cutis 1989; 43(6): 599-601.
[PMID: 2501071]

[99]   Kim SY, Lee Y-S, Kang T, Kim S, Lee J. Pharmacophore-based virtual screening: the discovery of novel methionyl-tRNA synthetase inhibitors. Bioorg Med Chem Lett 2006; 16(18): 4898-907.

[http://dx.doi.org/10.1016/j.bmcl.2006.06.057] [PMID: 16824759]

[100] Tandon M, Coffen DL, Gallant P, Keith D, Ashwell MA. Potent and selective inhibitors of bacterial methionyl tRNA synthetase derived from an oxazolone-dipeptide scaffold. Bioorg Med Chem Lett 2004; 14(8): 1909-11.
[http://dx.doi.org/10.1016/j.bmcl.2004.01.094] [PMID: 15050625]

[101] Lee J, Kang SU, Kang MK, *et al.* Methionyl adenylate analogues as inhibitors of methionyl-tRNA synthetase. Bioorg Med Chem Lett 1999; 9(10): 1365-70.
[http://dx.doi.org/10.1016/S0960-894X(99)00206-1] [PMID: 10360737]

[102] Finn J, Stidham M, Hilgers M, G C K. Identification of novel inhibitors of methionyl-tRNA synthetase (MetRS) by virtual screening. Bioorg Med Chem Lett 2008; 18(14): 3932-7.
[http://dx.doi.org/10.1016/j.bmcl.2008.06.032] [PMID: 18590962]

[103] Liu C, He G, Jiang Q, Han B, Peng C. Novel hybrid virtual screening protocol based on molecular docking and structure-based pharmacophore for discovery of methionyl-tRNA synthetase inhibitors as antibacterial agents. Int J Mol Sci 2013; 14(7): 14225-39.
[http://dx.doi.org/10.3390/ijms140714225] [PMID: 23839093]

[104] Martí-Renom MA, Stuart AC, Fiser A, Sánchez R, Melo F, Sali A. Comparative protein structure modeling of genes and genomes. Annu Rev Biophys Biomol Struct 2000; 29: 291-325.
[http://dx.doi.org/10.1146/annurev.biophys.29.1.291] [PMID: 10940251]

[105] Elbaramawi SS, Ibrahim SM, Lashine EM, El-Sadek ME, Mantzourani E, Simons C. Exploring the binding sites of *Staphylococcus aureus* phenylalanine tRNA synthetase: A homology model approach. J Mol Graph Model 2017; 73: 36-47.
[http://dx.doi.org/10.1016/j.jmgm.2017.02.002] [PMID: 28235746]

[106] Molecular Operating Environment (MOE). 2013.08; Chemical Computing Group ULC, 1010 Sherbooke St. West, Suite #910, Montreal, QC, Canada, H3A 2R7, 2017

[107] Patrick GL. An introduction to medicinal chemistry; Oxford University Press: Oxford, cop. 2013; pp xxiii, 789 s

[108] Ewing TJ, Makino S, Skillman AG, Kuntz ID. DOCK 4.0: search strategies for automated molecular docking of flexible molecule databases. J Comput Aided Mol Des 2001; 15(5): 411-28.
[http://dx.doi.org/10.1023/A:1011115820450] [PMID: 11394736]

[109] Goodsell DS, Olson AJ. Automated docking of substrates to proteins by simulated annealing. Proteins 1990; 8(3): 195-202.
[http://dx.doi.org/10.1002/prot.340080302] [PMID: 2281083]

[110] Rarey M, Kramer B, Lengauer T, Klebe G. A fast flexible docking method using an incremental construction algorithm. J Mol Biol 1996; 261(3): 470-89.
[http://dx.doi.org/10.1006/jmbi.1996.0477] [PMID: 8780787]

[111] Friesner RA, Banks JL, Murphy RB, *et al.* Glide: a new approach for rapid, accurate docking and scoring. 1. Method and assessment of docking accuracy. J Med Chem 2004; 47(7): 1739-49.
[http://dx.doi.org/10.1021/jm0306430] [PMID: 15027865]

[112] Jones G, Willett P, Glen RC, Leach AR, Taylor R. Development and validation of a genetic algorithm for flexible docking. J Mol Biol 1997; 267(3): 727-48.
[http://dx.doi.org/10.1006/jmbi.1996.0897] [PMID: 9126849]

[113] Gagnon JK, Law SM, Brooks CL III. Flexible CDOCKER: Development and application of a pseudo-explicit structure-based docking method within CHARMM. J Comput Chem 2016; 37(8): 753-62.
[http://dx.doi.org/10.1002/jcc.24259] [PMID: 26691274]

[114] Guedes IA, de Magalhães CS, Dardenne LE. Receptor-ligand molecular docking. Biophys Rev 2014; 6(1): 75-87.
[http://dx.doi.org/10.1007/s12551-013-0130-2] [PMID: 28509958]

[115]   Irwin JJ, Shoichet BK. ZINC-a free database of commercially available compounds for virtual screening. J Chem Inf Model 2005; 45(1): 177-82.
[http://dx.doi.org/10.1021/ci049714+] [PMID: 15667143]

[116]   http://www.asinex.com/libraries.html

[117]   Taylor JS, Burnett RM. DARWIN: a program for docking flexible molecules. Proteins 2000; 41(2): 173-91.
[http://dx.doi.org/10.1002/1097-0134(20001101)41:2<173::AID-PROT30>3.0.CO;2-3]   [PMID: 10966571]

[118]   Connolly ML. Analytical molecular surface calculation. J Appl Cryst 1983; 16: 548-58.
[http://dx.doi.org/10.1107/S0021889883010985]

[119]   Goodford PJ. A computational procedure for determining energetically favorable binding sites on biologically important macromolecules. J Med Chem 1985; 28(7): 849-57.
[http://dx.doi.org/10.1021/jm00145a002] [PMID: 3892003]

[120]   Miller MD, Kearsley SK, Underwood DJ, Sheridan RP. FLOG: a system to select 'quasi-flexible' ligands complementary to a receptor of known three-dimensional structure. J Comput Aided Mol Des 1994; 8(2): 153-74.
[http://dx.doi.org/10.1007/BF00119865] [PMID: 8064332]

[121]   Welch W, Ruppert J, Jain AN. Hammerhead: fast, fully automated docking of flexible ligands to protein binding sites. Chem Biol 1996; 3(6): 449-62.
[http://dx.doi.org/10.1016/S1074-5521(96)90093-9] [PMID: 8807875]

[122]   Osguthorpe DJ, Sherman W, Hagler AT. Exploring protein flexibility: incorporating structural ensembles from crystal structures and simulation into virtual screening protocols. J Phys Chem B 2012; 116(23): 6952-9.
[http://dx.doi.org/10.1021/jp3003992] [PMID: 22424156]

[123]   Kumari I, Sandhu P, Ahmed M, Akhter Y. Molecular dynamics simulations, challenges and opportunities: a biologist's prospective. Curr Protein Pept Sci 2017; 18(11): 1163-79.
[http://dx.doi.org/10.2174/1389203718666170622074741] [PMID: 28637405]

[124]   Xu M, Lill MA. Induced fit docking, and the use of QM/MM methods in docking. Drug Discov Today Technol 2013; 10(3): e411-8.
[http://dx.doi.org/10.1016/j.ddtec.2013.02.003] [PMID: 24050138]

[125]   Cozzini P, Kellogg GE, Spyrakis F, *et al.* Target flexibility: an emerging consideration in drug discovery and design. J Med Chem 2008; 51(20): 6237-55.
[http://dx.doi.org/10.1021/jm800562d] [PMID: 18785728]

[126]   Jiang F, Kim SH. "Soft docking": matching of molecular surface cubes. J Mol Biol 1991; 219(1): 79-102.
[http://dx.doi.org/10.1016/0022-2836(91)90859-5] [PMID: 2023263]

[127]   Leach AR, Lemon AP. Exploring the conformational space of protein side chains using dead-end elimination and the A* algorithm. Proteins 1998; 33(2): 227-39.
[http://dx.doi.org/10.1002/(SICI)1097-0134(19981101)33:2<227::AID-PROT7>3.0.CO;2-F]   [PMID: 9779790]

[128]   Liu J, Wang R. Classification of current scoring functions. J Chem Inf Model 2015; 55(3): 475-82.
[http://dx.doi.org/10.1021/ci500731a] [PMID: 25647463]

[129]   Yin S, Biedermannova L, Vondrasek J, Dokholyan NV. MedusaScore: an accurate force field-based scoring function for virtual drug screening. J Chem Inf Model 2008; 48(8): 1656-62.
[http://dx.doi.org/10.1021/ci8001167] [PMID: 18672869]

[130]   Ishchenko AV, Shakhnovich EI. SMall Molecule Growth 2001 (SMoG2001): an improved knowledge-based scoring function for protein-ligand interactions. J Med Chem 2002; 45(13): 2770-80.

[http://dx.doi.org/10.1021/jm0105833] [PMID: 12061879]

[131] Ain QU, Aleksandrova A, Roessler FD, Ballester PJ. Machine-learning scoring functions to improve structure-based binding affinity prediction and virtual screening. Wiley Interdiscip Rev Comput Mol Sci 2015; 5(6): 405-24.
[http://dx.doi.org/10.1002/wcms.1225] [PMID: 27110292]

[132] Wójcikowski M, Ballester PJ, Siedlecki P. Performance of machine-learning scoring functions in structure-based virtual screening. Sci Rep 2017; 7: 46710.
[http://dx.doi.org/10.1038/srep46710] [PMID: 28440302]

[133] Ballester PJ, Mangold M, Howard NI, *et al.* Hierarchical virtual screening for the discovery of new molecular scaffolds in antibacterial hit identification. J R Soc Interface 2012; 9(77): 3196-207.
[http://dx.doi.org/10.1098/rsif.2012.0569] [PMID: 22933186]

[134] Wang R, Lai L, Wang S. Further development and validation of empirical scoring functions for structure-based binding affinity prediction. J Comput Aided Mol Des 2002; 16(1): 11-26.
[http://dx.doi.org/10.1023/A:1016357811882] [PMID: 12197663]

[135] Terp GE, Johansen BN, Christensen IT, Jørgensen FS. A new concept for multidimensional selection of ligand conformations (MultiSelect) and multidimensional scoring (MultiScore) of protein-ligand binding affinities. J Med Chem 2001; 44(14): 2333-43.
[http://dx.doi.org/10.1021/jm001090l] [PMID: 11428927]

[136] Bar-Haim S, Aharon A, Ben-Moshe T, Marantz Y, Senderowitz H. SeleX-CS: a new consensus scoring algorithm for hit discovery and lead optimization. J Chem Inf Model 2009; 49(3): 623-33.
[http://dx.doi.org/10.1021/ci800335j] [PMID: 19231809]

[137] Booth IR, Blount P. The MscS and MscL families of mechanosensitive channels act as microbial emergency release valves. J Bacteriol 2012; 194(18): 4802-9.
[http://dx.doi.org/10.1128/JB.00576-12] [PMID: 22685280]

[138] Deplazes E, Louhivuori M, Jayatilaka D, Marrink SJ, Corry B. Structural investigation of MscL gating using experimental data and coarse grained MD simulations. PLOS Comput Biol 2012; 8(9): e1002683.
[http://dx.doi.org/10.1371/journal.pcbi.1002683] [PMID: 23028281]

[139] Nguyen T, Clare B, Guo W, Martinac B. The effects of parabens on the mechanosensitive channels of E. coli. Eur Biophys J 2005; 34(5): 389-95.
[http://dx.doi.org/10.1007/s00249-005-0468-x] [PMID: 15770478]

[140] Iscla I, Wray R, Wei S, Posner B, Blount P. Streptomycin potency is dependent on MscL channel expression. Nat Commun 2014; 5: 4891.
[http://dx.doi.org/10.1038/ncomms5891] [PMID: 25205267]

[141] Iscla I, Wray R, Blount P, *et al.* A new antibiotic with potent activity targets MscL. J Antibiot 2015; 68(7): 453-62.
[http://dx.doi.org/10.1038/ja.2015.4] [PMID: 25649856]

[142] Rao S, Prestidge CA, Miesel L, Sweeney D, Shinabarger DL, Boulos RA. Preclinical development of Ramizol, an antibiotic belonging to a new class, for the treatment of Clostridium difficile colitis. J Antibiot 2016; 69(12): 879-84.
[http://dx.doi.org/10.1038/ja.2016.45] [PMID: 27189122]

[143] Nakama T, Nureki O, Yokoyama S. Structural basis for the recognition of isoleucyl-adenylate and an antibiotic, mupirocin, by isoleucyl-tRNA synthetase. J Biol Chem 2001; 276(50): 47387-93.
[http://dx.doi.org/10.1074/jbc.M109089200] [PMID: 11584022]

[144] Hurdle JG, O'Neill AJ, Ingham E, Fishwick C, Chopra I. Analysis of mupirocin resistance and fitness in Staphylococcus aureus by molecular genetic and structural modeling techniques. Antimicrob Agents Chemother 2004; 48(11): 4366-76.
[http://dx.doi.org/10.1128/AAC.48.11.4366-4376.2004] [PMID: 15504866]

[145] Randall CP, Rasina D, Jirgensons A, O'Neill AJ. Targeting multiple aminoacyl-tRNA synthetases overcomes the resistance liabilities associated with antibacterial inhibitors acting on a single such enzyme. Antimicrob Agents Chemother 2016; 60(10): 6359-61.
[http://dx.doi.org/10.1128/AAC.00674-16] [PMID: 27431224]

[146] Arnér ES, Holmgren A. Physiological functions of thioredoxin and thioredoxin reductase. Eur J Biochem 2000; 267(20): 6102-9.
[http://dx.doi.org/10.1046/j.1432-1327.2000.01701.x] [PMID: 11012661]

[147] Lu J, Vlamis-Gardikas A, Kandasamy K, *et al.* Inhibition of bacterial thioredoxin reductase: an antibiotic mechanism targeting bacteria lacking glutathione. FASEB J 2013; 27(4): 1394-403.
[http://dx.doi.org/10.1096/fj.12-223305] [PMID: 23248236]

[148] Sweeney NL, Lipker L, Hanson AM, *et al.* Docking into mycobacterium tuberculosis thioredoxin reductase protein yields pyrazolone lead molecules for methicillin-resistant *Staphylococcus aureus.* Antibiot Basel Switz 2017; 6(1)
[http://dx.doi.org/10.3390/antibiotics6010004]

[149] Singh SB. Confronting the challenges of discovery of novel antibacterial agents. Bioorg Med Chem Lett 2014; 24(16): 3683-9.
[http://dx.doi.org/10.1016/j.bmcl.2014.06.053] [PMID: 25017034]

[150] Harbut MB, Vilchèze C, Luo X, *et al.* Auranofin exerts broad-spectrum bactericidal activities by targeting thiol-redox homeostasis. Proc Natl Acad Sci USA 2015; 112(14): 4453-8.
[http://dx.doi.org/10.1073/pnas.1504022112] [PMID: 25831516]

[151] Gustafsson TN, Osman H, Werngren J, Hoffner S, Engman L, Holmgren A. Ebselen and analogs as inhibitors of Bacillus anthracis thioredoxin reductase and bactericidal antibacterials targeting Bacillus species, Staphylococcus aureus and Mycobacterium tuberculosis. Biochim Biophys Acta 2016; 1860(6): 1265-71.
[http://dx.doi.org/10.1016/j.bbagen.2016.03.013] [PMID: 26971857]

[152] Liang W, Fernandes AP, Holmgren A, Li X, Zhong L. Bacterial thioredoxin and thioredoxin reductase as mediators for epigallocatechin 3-gallate-induced antimicrobial action. FEBS J 2016; 283(3): 446-58.
[http://dx.doi.org/10.1111/febs.13587] [PMID: 26546231]

[153] Blair JM, Webber MA, Baylay AJ, Ogbolu DO, Piddock LJ. Molecular mechanisms of antibiotic resistance. Nat Rev Microbiol 2015; 13(1): 42-51.
[http://dx.doi.org/10.1038/nrmicro3380] [PMID: 25435309]

[154] Brown ED, Wright GD. Antibacterial drug discovery in the resistance era. Nature 2016; 529(7586): 336-43.
[http://dx.doi.org/10.1038/nature17042] [PMID: 26791724]

[155] Gerdes K, Christensen SK, Løbner-Olesen A. Prokaryotic toxin-antitoxin stress response loci. Nat Rev Microbiol 2005; 3(5): 371-82.
[http://dx.doi.org/10.1038/nrmicro1147] [PMID: 15864262]

[156] Conlon BP, Nakayasu ES, Fleck LE, *et al.* Activated ClpP kills persisters and eradicates a chronic biofilm infection. Nature 2013; 503(7476): 365-70.
[http://dx.doi.org/10.1038/nature12790] [PMID: 24226776]

[157] Page R, Peti W. Toxin-antitoxin systems in bacterial growth arrest and persistence. Nat Chem Biol 2016; 12(4): 208-14.
[http://dx.doi.org/10.1038/nchembio.2044] [PMID: 26991085]

[158] Połom D, Boss L, Węgrzyn G, Hayes F, Kędzierska B. Amino acid residues crucial for specificity of toxin-antitoxin interactions in the homologous Axe-Txe and YefM-YoeB complexes. FEBS J 2013; 280(22): 5906-18.
[http://dx.doi.org/10.1111/febs.12517] [PMID: 24028219]

[159] Zheng C, Xu J, Ren S, *et al.* Identification and characterization of the chromosomal yefM-yoeB toxin-antitoxin system of Streptococcus suis. Sci Rep 2015; 5: 13125.
[http://dx.doi.org/10.1038/srep13125] [PMID: 26272287]

[160] Grady R, Hayes F. Axe-Txe, a broad-spectrum proteic toxin-antitoxin system specified by a multidrug-resistant, clinical isolate of Enterococcus faecium. Mol Microbiol 2003; 47(5): 1419-32.
[http://dx.doi.org/10.1046/j.1365-2958.2003.03387.x] [PMID: 12603745]

[161] Barnoud J, Monticelli L. Coarse-grained force fields for molecular simulations. Methods Mol Biol 2015; 1215: 125-49.
[http://dx.doi.org/10.1007/978-1-4939-1465-4_7] [PMID: 25330962]

[162] Kokhan O, Shinkarev VP. All-atom molecular dynamics simulations reveal significant differences in interaction between antimycin and conserved amino acid residues in bovine and bacterial bc1 complexes. Biophys J 2011; 100(3): 720-8.
[http://dx.doi.org/10.1016/j.bpj.2010.12.3705] [PMID: 21281587]

[163] Hamelberg D, Mongan J, McCammon JA. Accelerated molecular dynamics: a promising and efficient simulation method for biomolecules. J Chem Phys 2004; 120(24): 11919-29.
[http://dx.doi.org/10.1063/1.1755656] [PMID: 15268227]

[164] Case DA, Berryman JT, Betz RM, *et al.* AMBER 2015. University of California, San Francisco; 2015

[165] Vanommeslaeghe K, Hatcher E, Acharya C, *et al.* CHARMM general force field: A force field for drug-like molecules compatible with the CHARMM all-atom additive biological force fields. J Comput Chem 2010; 31(4): 671-90.
[PMID: 19575467]

[166] Kaminski GA, Friesner RA, Tirado-Rives J, Jorgensen WL. Evaluation and reparametrization of the OPLS-AA force field for proteins *via* comparison with accurate quantum chemical calculations on peptides. J Phys Chem B 2001; 105(28): 6474-87.
[http://dx.doi.org/10.1021/jp003919d]

[167] Jämbeck JPM, Lyubartsev AP. Another piece of the membrane puzzle: Extending slipids further. J Chem Theory Comput (Stycze) 2013; 9(1): 774-84.

[168] Klauda JB, Venable RM, Freites JA, *et al.* Update of the CHARMM all-atom additive force field for lipids: Validation on six lipid types. J Phys Chem B 2010; 114(23): 7830-43.
[http://dx.doi.org/10.1021/jp101759q] [PMID: 20496934]

[169] Dickson CJ, Madej BD, Skjevik ÅA, *et al.* Lipid14: The amber lipid force field. J Chem Theory Comput 2014; 10(2): 865-79.
[http://dx.doi.org/10.1021/ct4010307] [PMID: 24803855]

[170] Lyubartsev AP, Rabinovich AL. Force field development for lipid membrane simulations. Biochim Biophys Acta 2016; 1858(10): 2483-97.
[http://dx.doi.org/10.1016/j.bbamem.2015.12.033] [PMID: 26766518]

[171] Home | Lipid builder. 2017.http://lipidbuilder.epfl.ch/home

[172] Berglund NA, Piggot TJ, Jefferies D, Sessions RB, Bond PJ, Khalid S. Interaction of the antimicrobial peptide polymyxin B1 with both membranes of *E. coli*: A molecular dynamics study. PLoS Comput Biol 2015.http://www.ncbi.nlm.nih.gov/pmc/articles/PMC4401565/

[173] YASARA. 2016. http://www.yasara.org

[174] SCIGRESS - Molecular modeling software. 2017. http://www.fqs.pl/chemistry_materials_life_science/products/scigress

[175] Dassault Systèmes BI. Discovery Studio, version 35. San Diego: Dassault Systèmes 2016.

[176] Desmond Molecular Dynamics System. D. E. Shaw Research, New York, NY, 2017. Maestro-Desmond Interoperability Tools, Schrödinger, New York, NY, 2017

[177] Hynninen A-P, Crowley MF. New faster CHARMM molecular dynamics engine. J Comput Chem 2014; 35(5): 406-13.
[http://dx.doi.org/10.1002/jcc.23501] [PMID: 24302199]

[178] Phillips JC, Braun R, Wang W, *et al.* Scalable molecular dynamics with NAMD. J Comput Chem 2005; 26(16): 1781-802.
[http://dx.doi.org/10.1002/jcc.20289] [PMID: 16222654]

[179] Humphrey W, Dalke A, Schulten K. VMD: visual molecular dynamics. J Mol Graph 1996. 14(1):33–8, 27–8

[180] Pronk S, Páll S, Schulz R, *et al.* GROMACS 4.5: a high-throughput and highly parallel open source molecular simulation toolkit. Bioinformatics 2013; 29(7): 845-54.
[http://dx.doi.org/10.1093/bioinformatics/btt055] [PMID: 23407358]

[181] Altuntaş S, Bozkus Z, Fraguela BB. GPU accelerated molecular docking simulation with genetic algorithms. 2016. In: Squillero G, Burelli P, editors Applications of Evolutionary Computation (Internet) Switzerland: Springer International Publishing; 2016 (cited 2016 Dec 12) p 134–46 (Lecture Notes in Computer Science) http://link.springer.com/chapter/10.1007/978-3-319-31153-1_10
[http://dx.doi.org/10.1007/978-3-319-31153-1_10]

[182] McClendon CL, Friedland G, Mobley DL, Amirkhani H, Jacobson MP. Quantifying correlations between allosteric sites in thermodynamic ensembles. J Chem Theory Comput Wrzesie 2009; 5(9): 2486-502.

[183] LeVine MV, Weinstein H. NbIT--a new information theory-based analysis of allosteric mechanisms reveals residues that underlie function in the leucine transporter LeuT. PLOS Comput Biol 2014; 10(5): e1003603.
[http://dx.doi.org/10.1371/journal.pcbi.1003603] [PMID: 24785005]

[184] Kuttel MM, Cescutti P, Distefano M, Rizzo R. Fluorescence and NMR spectroscopy together with molecular simulations reveal amphiphilic characteristics of a Burkholderia biofilm exopolysaccharide. J Biol Chem 2017; 292(26): 11034-42.
[http://dx.doi.org/10.1074/jbc.M117.785048] [PMID: 28468829]

[185] Gupta A, Mishra S, Singh S, Mishra S. Prevention of IcaA regulated poly N-acetyl glucosamine formation in Staphylococcus aureus biofilm through new-drug like inhibitors: In silico approach and MD simulation study. Microb Pathog 2017; 110: 659-69.
[http://dx.doi.org/10.1016/j.micpath.2017.05.025] [PMID: 28579399]

[186] Luo H, Liang D-F, Bao M-Y, *et al. In silico* identification of potential inhibitors targeting Streptococcus mutans sortase A. Int J Oral Sci 2017; 9(1): 53-62.
[http://dx.doi.org/10.1038/ijos.2016.58] [PMID: 28358034]

[187] Cho H, Huang X, Lan Piao Y, *et al.* Molecular modeling and redesign of alginate lyase from Pseudomonas aeruginosa for accelerating CRPA biofilm degradation. Proteins 2016; 84(12): 1875-87.
[http://dx.doi.org/10.1002/prot.25171] [PMID: 27676452]

[188] Rajamanikandan S, Srinivasan P. Pharmacophore modeling and structure-based virtual screening to identify potent inhibitors targeting LuxP of Vibrio harveyi. J Recept Signal Transduct Res 2016; 36(6): 617-32.
[http://dx.doi.org/10.3109/10799893.2016.1155063] [PMID: 27049472]

[189] Rajamanikandan S, Jeyakanthan J, Srinivasan P. Molecular docking, molecular dynamics simulations, computational screening to design quorum sensing inhibitors targeting luxP of vibrio harveyi and its biological evaluation. Appl Biochem Biotechnol 2017; 181(1): 192-218.
[http://dx.doi.org/10.1007/s12010-016-2207-4] [PMID: 27535409]

[190] Blasco P, Patel DS, Engström O, Im W, Widmalm G. Conformational dynamics of the lipopolysaccharide from *Escherichia coli* O91 revealed by NMR spectroscopy and molecular simulations. Biochemistry (Mosc) 2017.

[191] Nidhi , Siddiqi MI. Recent advances in QSAR-based identification and design of anti-tubercular agents. Curr Pharm Des 2014; 20(27): 4418-26.
[http://dx.doi.org/10.2174/1381612819666131118165059] [PMID: 24245761]

[192] Damale MG, Harke SN, Kalam Khan FA, Shinde DB, Sangshetti JN. Recent advances in multidimensional QSAR (4D-6D): a critical review. Mini Rev Med Chem 2014; 14(1): 35-55.
[http://dx.doi.org/10.2174/1389557511313660104] [PMID: 24195665]

[193] Polanski J. Receptor dependent multidimensional QSAR for modeling drug--receptor interactions. Curr Med Chem 2009; 16(25): 3243-57.
[http://dx.doi.org/10.2174/092986709788803286] [PMID: 19548875]

[194] Myint KZ, Xie X-Q. Recent advances in fragment-based QSAR and multi-dimensional QSAR methods. Int J Mol Sci 2010; 11(10): 3846-66.
[http://dx.doi.org/10.3390/ijms11103846] [PMID: 21152304]

[195] Cherkasov A, Muratov EN, Fourches D, et al. QSAR modeling: where have you been? Where are you going to? J Med Chem 2014; 57(12): 4977-5010.
[http://dx.doi.org/10.1021/jm4004285] [PMID: 24351051]

[196] Martins F, Ventura C, Santos S, Viveiros M. QSAR based design of new antitubercular compounds: improved isoniazid derivatives against multidrug-resistant TB. Curr Pharm Des 2014; 20(27): 4427-54.
[http://dx.doi.org/10.2174/1381612819666131118164434] [PMID: 24245762]

[197] Rajkhowa S, Deka RC. DFT based QSAR/QSPR models in the development of novel anti-tuberculosis drugs targeting Mycobacterium tuberculosis. Curr Pharm Des 2014; 20(27): 4455-73.
[http://dx.doi.org/10.2174/1381612819666131118165824] [PMID: 24245759]

[198] Bueno RV, Braga RC, Segretti ND, Ferreira EI, Trossini GH, Andrade CH. New tuberculostatic agents targeting nucleic acid biosynthesis: drug design using QSAR approaches. Curr Pharm Des 2014; 20(27): 4474-85.
[http://dx.doi.org/10.2174/1381612819666131118170238] [PMID: 24245758]

[199] Friggeri L, Ballante F, Ragno R, et al. Pharmacophore assessment through 3-D QSAR: evaluation of the predictive ability on new derivatives by the application on a series of antitubercular agents. J Chem Inf Model 2013; 53(6): 1463-74.
[http://dx.doi.org/10.1021/ci400132q] [PMID: 23617317]

[200] Lee S-H, Choi M, Kim P, Myung PK. 3D-QSAR and cell wall permeability of antitubercular nitroimidazoles against Mycobacterium tuberculosis. Molecules 2013; 18(11): 13870-85.
[http://dx.doi.org/10.3390/molecules181113870] [PMID: 24217328]

[201] Shah P, Saquib M, Sharma S, et al. 3D-QSAR and molecular modeling studies on 2,3-dideoxy hexenopyranosid-4-uloses as anti-tubercular agents targeting alpha-mannosidase. Bioorg Chem 2015; 59: 91-6.
[http://dx.doi.org/10.1016/j.bioorg.2015.02.001] [PMID: 25727263]

[202] Lee JY, Doddareddy MR, Cho YS, et al. Comparative QSAR studies on peptide deformylase inhibitors. J Mol Model 2007; 13(5): 543-58.
[http://dx.doi.org/10.1007/s00894-007-0175-x] [PMID: 17333308]

[203] Huang Z, Lin K, You Q. De novo design of novel DNA-gyrase inhibitors based on 2D molecular fingerprints. Bioorg Med Chem Lett 2013; 23(14): 4166-71.
[http://dx.doi.org/10.1016/j.bmcl.2013.05.033] [PMID: 23743285]

[204] Fang Y, Lu Y, Zang X, et al. 3D-QSAR and docking studies of flavonoids as potent Escherichia coli inhibitors. Sci Rep 2016; 6: 23634.
[http://dx.doi.org/10.1038/srep23634] [PMID: 27049530]

[205] Yu X, Zhang M, Annamalai T, et al. Synthesis, evaluation, and CoMFA study of fluoroquinophenoxazine derivatives as bacterial topoisomerase IA inhibitors. Eur J Med Chem 2017;

125: 515-27.
[http://dx.doi.org/10.1016/j.ejmech.2016.09.053] [PMID: 27689733]

[206] Kathiravan MK, Khilare MM, Chothe AS, Nagras MA. Design and development of topoisomerase inhibitors using molecular modelling studies. J Chem Biol 2012; 6(1): 25-36.
[http://dx.doi.org/10.1007/s12154-012-0079-9] [PMID: 24078835]

[207] Yanmaz E, Sarıpınar E, Şahin K, Geçen N, Çopur F. 4D-QSAR analysis and pharmacophore modeling: electron conformational-genetic algorithm approach for penicillins. Bioorg Med Chem 2011; 19(7): 2199-210.
[http://dx.doi.org/10.1016/j.bmc.2011.02.035] [PMID: 21419636]

[208] Wang D, Lin Z, Huo Z, Wang T, Yao Z, Cong Y. Mechanism-based QSAR models for the toxicity of quorum sensing inhibitors to gram-negative and gram-positive bacteria. Bull Environ Contam Toxicol 2016; 97(1): 145-50.
[http://dx.doi.org/10.1007/s00128-016-1801-z] [PMID: 27084097]

[209] Li M, Wei D, Du Y. Genotoxicity of quinolone antibiotics in chlorination disinfection treatment: formation and QSAR simulation. Environ Sci Pollut Res Int 2016; 23(20): 20637-45.
[http://dx.doi.org/10.1007/s11356-016-7246-4] [PMID: 27470245]

[210] Zanni R, Galvez-Llompart M, Machuca J, et al. Molecular topology: A new strategy for antimicrobial resistance control. Eur J Med Chem 2017; 137: 233-46.
[http://dx.doi.org/10.1016/j.ejmech.2017.05.055] [PMID: 28595068]

[211] Bojarska-Dahlig H, Simon Z, Głabski T. Quantitative structure-activity relationships in erythromycin group with MTD technique. Pol J Pharmacol Pharm 1981; 33(3): 359-63.
[PMID: 7322948]

[212] Tanaka H, Moriguchi I, Hirono S, Omura S. Quantitative structure-activity relationships of O-acyl derivatives of leucomycin for antimicrobial and ribosome-binding activities. Chem Pharm Bull (Tokyo) 1985; 33(7): 2803-8.
[http://dx.doi.org/10.1248/cpb.33.2803] [PMID: 4085039]

[213] Setny P, Trylska J. Search for novel aminoglycosides by combining fragment-based virtual screening and 3D-QSAR scoring. J Chem Inf Model 2009; 49(2): 390-400.
[http://dx.doi.org/10.1021/ci800361a] [PMID: 19434840]

[214] Vuorinen A, Schuster D. Methods for generating and applying pharmacophore models as virtual screening filters and for bioactivity profiling. Methods 2015; 71: 113-34.
[http://dx.doi.org/10.1016/j.ymeth.2014.10.013] [PMID: 25461773]

[215] Qing X, Lee XY, Raeymaecker JD, Tame JR, Zhang KY, Maeyer MD, et al. Pharmacophore modeling: advances, limitations, and current utility in drug discovery (Internet). Journal of Receptor, Ligand and Channel Research 2014. https://www.dovepress.com/pharmacophore-modeling-advanc-s-limitations-and-current-utility-in-dru-peer-reviewed-fulltext-article-JRLCR

[216] Wolber G, Seidel T, Bendix F, Langer T. Molecule-pharmacophore superpositioning and pattern matching in computational drug design. Drug Discov Today 2008; 13(1-2): 23-9.
[http://dx.doi.org/10.1016/j.drudis.2007.09.007] [PMID: 18190860]

[217] Yang S-Y. Pharmacophore modeling and applications in drug discovery: challenges and recent advances. Drug Discov Today 2010; 15(11-12): 444-50.
[http://dx.doi.org/10.1016/j.drudis.2010.03.013] [PMID: 20362693]

[218] Kaczor AA, Kronbach C, Unverferth K, et al. Novel non-competitive antagonists of kainate GluK1/GluK2 receptors Lett. Drug Des Discov 2012; 9(10): 891-8.
[http://dx.doi.org/10.2174/1570180811209050891]

[219] Khedkar SA, Malde AK, Coutinho EC, Srivastava S. Pharmacophore modeling in drug discovery and development: an overview. Med Chem 2007; 3(2): 187-97.
[http://dx.doi.org/10.2174/157340607780059521] [PMID: 17348856]

[220] Macalino SJ, Gosu V, Hong S, Choi S. Role of computer-aided drug design in modern drug discovery. Arch Pharm Res 2015; 38(9): 1686-701.
[http://dx.doi.org/10.1007/s12272-015-0640-5] [PMID: 26208641]

[221] Kaczor A, Matosiuk D. Structure-based virtual screening for novel inhibitors of Japanese encephalitis virus NS3 helicase/nucleoside triphosphatase. FEMS Immunol Med Microbiol 2010; 58(1): 91-101.
[http://dx.doi.org/10.1111/j.1574-695X.2009.00619.x] [PMID: 19863664]

[222] Lin S-K. Pharmacophore perception, development and use in drug design. Edited by Osman F. Güner. Molecules. 2000. 5(7): 987–9

[223] Patel Y, Gillet VJ, Bravi G, Leach AR. A comparison of the pharmacophore identification programs: Catalyst, DISCO and GASP. J Comput Aided Mol Des 2002; 16(8-9): 653-81.
[http://dx.doi.org/10.1023/A:1021954728347] [PMID: 12602956]

[224] Ananthula RS, Ravikumar M, Mahmood SK, Kumar MN. Insights from ligand and structure based methods in virtual screening of selective Ni-peptide deformylase inhibitors. J Mol Model 2012; 18(2): 693-708.
[http://dx.doi.org/10.1007/s00894-011-1068-6] [PMID: 21562829]

[225] Azam MA, Thathan J. Pharmacophore generation, atom-based 3D-QSAR and molecular dynamics simulation analyses of pyridine-3-carboxamide-6-yl-urea analogues as potential gyrase B inhibitors. SAR QSAR Environ Res 2017; 28(4): 275-96.
[http://dx.doi.org/10.1080/1062936X.2017.1310131] [PMID: 28399673]

[226] Radwan AA, Abdel-Mageed WM. *In silico* studies of quinoxaline-2-carboxamide 1,4-di-n-oxide derivatives as antimycobacterial agents. Molecules 2014; 19(2): 2247-60.
[http://dx.doi.org/10.3390/molecules19022247] [PMID: 24566302]

[227] Saha R, Tanwar O, Alam MM, Zaman MS, Khan SA, Akhter M. Pharmacophore based virtual screening, synthesis and SAR of novel inhibitors of Mycobacterium sulfotransferase. Bioorg Med Chem Lett 2015; 25(3): 701-7.
[http://dx.doi.org/10.1016/j.bmcl.2014.11.079] [PMID: 25541388]

[228] Tawari NR, Degani MS. Predictive models for nucleoside bisubstrate analogs as inhibitors of siderophore biosynthesis in Mycobacterium tuberculosis: pharmacophore mapping and chemometric QSAR study. Mol Divers 2011; 15(2): 435-44.
[http://dx.doi.org/10.1007/s11030-010-9243-8] [PMID: 20306296]

[229] Uddin R, Lodhi MU, Ul-Haq Z. Combined pharmacophore and 3D-QSAR study on a series of Staphylococcus aureus Sortase A inhibitors. Chem Biol Drug Des 2012; 80(2): 300-14.
[http://dx.doi.org/10.1111/j.1747-0285.2012.01403.x] [PMID: 22553957]

[230] Yilmaz S, Altinkanat-Gelmez G, Bolelli K, *et al.* Pharmacophore generation of 2-substituted benzothiazoles as AdeABC efflux pump inhibitors in A. baumannii. SAR QSAR Environ Res 2014; 25(7): 551-63.
[http://dx.doi.org/10.1080/1062936X.2014.919357] [PMID: 24905472]

[231] Fengxian C, Reti H. Analysis of positions and substituents on genotoxicity of fluoroquinolones with quantitative structure-activity relationship and 3D Pharmacophore model. Ecotoxicol Environ Saf 2017; 136: 111-8.
[http://dx.doi.org/10.1016/j.ecoenv.2016.10.036] [PMID: 27835744]

[232] Ghorab MM, Ismail ZH, Abdalla M, Radwan AA. Synthesis, antimicrobial evaluation and molecular modelling of novel sulfonamides carrying a biologically active quinazoline nucleus. Arch Pharm Res 2013; 36(6): 660-70.
[http://dx.doi.org/10.1007/s12272-013-0094-6] [PMID: 23529860]

[233] Tawari NR, Degani MS. Pharmacophore modeling and density functional theory analysis for a series of nitroimidazole compounds with antitubercular activity. Chem Biol Drug Des 2011; 78(3): 408-17.
[http://dx.doi.org/10.1111/j.1747-0285.2011.01161.x] [PMID: 21689377]

[234] Yang N, Wang J, Li J, Wang Q-H, Wang Y, Cheng M-S. A three-dimensional pharmacophore model for IMPDH inhibitors. Chem Biol Drug Des 2011; 78(1): 175-82.
[http://dx.doi.org/10.1111/j.1747-0285.2011.01128.x] [PMID: 21507206]

[235] Agarwal AK, Fishwick CW. Structure-based design of anti-infectives. Ann N Y Acad Sci 2010; 1213: 20-45.
[http://dx.doi.org/10.1111/j.1749-6632.2010.05859.x] [PMID: 21175675]

[236] Bartuzi D, Kaczor AA, Targowska-Duda KM, Matosiuk D. Recent Advances and Applications of Molecular Docking to G Protein-Coupled Receptors. Mol Basel Switz 2017. 22(2)

[237] Shoichet BK, Kobilka BK. Structure-based drug screening for G-protein-coupled receptors. Trends Pharmacol Sci 2012; 33(5): 268-72.
[http://dx.doi.org/10.1016/j.tips.2012.03.007] [PMID: 22503476]

[238] Sliwoski G, Kothiwale S, Meiler J, Lowe EW Jr. Computational methods in drug discovery. Pharmacol Rev 2013; 66(1): 334-95.
[http://dx.doi.org/10.1124/pr.112.007336] [PMID: 24381236]

[239] Voet A, Zhang KY. Pharmacophore modelling as a virtual screening tool for the discovery of small molecule protein-protein interaction inhibitors. Curr Pharm Des 2012; 18(30): 4586-98.
[http://dx.doi.org/10.2174/138161212802651616] [PMID: 22650262]

[240] Price AJ, Howard S, Cons BD. Fragment-based drug discovery and its application to challenging drug targets. Essays Biochem 2017; 61(5): 475-84.
[http://dx.doi.org/10.1042/EBC20170029] [PMID: 29118094]

[241] Wang T, Wu M-B, Chen Z-J, Chen H, Lin J-P, Yang L-R. Fragment-based drug discovery and molecular docking in drug design. Curr Pharm Biotechnol 2015; 16(1): 11-25.
[http://dx.doi.org/10.2174/1389201015666141122204532] [PMID: 25420726]

[242] Martí Solano M, Kaczor AA, Guixà-González R, Selent J. Computational strategies to incorporate GPCR complexity in drug design. W: Frontiers in Computational Chemistry. Vol. 1. Eds. Zaheer Ul-Haq, Jeffry D. Madura, 2015, Bentham Science Publishers, s. 3-43

[243] Tomašić T, Kovač A, Klebe G, et al. Virtual screening for potential inhibitors of bacterial MurC and MurD ligases. J Mol Model 2012; 18(3): 1063-72.
[http://dx.doi.org/10.1007/s00894-011-1139-8] [PMID: 21667288]

[244] Samal HB, Das JK, Mahapatra RK, Suar M. Molecular modeling, simulation and virtual screening of MurD ligase protein from Salmonella typhimurium LT2. J Pharmacol Toxicol Methods 2015; 73: 34-41.
[http://dx.doi.org/10.1016/j.vascn.2015.03.005] [PMID: 25841669]

[245] Howard MH, Cenizal T, Gutteridge S, et al. A novel class of inhibitors of peptide deformylase discovered through high-throughput screening and virtual ligand screening. J Med Chem 2004; 47(27): 6669-72.
[http://dx.doi.org/10.1021/jm049222o] [PMID: 15615515]

[246] Gao J, Liang L, Zhu Y, Qiu S, Wang T, Zhang L. Ligand and Structure-Based Approaches for the Identification of Peptide Deformylase Inhibitors as Antibacterial Drugs. Int J Mol Sci 2016; 17(7): E1141.
[http://dx.doi.org/10.3390/ijms17071141] [PMID: 27428963]

[247] Ghosh P, Bagchi MC. Anti-tubercular drug designing by structure based screening of combinatorial libraries. J Mol Model 2011; 17(7): 1607-20.
[http://dx.doi.org/10.1007/s00894-010-0861-y] [PMID: 20953648]

[248] Kolaric A, Minovski N. Structure-based design of novel combinatorially generated NBTIs as potential DNA gyrase inhibitors against various Staphylococcus aureus mutant strains. Mol Biosyst 2017; 13(7): 1406-20.
[http://dx.doi.org/10.1039/C7MB00168A] [PMID: 28590495]

[249]   Maharaj Y, Soliman ME. Identification of novel gyrase B inhibitors as potential anti-TB drugs: homology modelling, hybrid virtual screening and molecular dynamics simulations. Chem Biol Drug Des 2013; 82(2): 205-15.
[http://dx.doi.org/10.1111/cbdd.12152] [PMID: 23614896]

[250]   Islam MA, Pillay TS. Identification of promising DNA GyrB inhibitors for Tuberculosis using pharmacophore-based virtual screening, molecular docking and molecular dynamics studies. Chem Biol Drug Des 2017; 90(2): 282-96.
[http://dx.doi.org/10.1111/cbdd.12949] [PMID: 28109130]

[251]   Saxena S, Renuka J, Jeankumar VU, Yogeeswari P, Sriram D. Mycobacterial DNA gyrB inhibitors: Ligand based pharmacophore modelling and *in vitro* enzyme inhibition studies. Curr Top Med Chem 2014; 14(17): 1990-2005.
[http://dx.doi.org/10.2174/1568026613666140929123833] [PMID: 25262795]

[252]   Saxena S, Renuka J, Yogeeswari P, Sriram D. Discovery of novel mycobacterial DNA gyrase B inhibitors: *In silico* and *in vitro* biological evaluation. Mol Inform 2014; 33(9): 597-609.
[http://dx.doi.org/10.1002/minf.201400058] [PMID: 27486079]

[253]   Werner MM, Li Z, Zauhar RJ. Computer-aided identification of novel 3,5-substituted rhodanine derivatives with activity against Staphylococcus aureus DNA gyrase. Bioorg Med Chem 2014; 22(7): 2176-87.
[http://dx.doi.org/10.1016/j.bmc.2014.02.020] [PMID: 24629449]

[254]   Sridevi JP, Suryadevara P, Janupally R, *et al.* Identification of potential *Mycobacterium tuberculosis* topoisomerase I inhibitors: a study against active, dormant and resistant tuberculosis. Eur J Pharm Sci 2015; 72: 81-92.
[http://dx.doi.org/10.1016/j.ejps.2015.02.017] [PMID: 25769524]

[255]   Chan F-Y, Sun N, Neves MA, *et al.* Identification of a new class of FtsZ inhibitors by structure-based design and *in vitro* screening. J Chem Inf Model 2013; 53(8): 2131-40.
[http://dx.doi.org/10.1021/ci400203f] [PMID: 23848971]

[256]   Vijayalakshmi P, Nisha J, Rajalakshmi M. Virtual screening of potential inhibitor against FtsZ protein from Staphylococcus aureus. Interdiscip Sci 2014; 6(4): 331-9.
[http://dx.doi.org/10.1007/s12539-012-0229-3] [PMID: 25519150]

[257]   Pérez-Castillo Y, Cruz-Monteagudo M, Lazar C, *et al.* Toward the computer-aided discovery of FabH inhibitors. Do predictive QSAR models ensure high quality virtual screening performance? Mol Divers 2014; 18(3): 637-54.
[http://dx.doi.org/10.1007/s11030-014-9513-y] [PMID: 24671521]

[258]   Kumari S, Mohana Priya A, Lulu S, Tauqueer M. Molecular modeling, simulation and virtual screening of ribosomal phosphoprotein P1 from Plasmodium falciparum. J Theor Biol 2014; 343: 113-9.
[http://dx.doi.org/10.1016/j.jtbi.2013.10.014] [PMID: 24211527]

[259]   Walters WP, Murcko MA. Prediction of 'drug-likeness'. Adv Drug Deliv Rev 2002; 54(3): 255-71.
[http://dx.doi.org/10.1016/S0169-409X(02)00003-0] [PMID: 11922947]

[260]   Dougherty TJ, Pucci MJ, Eds. Antibiotic discovery and development. Boston, MA, Springer.
[http://dx.doi.org/10.1007/978-1-4614-1400-1]

CHAPTER 5

Nucleic Acid Aptamers Against Virulence Factors of Drug Resistant Pathogens

Canan Ozyurt, Ozge Ugurlu, Burhan Bora and **Serap Evran**[*]

Department of Biochemistry, Faculty of Science, Ege University, 35100, Bornova-Izmir, Turkey

Abstract: Aptamers are single-stranded DNA or RNA molecules, which can bind their targets with high affinity and specificity. SELEX (Systematic Evolution of Ligands by Exponential Enrichment) is the technology that allows to select aptamers from a random oligonucleotide library. Binding properties of aptamers are comparable to those of antibodies. But, unlike antibodies, aptamer production is a more rapid and less expensive process. One remarkable application is aptamer-based biosensors for specific and sensitive detection of bacterial toxins. In addition, a few aptamers have been shown to inhibit pathogens by blocking the activity of virulence factors. The chapter mainly covers aptamers that target virulence factors, rather than pathogen cells. First, general methodology for selection of aptamers is described. Then, aptamers developed against toxins, protein virulence factors and quorum sensing molecules are reviewed. In addition, chemical modification strategies to improve drug potential of aptamers are addressed. Although aptamers are excellent antimicrobial drug candidates, there are only a few studies that describe functional cell-based assays and potential therapeutic use. In this chapter, analytical applications of aptamers, as well as limited studies on their antimicrobial effect are reviewed.

Keywords: Antimicrobial resistance, Antibacterial aptamers, Aptamers, *In vitro* selection, Modified aptamers, Multi-drug resistant pathogens, SELEX, Therapeutic aptamers, Virulence factors.

INTRODUCTION

Aptamers are single stranded DNA (ssDNA) or RNA molecules that are capable of folding into complex three dimensional structures and bind to their targets with high affinity and specificity. The term "aptamer" originates from the words "aptus" and "meros", which together mean "fitting particle" [1].

Since first introduction of aptamers to scientific community by the laboratories of Szostak and Gold [1, 2], more than 1000 well-characterized aptamers for at least

---

[*] **Corresponding authors Serap Evran:** Department of Biochemistry, Faculty of Science, Ege University, 35100, Bornova-Izmir, Turkey; Tel: +90 232 3112304; Fax: +90 232 3115485; E-mail: serap.evran@ege.edu.tr

Atta-ur-Rahman & M. Iqbal Choudhary (Eds.)

550 target molecules have been reported by several research groups. Aptamers are promising alternatives to antibodies; hence they are defined as chemical antibodies [3, 4]. Understanding the nature of aptamers, their characteristics and advantages over antibodies will be helpful for understanding the reason of great interest in aptamers. Aptagen "Apta-Index" database [http://www.aptagen.com/aptamer-index/aptamer-list.aspx] is a comprehensive source that includes more than 500 aptamers.

Before the discovery of novel functionalities, it was assumed that the sole function of nucleic acids was to carry the genetic information. In the beginning of 1990s, it was observed that short RNA molecules could fold into specific three dimensional structures and bind to non-nucleic acid targets [5]. This revolutionary observation encouraged researchers to investigate RNA-ligand interactions. Those efforts resulted in identification of RNA aptamers for bacteriophage T4 DNA polymerase and organic dyes [1, 2]. Moreover, ssDNA-cleaving RNA was selected [6]. Then, this pioneering discovery was followed by identification of ssDNA aptamers against different targets [7]. Specific three dimensional structure of aptamer is formed by stems, loops, bulges, hairpins, pseudoknots, triplexes or G-quadruplexes. The complex structure forms the basis for conformational adaptation in aptamer-ligand interaction [8]. Hydrogen bonds, van der Waals interactions, electrostatic interactions and base stacking of aromatic groups enable the aptamer to fold into a specific 3D structure. These forces also contribute to aptamer-ligand interactions [9 - 11]. Structural diversity and nature of chemical interactions make it possible to develop nucleic acid aptamers to almost any target. However, natural nucleobases restrict structural and chemical diversity of aptamers. To overcome this limitation, researchers introduced a variety of modified bases to expand the chemical diversity [12]. The great reputation of nucleic acid aptamers can not only be attributed to their structural diversity and their ability to bind different ligands. Intrinsic properties, such as chemical and temperature stability, ease of chemical production, non-immunogenic property, the possibility to attach dyes or functional groups during synthesis make aptamers superior to antibodies [13]. Aptamers can be chemically modified to provide nuclease resistance, which is needed in therapeutic applications.

Selection of Aptamers

DNA or RNA aptamers are selected from random libraries using a process called SELEX (Systematic Evolution of Ligands by EXponential Enrichment) [2]. The flexibility of SELEX technology allows to identify aptamers that bind to ligands under pre-determined conditions [14]. Since the discovery of SELEX methodology, numerous novel techniques have been introduced and used to identify new DNA or RNA aptamers against different targets ranging from metal ions to complex cellular targets, or even whole cells. These techniques have been comprehensively reviewed elsewhere [14 - 16]. SELEX can be summarized as iterative cycles of binding, partitioning, amplification and re-introduction of nucleic acid pool with the target until target-binders are enriched (Fig. **1**). A very large combinatorial library of oligonucleotides is screened through SELEX process. Oligonucleotide library represents $\sim 10^{14}$-10^{15} different sequences containing a random region of 20-80 bases. Random sequences are flanked by primer binding sites, which are required for polymerase chain reaction (PCR). Design and diversity of starting nucleic acid library is the critical point that determines not only the success of SELEX process, but also functional characteristics of aptamers. Therefore, bioinformatic analysis of next-generation sequencing data allows deeper analysis and optimization of random library [15, 17].

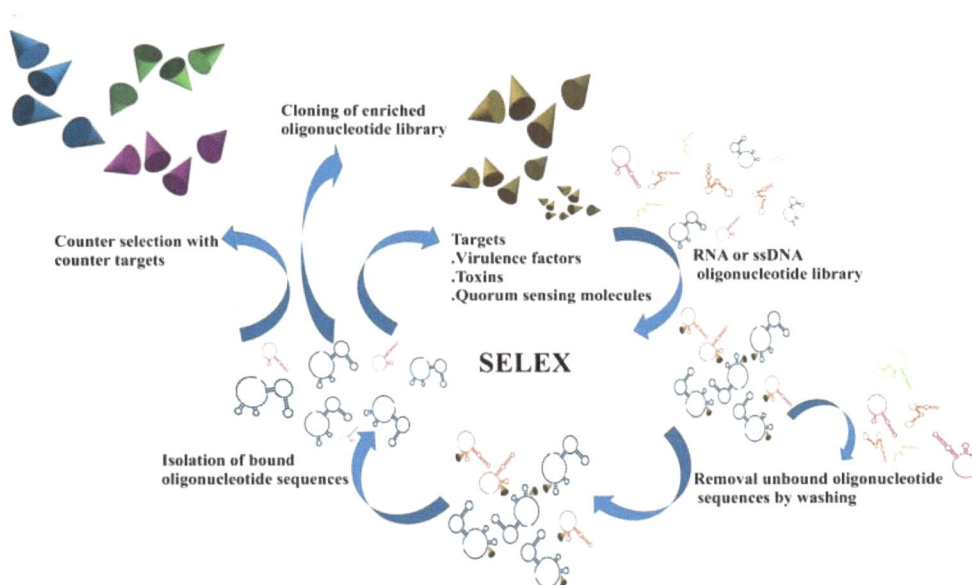

Fig. (1). Basic flow diagram of SELEX process.

In SELEX process, nucleic acid library is first incubated with target molecule under pre-determined conditions. The next step is partitioning of binding aptamer pool from unbound sequences. Unbound sequences are removed, and bound ones are eluted from the target. Eluted DNA is used as template in PCR, which allows enrichment of binder sequences. Unlike the starting nucleic acid library, PCR amplification gives double-stranded DNA product. In order to obtain ssDNA from PCR product, different methods can be used. Asymmetric PCR is based on using excessive amount of one primer to obtain an experimentally pre-determined forward/reverse primer ratio [18]. This primer ratio results in over-amplification of one strand, which is then used in the next round of SELEX. Another method relies on biotin-streptavidin separation. In this method, one of the primers is obtained in biotinylated form. Double-stranded DNA product is incubated with streptavidin beads, and then non-biotinylated strand is separated *via* NaOH treatment [19]. If PCR product contains a phosphorylated end at one strand, lambda exonuclease digestion can be another option to generate ssDNA. Selectivity of lambda exonuclease for phosphorylated strand allows protection of non-phosphorylated strand against digestion under carefully controlled conditions [20]. Denaturing urea polyacrylamide gel electrophoresis is another method to generate ssDNA. In this method, one PCR primer is designed to contain a PCR terminator group. After performing PCR, strands with different sizes can be readily separated using denaturing urea polyacrylamide gel electrophoresis [21]. Combination of lambda exonuclease digestion and asymmetric PCR was shown to be the most effective method with the highest yield of ssDNA [22].

Effective partitioning of binder sequences from unbound ones is dependent on selection platform. Magnetic beads are often used due to the ease of use, efficient partitioning and great diversity of ligand coupling chemistry. Magnetic SELEX was developed in early 2000s [23, 24], and then it was modified as FluMag SELEX [25]. Other selection platforms are capillary electrophoresis microarray, graphene oxide, and nitrocellulose filter [16]. Selectivity and affinity of selected aptamers is dependent on conditions and stringency of SELEX process. In order to improve binding properties of aptamers, negative SELEX and counter SELEX are employed. Negative selection step is performed in order to eliminate sequences that bind to target in a non-specific manner [26, 27]. Negative SELEX is useful to eliminate the sequences adsorbed onto immobilization matrix. For example, if target is immobilized onto magnetic beads, nucleic acid pool is treated with empty magnetic beads, and then unbound sequences are incubated with the target. Counter SELEX is another way to improve the binding properties of aptamer. Nucleic acid sequences that bind to molecules that are closely related to target molecule can be eliminated during counter selection step. That allows to eliminate the sequences that bind to structurally-similar non-target molecules. For this aim, nucleic acid pool is incubated with non-target molecule first, and then unbound sequences are incubated with the target. This step results in further improvement of selectivity [28]. Moreover, a careful and smart control of the ratio of nucleic acid to ligand, addition of competitors such as yeast tRNA or salmon sperm DNA, decreasing the amount of target, increasing the number of washing steps, and shortening the incubation time eliminate weak-binding aptamers. Final step of SELEX is to clone and sequence the enriched library. Conventionally, enriched DNA library can be cloned using standard restriction endonuclease cleavage and DNA ligation. Alternatively, TA cloning method can be used in order to improve cloning efficiency. While traditional Sanger sequencing is still the most widely used method, high-throughput sequencing attracts interest due to reduced cost and increased availability [29 - 32, 4]. Meme Suite is a powerful web-based program that allows users to enter the sequences of aptamers and discover enriched motifs [33]. Enriched motifs can then be characterized in terms of secondary structure and relative Gibbs free energy parameters, which are predicted by mfold web server [34]. Aptamer candidates can be further characterized for their selectivity and affinity using different methods, such as flow cytometry [35] radioactive labeling [36], filter retention assay [37], surface plasmon resonance (SPR) [38], isothermal titration calorimetry [39], fluorescence polarization [40], enzyme linked oligonucleotide assay (ELONA) [41 - 44], and electromobility shift assay [45]. In addition, gold nanoparticle and graphene oxide-based assays, as well as direct fluorophore labeling and fluorescence quenching can be used to characterize binding properties [46]. Each assay has its unique advantages and disadvantages over others, and there is no currently available gold standard method that can be adapted to all aptamers. This limitation can be explained by large repertoire of aptamer targets, ranging from small molecules to proteins or even cells. Therefore, each target could require a specific method for characterization of aptamer-ligand interaction.

Aptamers Against Toxins and Protein Virulence Factors

Aptamers are attractive molecules for diagnostic applications. For this purpose, several aptamers have been developed against pathogen cells. In this approach, target is directly the pathogen cell itself, and the whole process is called Cell-SELEX [47]. There are many studies on pathogen-specific aptamers and their use in biosensors [48 - 50]. In addition to their function as sensing components of biosensors, aptamers also display great potential as alternative drugs. For this aim, several virulence factors are targeted by nucleic acid aptamers.

Aptamers Against Staphylococcal Toxins

DNA aptamer against α-toxin of *Staphylococcus aureus* was developed by Vivekananda *et al.* [51]. In this study, inhibition of the lethal activity of α-toxin was aimed. The authors identified aptamer sequences that were able to inhibit the toxin-induced death of Jurkat T cells. Related with this study, the authors also hold a patent on drug development using AT-27, AT-33, AT-36, or AT-49 aptamers [52]. The first aptamer for staphylococcal enterotoxin B (SEB) was developed by Bruno and Kiel [53]. Development of aptamers against SEB was one of the pioneering work in this field [53], and it was followed by different studies [54, 55]. Since the first aptamer sequence for SEB was non-disclosed,

DeGrasse performed SELEX again and developed a novel aptamer that was called APT[SEB1] [54]. Purschke *et al.* developed a Spiegelmer DNA aptamer, but its selectivity among other staphylococcal enterotoxins was not good enough [56]. SEB-binding aptamer was used in different detection systems [57, 58]. In another study, CNBr-activated sepharose 4B affinity chromatography based aptamer selection method was introduced for SEB [59]. As reviewed elsewhere [57], Huang *et al.* developed a DNA aptamer for staphylococcal enterotoxin C1 (SEC1) [60].

Aptamers Against Clostridium Toxins

Clostridium difficile toxins are associated with colitis and diarrhea. Aptamers were selected for those toxins [61, 62]. Slow off-rate modified aptamers (SOMAmers) were developed against *C. difficile* toxins A, B and binary toxin using magnetic-bead SELEX [61]. In this study, recombinant *C. difficile* toxins were obtained in soluble fraction, and they were purified by affinity chromatography. Hong *et al.* used carboxylic acid-coated magnetic beads to immobilize the lyophilized toxin B from *C. difficile* [62]. During SELEX, bovine serum albumin, alpha toxin from *S. aureus*, exotoxin A from *Pseudomonas aeruginosa*, and cholera toxin from *Vibrio cholera* were used as negative targets. Binding affinity was characterized using SPR, and the selected aptamer had a K_d value of 47.3 ± 13.7 nM.

SOMAmers were firstly described by Gold *et al.* in a study funded by SomaLogic [63]. SOMAmers were designed to include chemical modifications at 5-position of uridine (dUTP). SELEX was performed using random libraries containing modified nucleotides, such as 5-benzylaminocarbonyl-dU (BndU), 5-naphthylmethylaminocarbonyl-dU (NapdU), 5-tryptaminocarbonyl-dU (TrpdU), and 5-isobutylaminocarbonyl-dU (iBudU). Establishment of SOMAmer technology provided SOMAmers with more diversity, stability and affinity, and they were used in further studies [48, 64]. Recently, new SOMAmers with additional modification at 5-position of deoxycytidine (dC) were obtained [65].

Correct and rapid diagnosis of *C. difficile* infections is critical to get disease under control [66, 67]. Toxin A and toxin B are two major toxins secreted by *C. difficile* [48, 67]. Aptamer-based toxin B analysis was achieved in human fecal samples at nanomolar concentrations [62]. In this study, Hong *et al.* used aptamer-modified sandwich ELISA assay. The amino-modified aptamer was used to capture toxin B on the surface of microwell, and then primary anti-toxin B antibody was bound to the toxin. Addition of secondary antibody conjugated to horseradish peroxidase generated the colorimetric signal. In another study, Luo *et al.* developed an aptamer specific for toxin A. The authors designed an electrochemical aptamer-based biosensor to detect the toxin with a detection limit of 1 nM [68].

Botulinum neurotoxins (BoNTs) produced by anaerobic *Clostridium botulinum* are lethal and they cause botulism [69, 70]. BoNT consists of light chain (LC) and heavy chain (HC), which are held together *via* a single disulfide bond [71]. In an attempt to develop aptamers against the neurotoxin, Bruno *et al.* immobilized LC and used it for SELEX. In this study, aptamer beacon was constructed by labeling the aptamer sequence with 5'-TYE 665 and 3'-Iowa Black quencher. The authors observed a fluorescence response to increasing levels of LC with a detection limit of 1 ng/mL. The designed beacon also responded to BoNT type B, type E holotoxins, HC or LC components in diluted soil sample [72]. In another study, Chang *et al.* developed two RNA aptamers against LC of type A BoNT. It was reported that the aptamers showed strong binding affinity for their targets. The calculated K_d values were 31.4 nM and 27.9 nM. Moreover, endopeptidase activity of LC was considerably inhibited by the aptamers. It was concluded that the selected aptamers could be promising as potential therapeutic agents against botulism [73].

Tok and Fischer performed a single microbead SELEX to select DNA aptamers against BoNT/A Hc-peptide and toxoid. In this study, BoNT/A Hc-peptide and toxoid were immobilized onto Ni-NTA agarose and amine-functionalized polystyrene TentaGel beads, respectively. The functionalized microbeads were incubated with aptamer library, and after only two SELEX rounds aptamers could be selected. The K_d values were determined using fluorescence anisotropy measurements. The K_d values ranged between 3-51 nM for toxoid aptamers, and 1-4 μM for HC peptide-specific aptamers [71].

Ren *et al.* identified DNA aptamers against BoNT type E toxoid (BoNTE) using a porous silicon-sol–gel (PS-SG) SELEX approach. The bound aptamers were selected after five SELEX rounds. The selected aptamers were analyzed using next-generation sequencing and biolayer interferometry. In addition, the selected aptamer was used to develop a graphene oxide-based fluorimetric assay. The characterized aptamer showed a binding affinity at low nanomolar range with a K_d value of 53.3 nM [69].

Aptamers Against E. coli Toxins

Shiga toxin is one of the most common and dangerous foodborne toxins. Two members of the Shiga toxins (Stx 1 and Stx 2) were targeted, and SELEX rounds were performed using unmodified and modified nuclease-resistant RNA libraries [74]. In this study, the relevant toxins were immobilized onto a microtiter plate *via* their respective antibodies and then incubated with RNA library in binding buffer. It was observed that the aptamers developed against Stx2 could inhibit binding of the toxin to the cell surface. This was attributed to binding of the aptamers to Stx2 B subunit, as well as to the corresponding antibody. Although aptamers were successfully selected for Stx2, specific aptamers could not be obtained for Stx1. The authors concluded that Stx1 was not a good candidate for SELEX. However, the results were not fully explained. Another aptamer selection study against *E. coli* virulence factors was carried out by Bruno *et al.* [75]. In this study, DNA aptamers were developed against lipopolysaccharide (LPS), intimin, and Stx1.

Aptamers Against Aspergillus and Penicillium Toxins

Ochratoxin A (OTA) is produced by fungal species, such as *Aspergillus* and *Penicillium*. Aptamers against OTA were developed using SELEX [76]. As reviewed elsewhere [77], OTA-specific aptamer was used as the sensing component of several biosensor constructs. Aflatoxin is one of the major foodborne mycotoxins, which has genotoxic and carcinogenic effects. The mycotoxin is produced by molds, such as *Aspergillus flavus* and *Aspergillus parasiticus* [78]. One of the first attempts to generate DNA aptamer against Aflatoxin B1 (AFB1) was performed by Ma *et al.* [79]. In this study, magnetic nanoparticle-based SELEX process was employed. In order to improve the specificity of aptamer, other toxins (AFB2, AFG1, AFG2, OTA, and FB1) were used as counter targets. The aptamer was used as the sensing component, and aptamer-based fluorescent sensing was performed with a detection limit of 35 ng/L AFB1. In another study, AFB1 aptamer was generated using immunoaffinity SELEX [80]. The K_d values of three aptamer candidates, namely AFLA5, AFLA53, and AFLA71 were determined. The aptamer AFLA 53 showed the best affinity with a K_d of 48.29 ± 9.45 nM. Detection limit was determined using the same method, and it was found to be 20 ng/mL and 40 ng/mL for AFLA5 and AFLA71, respectively.

Aptamers Against Mycobacterium Tuberculosis Toxins

The emergence of drug-resistant *Mycobacterium tuberculosis* is one major problem, and therefore novel therapeutic agents are urgently needed [50]. In order to overcome this problem, Shum *et al.* attempted to target the bacterial enzyme polyphosphate kinase 2 (PPK2). PPK2 plays a critical role in synthesis of some molecules, which are important for bacterial survival. The authors performed SELEX and the selected aptamer had a K_d value of 870 nM. Moreover, the aptamer was able to inhibit the enzyme activity by 50% [81].

EsxG is another protein secreted by the ESX-3 secretion system of *M. tuberculosis*. This system is an essential mechanism providing pathogenicity in low iron environments. For that reason, Nqobile *et al.* aimed to develop aptamers against

EsxG. In this study, two aptamers (G43 and G78) were characterized using SPR-based SELEX. The results showed that binding affinity of G43 and G78 against EsxG was 8.04 ± 1.90 nM and 78.85 ± 9.40 nM, respectively. The aptamer G43 could specifically bind to EsxG, but no significant binding was observed for the homologous protein EsxA [82].

Qin *et al.* aimed to develop an aptamer-based detection system for the biomarker protein MPT64. In order to monitor tuberculosis infection, they designed a sandwich assay based on the complex between aptamer and MPT64. Detection of the biomarker in culture samples was achieved with 86.3% sensitivity and 88.5% specificity [83]. In a similar study, Sypabekova *et al.* developed and analyzed MPT64-specific DNA aptamers. In this study, a different SELEX approach based on capturing the protein-aptamer complex on nitrocellulose membrane was employed. The aptamer with the highest binding affinity was identified using SPR and ELONA. Sensitivity and specificity of the selected aptamer was found to be 91.3% and 90%, respectively. Moreover, other mycobacterial secreted proteins (ESAT-6 and CFP-10) were used as non-target controls and the selected aptamer could recognize MPT64 protein among others. The authors concluded that the developed aptamer could be used in further medical diagnostics to detect tuberculosis infection [41].

Rotherham *et al.* targeted the heterodimer CFP-10-ESAT-6 to design aptamer-based monitoring assay for tuberculosis infection. One of the developed aptamers was analyzed using ELONA. The results showed that 100% sensitivity and 68.75% specificity were achieved in analysis of sputum samples from patients. On the other hand, the authors reported that time-consuming aptamer-based assay had some limitations due to antigenic cross-reactivity [84]. In another study, the heterodimer CFP-10-ESAT-6 was re-targeted by Tang *et al.* [85]. The authors selected two DNA aptamers, namely CE24 and CE15. A novel and improved aptamer-based ELONA assay was designed to detect CFP10 and ESAT6 proteins in serum samples from patients. The aptamer CE24 showed better performance in terms of sensitivity and specificity.

Aptamers Against Other Toxins

Aptamers against cholera toxin were developed by Bruno and Kiel [53]. The authors determined the limit of detection (LOD) using two different methods. Enzyme-linked aptamer assay and electrochemiluminescence assay resulted in LOD values of 10 ng and 40 ng, respectively.

Bruno *et al.* targeted the outer membrane protein of *E. coli* strain 8739, and they developed aptamers against the target protein [86]. For this purpose, they extracted the target protein and then immobilized it onto magnetic beads. The developed aptamers were used in different sensing applications [87, 88].

Protective antigen toxin of *Bacillus anthracis* is an important virulence factor [89]. Capillary electrophoresis based SELEX process was applied to generate specific aptamers for the protective antigen. The selected aptamer had a K_d value of 112 nM [90]. Oh *et al*. developed a 29-mer DNA aptamer against the anthrax protective antigen [91]. A different SELEX approach called artificially expanded genetic information system was employed to develop aptamers against the protective antigen of *B. anthracis* [92]. Since lethal factor of *B. anthracis* conjugates with protective antigen to form the lethal toxin, Ryabko *et al*. developed a DNA aptamer to block the activity of lethal toxin [93].

Internalin (InlA) is the invasive protein of *Listeria* species and it is known to complex with human E-cadherin receptor [94]. The aptamer against InlA was developed for recognition and biosensing of *Listeria* spp [95]. Another research group also developed aptamers against Internalin A, B and E proteins, as well as protein 0610 [96, 97].

Type IVB pili is one of the virulence factors of *Salmonella enterica* Serovar Typhi [98]. Pan *et al*. developed aptamers against Type IVB pili protein using SELEX [99]. For this aim, the protein was produced in fusion with glutathione S-transferase (GST), which was expressed in *E. coli* cells and then purified using glutathione-Sepharose 4B column. The purified protein was immobilized on glutathione-Sepharose 4B *via* its GST fusion partner and then incubated with random RNA library. Inhibitory effect of the aptamers on adhesion and invasion of THP-1 cells was studied. The authors showed that treatment with the aptamer pool efficiently inhibited the invasion of *S. enterica* Typhi into THP-1 cells. It was concluded that this result was promising for developing drugs.

Aptamers Against Quorum Sensing Molecules

Quorum sensing is a key mechanism for cell-cell communication [100]. Bacterial species can regulate the expression of quorum sensing signal molecules according to the density of cell-population. These signal molecules are called autoinducers. Gram-negative bacteria use acylated homoserine lactones as autoinducers. Acyl-homoserine lactones (AHLs) are secreted by gram-positive and gram-negative bacteria. *Pseudomonas aeruginosa* produces this kind of signaling molecules, namely C4-HSL and 3O-C12-HSL [101, 102]. Some strains of *P. aeruginosa* are resistant to nearly all antibiotics [103]. For that reason, any alternative system is important to prevent diseases caused by drug-resistant pathogens. *P. aeruginosa* has two quorum sensing systems: las and rhl system. Las system is composed of LasR transcriptional regulator and LasI synthase that is responsible for production of AHL signal molecule N-(3-oxododecanoyl)-L homoserine lactone (3O-C1-

-HSL). Rhl system is composed of RhlR that functions as a transcriptional regulator and RhlI that produces N-butyryl-L-homoserine lactone (C4-HSL) [104].

Zhao *et al.* developed specific DNA aptamers for N-acyl homoserine lactones. The aim of this study was to inhibit biofilm formation and secretion of LasA protease, LasB elastase and pyocyanin using aptamers. The C4-HSL-specific aptamer was effective on rhl system and it was able to inhibit the secretion of pyocyanin. The 3O-C12-HSL-specific aptamer inhibited both biofilm formation and release of virulence factors such as LasA protease, pyocyanin and LasB elastase [105]. Table **1** summarizes some aptamers developed against virulence factors, as well as their use for different applications.

Table 1. Aptamers developed against some virulence factors, applications and outputs.

Target	K_d	Application/Outcomes
Clostridium difficile toxin B	47.3 nM	Modified ELISA [62]
Clostridium difficile toxin A	-	Electrochemical biosensor [64]
Clostridium difficile binary toxin	0.02–2.7 nM	Sandwich assays [106]
Clostridium toxin A, B and binary toxin	low nM range	Sandwich assays Dot blot assays Pull-down assays [61]
Clostridium botulinum neurotoxin Type A LC	31.4-27.9 nM	Inhibition of endopeptidase activity [73]
Clostridium botulinum neurotoxin type A HC peptide/toxoid	low nM range	Inhibition of interaction between the peptide and anti-BoNT Ab [71]
Clostridium botulinum Neurotoxin E	53.3 nM	Graphene oxide (GO)-based fluorimetric detection [69]
Pseudomonas aeruginosa 3O-C12-HSL C4- HSL	20-35 nM 25-50 nM	Inhibition of biofilm formation and secretion of virulence factors [105]
Mycobacterium tuberculosis MPT64 protein	8.92 nM	ELONA [41]
Mycobacterium tuberculosis CFP-10-ESAT-6 heterodimer	low nanomolar range	ELONA [84]
Mycobacterium tuberculosis CFP-10 ESAT-6	3.75×10^{-7} M 1.6×10^{-7} M	ELONA [85]
Mycobacterium tuberculosis polyphosphate kinase 2	870 nM	Inhibition of the enzyme activity [81]
Mycobacterium tuberculosis MPT64 protein	-	Sandwich assay [83]

(Table 1) contd.....

Target	K_d	Application/Outcomes
Mycobacterium tuberculosis EsxG protein	8.04-78.85 nM	Molecular probes to study EsxG [82]
Staphylococcus aureus α-toxin	unspecified	Inhibition of α-toxin and drug development [51, 52]
Staphylococcus aureus enterotoxin B	unspecified	Biosensor studies [54]
Staphylococcus aureus enterotoxin B	64 nM	Neutralization of staphylococcal enterotoxin B [55]
Staphylococcus aureus enterotoxin B	2.3×10^{-11} M	SEB detection in human serum [59]
Staphylococcus aureus enterotoxin C1	49.43 nM, 65.14 nM, 154.9 nM	SEC1 analysis in milk samples [60]
Escherichia coli Shiga toxins	unspecified	Neutralization of Stx2-mediated HeLa cell cytotoxicity [74]
Ochratoxin A produced by *Aspergillus* spp. and *Penicillium* spp.	370 nM, 290 nM, 110 nM	SYBR® Green I fluorescence-based OTA biosensing [76]
Ochratoxin A produced by *Aspergillus* spp. and *Penicillium* spp.	360 nM	OTA detections in foods [107]
Aflatoxin B1	11.39 nM	AFB1 detection in peanut oil sample [79]
Aflatoxin B1	50.45 nM, 48.29 nM, 85.02 nM	AFB1 detection in corn sample [80]
Escherichia coli strain 8739 outer membrane protein	unspecified	FRET-based detection systems [86]
Bacillus anthracis protective antigen toxin	112 nM	Aptamer-functionalized single-walled carbon nanotube (SWNT) conjugate [90]
Bacillus anthracis protective antigen toxin	35 nM	Inhibition of LF binding [92]
Bacillus anthracis lethal factor	unspecified	Inhibition of the lethal toxin activity [93]
Listeria monocytogenes Internalin (InlA)	unspecified	Fiber-optic biosensor [95]
Salmonella enterica Serovar Typhi Type IVB Pili	8.56 nM	Inhibition effect on adhesion [99]

Modifications of Aptamers for Improving Therapeutic Potential

Aptamers have unique and valuable advantages, which make them attractive to be studied by various fields of life sciences. However, their degradation by nucleases is a major problem that should be taken into consideration when planning their use in therapeutic applications [13, 108]. Serum half-life of unmodified aptamers can be as low as seconds. Improving nuclease resistance is not the only reason that makes aptamer modifications promising. Modifications also allow enhanced binding affinity and higher repertoire of ligands [12, 109, 110]. This is because of that chemical modifications provide expanded sequence space and functionalities. Chemical modifications of aptamer library can be grouped into three classes; i) sugar modifications, ii) phosphate backbone modifications, and iii) nucleobase modifications. While chemically modified nucleic acid library can be a good starting point for aptamer selection in most cases, some groups reported aptamer libraries with expanded genetic alphabet and obtained improved binding affinity against novel ligands [111 - 113]. Regarding aptamer modifications, there are some recent excellent reviews [3, 12, 114]. In Fig. (**2**), possible modifications to solve some problems of aptamer-based applications are summarized.

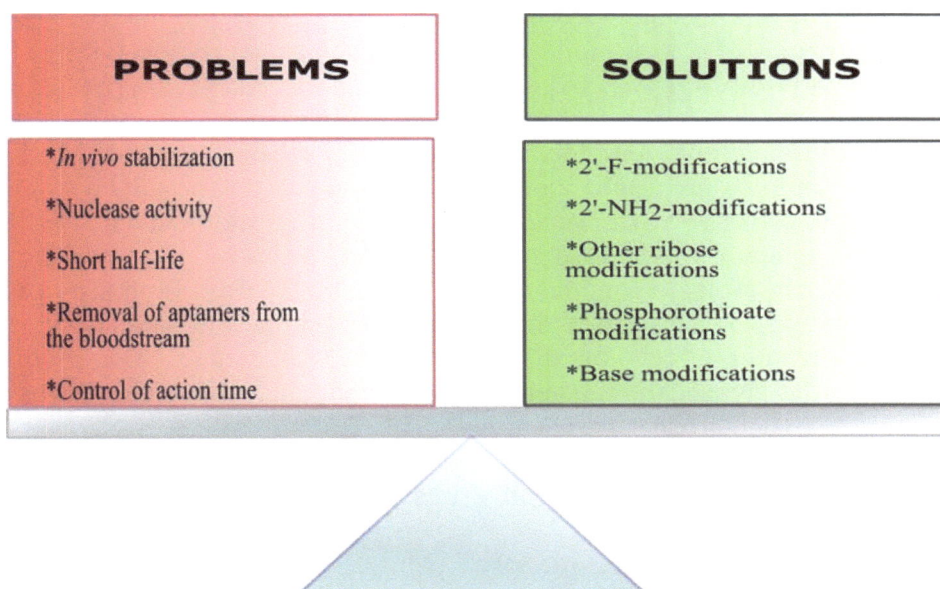

PROBLEMS

* *In vivo* stabilization

* Nuclease activity

* Short half-life

* Removal of aptamers from the bloodstream

* Control of action time

SOLUTIONS

* 2'-F-modifications

* 2'-NH_2-modifications

* Other ribose modifications

* Phosphorothioate modifications

* Base modifications

Fig. (2). Possible problems and solutions in aptamer-based applications.

2'-F-Modified RNA Aptamers

2'-Fluoro modification of nucleic acids is one of the most widely used chemical modifications. In most cases, only slight alteration or no change of binding affinity have been reported. Besides, 2'-F modification has the advantage of being compatible to be synthesized by reverse transcriptase, while increasing resistance against attack by nucleases. Ulrich *et al.* designed several 2'-F modified RNA aptamers against the protein targets from *Trypanosoma cruzi* [115]. Even though *in vivo* characterization of the developed aptamers was not performed, the authors successfully proved that chemically modified aptamers were able to inhibit parasite invasion into mammalian cells to some degree. The chemically modified and truncated RNA aptamer was introduced by Dey *et al.* [116]. They showed that 2'-F modified RNA aptamers were able to bind and neutralize the surface glycoprotein gp120 of HIV-1. Substitution of 2'-F bases with their natural analogs resulted in complete loss of affinity, clearly showing the role of 2'-F modification in aptamer-ligand interaction. In addition, the truncated minimal version of RNA aptamer B40t77 was able to bind and neutralize gp120 with a similar affinity to the parental RNA aptamer. Truncation of nucleic acid aptamers enables researchers to synthesize aptamers *via* phosphoramidite chemistry in large quantities. Synthesis scale is particularly important to evaluate the success of modification. 2'-Fluoropyrimidine modified RNA aptamer for the erythrocyte membrane protein 1 of *Plasmodium falciparum* was shown to be effective as a putative anti-rosetting agent [117]. A partially modified RNA aptamer was developed against Herpes Simplex Virus Type 1, and the aptamer was able to inhibit the antiviral activity *via* blocking the interaction between gD-HVEM and gD-nectin 1. Moreover, a 44-nucleotide minimal aptamer was designed from the parental aptamer consisting of 113 bases by both mapping and boundary analysis. The truncated aptamer was shown to have almost the same characteristics as parental aptamer in terms of binding affinity and functionality. In this study, 2'-fluoro modification was performed and it was observed that the modification had different stabilization effects on different aptamer sequences. The modified aptamer-1 showed significant resistance against endonuclease, while it was not stable against exonuclease. This study is interesting, since it shows that exonuclease degradation of RNA sequences should also be taken into consideration, if the purpose is to investigate therapeutic potential of RNA aptamers [118].

2'-NH₂ Modification of Aptamers

2'-NH$_2$ modification is another popular chemical modification used widely for increasing nuclease resistance. Wang *et al.* developed 2'-NH$_2$ modified RNA aptamers against the glycoproteins B and H of human cytomegalovirus [119]. Ribonuclease-resistant RNA aptamers showed antiviral activity primarily due to inhibition of the viral genome entry into cells.

In another study, it was aimed to develop RNA aptamers to an invariant surface domain of live African trypanosome. The authors showed that RNA aptamer was capable of binding to flagellar attachment zone with high affinity [120]. 2'-NH$_2$ modification of RNA aptamer was shown to increase serum half-life from seconds to ≥ 30 h in human serum, compared to its 2'-OH analog. Indirect *in situ* fluorescence labeling was performed using the biotinylated RNA aptamer and fluorophore-conjugated anti-biotin antibody. As a potential therapeutic approach, the results clearly showed that the biotinylated aptamer could be used to re-direct immunoglobulins against live parasite cells.

Bugaut *et al.* introduced the combination of dynamic combinatorial chemistry and SELEX for selection of modified aptamers conjugated to various small molecules [121]. In this proof of principle study, $2'-NH_2$ modified uridine bases were used to create the starting combinatorial nucleic acid library. In order to create dynamic combinatorial library of $2'$-imino conjugated oligonucleotides, the library was incubated with target in the presence of various aldehydes. In this study, the target was the transactivation-response element of HIV-1. The target-bound $2'$-imino modified sequences were eluted, which resulted in concomitant hydrolysis of imine linkages. By this way, several aptamers were identified and $2'$-imino modification sites were determined.

Other Ribose Modified Aptamers

Synthetic nucleic acid analogs with altered sugar backbones are known as xeno-nucleic acids or XNAs. $2'$-deoxy-$2'$-fluoroarabinonucleotides (FANAs) also belong to XNAs, which are typically less susceptible to nuclease degradation because of unnatural nucleoside structure. Ferreira-Bravo *et al.* developed FANA aptamers against HIV-1RT. The authors showed that the aptamer completely lost the target-binding ability and concluded that FANA modification was critical for binding [122]. The developed FANA aptamer, namely FA1, was also capable of inhibiting HIV-1RT. It was shown that binding affinity of FA1 was comparable to those aptamers developed earlier.

L-aptamers or Spiegelmers are enantiomers of D-aptamers, and they are completely resistant to nuclease degradation. *In vitro* selection of L-aptamers is performed using D-nucleic acid library and enantiomer (mirror image-spiegel) of the target molecule. Sczepanski and Joyce developed a Spiegelmer against HIV TAR RNA and showed that the Spiegelmer could inhibit formation of Tat-TAR ribonucleoprotein, the complex essential for TAR function [123]. One limiting feature of Spiegelmers is that the enantiomer of target needs to be synthesized. If the target is a complex protein, this process becomes more complicated. Purschke *et al.* showed that Spiegelmers could be developed against large protein targets using a domain approach [56]. They identified a stable domain of 25 amino acids as an appropriate target, and synthesized the D-enantiomer of this domain. Mirror image of the target was incubated with D-deoxyribose nucleic acid library during SELEX process. Post-SELEX characterization studies revealed the binding of L-DNA Spiegelmer to the L-peptide domain.

Locked nucleic acids (LNA) are conformationally restricted nucleotide analogs, and they show great resistance against nuclease degradation. HIV-1 TAR RNA aptamer was modified as LNA/DNA chimera, and it was shown that binding affinity of the modified aptamer was comparable to the parental aptamer. Furthermore, nuclease resistance of modified LNA/DNA chimera was tested in bovine serum. No difference in gel shift was observed, indicating an excellent nuclease resistance.

Phosphorothioate Modification

Phosphorothioate modification is another kind of modification that provides nuclease resistance. It was shown that thioanalogs of thrombin-binding DNA aptamers had greater nuclease stability in plasma [108]. Recently, some studies clearly demonstrated *in vivo* stability of phosphorothioate-modified aptamers. Phosphorothioate-modified DNA aptamers were developed against advanced glycation end products (AGE). Modified AGE aptamer was still detected in the kidney of rats even at 14th day after stopping intraperitoneal infusion [124]. Similarly, modified DNA aptamers that were raised against the receptor of AGEs could be detected in the kidney of rats 3 days after stopping injection [125]. These studies clearly demonstrate the efficiency of phosphorothioate modification when *in vivo* stability of aptamers is a concern. Wyatt et al. developed a DNA aptamer modified with phosphorothioate backbone and investigated its potential use as an inhibitor of HIV envelope-mediated cell fusion [126]. In this study, it was shown that phosphodiester analog was not able to show antiviral activity. As a result, it was concluded that phosphorothioate backbone was mechanistically essential for the activity. Sheehan and Phan confirmed that phosphorothioate oligonucleotides were able to inhibit intrinsic tenase complex activity, but phosphodiester analogs did not have inhibition activity [127]. However, nuclease stability of phosphorothioate oligonucleotides was not investigated in the study. In conclusion, these studies clearly indicate that phosphorothioate modification can be used not only to increase the nuclease resistance of aptamers, but also to introduce novel functionalities to nucleic acid aptamers. While post-SELEX phosphorothioate modification can be performed to increase nuclease resistance of aptamers, selection of phosphorothioate oligonucleotides against specific targets is also possible [108, 128].

Nucleobase Modification of Aptamers

In addition to improved nuclease resistance, increasing the affinity of aptamers and introducing novel functionalities might also be desired. In order to select RNA aptamers against the Rev protein of HIV-1, Jensen *et al.* used a RNA pool substituted with the photoreactive chromophore 5-iodouracil [109]. 5-iodouracil has affinity to aromatic side chains and cysteine upon irradiation, and this ability results in cross-linking of RNA molecule with the protein of interest. The authors used a dual selection strategy, and SELEX rounds involving photocrosslinking selection were alternated with selection for high-affinity RNA sequences. The authors developed 5-iodouracil modified RNA aptamers with high affinity and photocrosslinking ability. Some of the developed aptamers had such a high affinity that strong RNA-protein interaction was observed even under denaturing gel electrophoresis conditions and without UV crosslinking. Escolana *et al.* developed SOMAmers against the surface-specific proteins of *Neisseria menengitis* and *Streptococcus pneumoniae*. The random library including 5-tryptaminocarbonyl-dU (TrpdU) modification was used. The developed SOMAmers were used to design potential aptasensors for detection of the pathogens [110].

CONCLUDING REMARKS

As pathogens use different strategies to overcome antimicrobial treatments, standard drugs become ineffective by time. Therefore, novel antimicrobial strategies are urgently needed. Nucleic acid aptamers hold promise as novel therapeutics against pathogens. There is an increasing interest in aptamers, which show comparable binding efficiency. Moreover, aptamers offer several advantages in terms of cost and ease of production. However, there are also some challenges that should be considered. One major problem is that aptamers are sensitive against serum nuclease degradation, which makes it difficult to use them as therapeutics. To overcome this problem, successful modification strategies have been introduced.

As summarized in this chapter, several nucleic acid aptamers against different pathogenic targets including toxins, surface components, quorum sensing molecules, invasion and adhesion factors are available. Aptamers have been widely used as recognition elements, and there are many immunobiosensor studies replacing antibodies with aptamers. The next question is implying aptamers as novel therapeutics, which needs continuous effort to improve some drawbacks of aptamers. The ever-increasing trend in the use of aptamers is promising for novel strategies in diagnosis and treatment of pathogens. However, it should be noted that animal studies are still needed to prove the therapeutic potential of antimicrobial aptamers.

CONSENT FOR PUBLICATION

Not applicable.

CONFLICT OF INTEREST

The editor declares no conflict of interest, financial or otherwise.

ACKNOWLEDGEMENT

We thank the Scientific and Technological Research Council of Turkey (TUBITAK) for financial support to develop aptamers against virulence factors (project number TUBITAK 214Z290 and TUBITAK 116Z024).

REFERENCES

[1]   Ellington AD, Szostak JW. *In vitro* selection of RNA molecules that bind specific ligands. Nature 1990; 346(6287): 818-22.
[http://dx.doi.org/10.1038/346818a0] [PMID: 1697402]

[2]   Tuerk C, Gold L. Systematic evolution of ligands by exponential enrichment: RNA ligands to bacteriophage T4 DNA polymerase. Science 1990; 249(4968): 505-10.
[http://dx.doi.org/10.1126/science.2200121] [PMID: 2200121]

[3]   Meek KN, Rangel AE, Heemstra JM. Enhancing aptamer function and stability *via in vitro* selection using modified nucleic acids. Methods 2016; 106(106): 29-36.
[http://dx.doi.org/10.1016/j.ymeth.2016.03.008] [PMID: 27012179]

[4]   Zhou J, Rossi J. Aptamers as targeted therapeutics: current potential and challenges. Nat Rev Drug Discov 2017; 16(3): 181-202.
[http://dx.doi.org/10.1038/nrd.2016.199] [PMID: 27807347]

[5]   Radom F, Jurek PM, Mazurek MP, Otlewski J, Jeleń F. Aptamers: molecules of great potential. Biotechnol Adv 2013; 31(8): 1260-74.
[http://dx.doi.org/10.1016/j.biotechadv.2013.04.007] [PMID: 23632375]

[6]   Robertson DL, Joyce GF. Selection *in vitro* of an RNA enzyme that specifically cleaves single-stranded DNA. Nature 1990; 344(6265): 467-8.
[http://dx.doi.org/10.1038/344467a0] [PMID: 1690861]

[7]   Ellington AD, Szostak JW. Selection *in vitro* of single-stranded DNA molecules that fold into specific ligand-binding structures. Nature 1992; 355(6363): 850-2.
[http://dx.doi.org/10.1038/355850a0] [PMID: 1538766]

[8]   Stoltenburg R, Reinemann C, Strehlitz B. SELEX--a (r)evolutionary method to generate high-affinity nucleic acid ligands. Biomol Eng 2007; 24(4): 381-403.
[http://dx.doi.org/10.1016/j.bioeng.2007.06.001] [PMID: 17627883]

[9]   Hermann T, Patel DJ. Adaptive recognition by aptamers nucleic acid. Science 2000; 287(5454): 820-5.
[http://dx.doi.org/10.1126/science.287.5454.820] [PMID: 10657289]

[10]   Aboul-ela F, Huang W, Abd Elrahman M, Boyapati V, Li P. Linking aptamer-ligand binding and expression platform folding in riboswitches: prospects for mechanistic modeling and design. Wiley Interdiscip Rev RNA 2015; 6(6): 631-50.
[http://dx.doi.org/10.1002/wrna.1300] [PMID: 26361734]

[11]   Perez-Gonzalez C, Lafontaine DA, Penedo JC. Fluorescence-based strategies to investigate the structure and dynamics of aptamer-ligand complexes. Front Chem 2016; 4(August): 33.
[PMID: 27536656]

[12]   Pfeiffer F, Rosenthal M, Siegl J, Ewers J, Mayer G. Customised nucleic acid libraries for enhanced aptamer selection and performance. Curr Opin Biotechnol 2017; 48: 111-8.
[http://dx.doi.org/10.1016/j.copbio.2017.03.026] [PMID: 28437710]

[13]   Keefe AD, Pai S, Ellington A. Aptamers as therapeutics. Nat Rev Drug Discov 2010; 9(7): 537-50.
        [http://dx.doi.org/10.1038/nrd3141] [PMID: 20592747]

[14]   Wu YX, Kwon YJ. Aptamers: The "evolution" of SELEX. Methods 2016; 106: 21-8.
        [http://dx.doi.org/10.1016/j.ymeth.2016.04.020] [PMID: 27109056]

[15]   Blind M, Blank M. Aptamer selection technology and recent advances. Mol Ther Nucleic Acids 2015;
        4: e223.
        [http://dx.doi.org/10.1038/mtna.2014.74] [PMID: 28110747]

[16]   Darmostuk M, Rimpelova S, Gbelcova H, Ruml T. Current approaches in SELEX: An update to
        aptamer selection technology. Biotechnol Adv 2015; 33(6 Pt 2): 1141-61.
        [http://dx.doi.org/10.1016/j.biotechadv.2015.02.008] [PMID: 25708387]

[17]   Blank M. Nucleic acid aptamers selection, characterization, and application. Springer. Chapter 7,
        Next-generation analysis of deep sequencing data: Bringing light into the black box of selex
        experiments. 2016; p. 85–95.

[18]   Marimuthu C, Tang T-H, Tominaga J, Tan S-C, Gopinath SC. Single-stranded DNA (ssDNA)
        production in DNA aptamer generation. Analyst (Lond) 2012; 137(6): 1307-15.
        [http://dx.doi.org/10.1039/c2an15905h] [PMID: 22314701]

[19]   Espelund M, Stacy RA, Jakobsen KS. A simple method for generating single-stranded DNA probes
        labeled to high activities. Nucleic Acids Res 1990; 18(20): 6157-8.
        [http://dx.doi.org/10.1093/nar/18.20.6157] [PMID: 2235518]

[20]   Avci-Adali M, Paul A, Wilhelm N, Ziemer G, Wendel HP. Upgrading SELEX technology by using
        lambda exonuclease digestion for single-stranded DNA generation. Molecules 2009; 15(1): 1-11.
        [http://dx.doi.org/10.3390/molecules15010001] [PMID: 20110867]

[21]   Williams KP, Bartel DP. PCR product with strands of unequal length. Nucleic Acids Res 1995;
        23(20): 4220-1.
        [http://dx.doi.org/10.1093/nar/23.20.4220] [PMID: 7479087]

[22]   Svobodová M, Pinto A, Nadal P, O' Sullivan CK. Comparison of different methods for generation of
        single-stranded DNA for SELEX processes. Anal Bioanal Chem 2012; 404(3): 835-42.
        [http://dx.doi.org/10.1007/s00216-012-6183-4] [PMID: 22733247]

[23]   Kikuchi K, Umehara T, Fukuda K, *et al.* RNA aptamers targeted to domain II of hepatitis C virus
        IRES that bind to its apical loop region. J Biochem 2003; 133(3): 263-70.
        [http://dx.doi.org/10.1093/jb/mvg036] [PMID: 12761160]

[24]   Murphy MB, Fuller ST, Richardson PM, Doyle SA. An improved method for the in vitro evolution of
        aptamers and applications in protein detection and purification. Nucleic Acids Res 2003; 31(18): e110.
        [http://dx.doi.org/10.1093/nar/gng110] [PMID: 12954786]

[25]   Stoltenburg R, Reinemann C, Strehlitz B. FluMag-SELEX as an advantageous method for DNA
        aptamer selection. Anal Bioanal Chem 2005; 383(1): 83-91.
        [http://dx.doi.org/10.1007/s00216-005-3388-9] [PMID: 16052344]

[26]   Blank M, Weinschenk T, Priemer M, Schluesener H. Systematic evolution of a DNA aptamer binding
        to rat brain tumor microvessels. selective targeting of endothelial regulatory protein pigpen. J Biol
        Chem 2001; 276(19): 16464-8.
        [http://dx.doi.org/10.1074/jbc.M100347200] [PMID: 11279054]

[27]   Vater A, Jarosch F, Buchner K, Klussmann S. Short bioactive Spiegelmers to migraine-associated
        calcitonin gene-related peptide rapidly identified by a novel approach: tailored-SELEX. Nucleic Acids
        Res 2003; 31(21): e130.
        [http://dx.doi.org/10.1093/nar/gng130] [PMID: 14576330]

[28]   Shangguan D, Li Y, Tang Z, *et al.* Aptamers evolved from live cells as effective molecular probes for
        cancer study. Proc Natl Acad Sci USA 2006; 103(32): 11838-43.

[http://dx.doi.org/10.1073/pnas.0602615103] [PMID: 16873550]

[29] Lou TF, Weidmann CA, Killingsworth J, Tanaka Hall TM, Goldstrohm AC, Campbell ZT. Integrated analysis of RNA-binding protein complexes using *in vitro* selection and high-throughput sequencing and sequence specificity landscapes (SEQRS). Methods 2017; 118-119: 171-81.
[http://dx.doi.org/10.1016/j.ymeth.2016.10.001] [PMID: 27729296]

[30] Dittmar KA, Jiang P, Park JW, *et al.* Genome-wide determination of a broad ESRP-regulated posttranscriptional network by high-throughput sequencing. Mol Cell Biol 2012; 32(8): 1468-82.
[http://dx.doi.org/10.1128/MCB.06536-11] [PMID: 22354987]

[31] Ditzler MA, Lange MJ, Bose D, *et al.* High-throughput sequence analysis reveals structural diversity and improved potency among RNA inhibitors of HIV reverse transcriptase. Nucleic Acids Res 2013; 41(3): 1873-84.
[http://dx.doi.org/10.1093/nar/gks1190] [PMID: 23241386]

[32] Ogawa N, Biggin MD. High-throughput SELEX determination of DNA sequences bound by transcription factors *in vitro*. Methods Mol Biol 2012; 786(786): 51-63.
[http://dx.doi.org/10.1007/978-1-61779-292-2_3] [PMID: 21938619]

[33] Bailey TL, Johnson J, Grant CE, Noble WS. The MEME Suite. Nucleic Acids Res 2015; 43(W1): W39-49.
[http://dx.doi.org/10.1093/nar/gkv416] [PMID: 25953851]

[34] Zuker M. Mfold web server for nucleic acid folding and hybridization prediction. Nucleic Acids Res 2003; 31(13): 3406-15.
[http://dx.doi.org/10.1093/nar/gkg595] [PMID: 12824337]

[35] Meyer M, Scheper T, Walter J-G. Aptamers: versatile probes for flow cytometry. Appl Microbiol Biotechnol 2013; 97(16): 7097-109.
[http://dx.doi.org/10.1007/s00253-013-5070-z] [PMID: 23838792]

[36] Carey J, Cameron V, de Haseth PL, Uhlenbeck OC. Sequence-specific interaction of R17 coat protein with its ribonucleic acid binding site. Biochemistry 1983; 22(11): 2601-10.
[http://dx.doi.org/10.1021/bi00280a002] [PMID: 6347247]

[37] Tolle F, Wilke J, Wengel J, Mayer G. By-product formation in repetitive PCR amplification of DNA libraries during SELEX. PLoS One 2014; 9(12): e114693.
[http://dx.doi.org/10.1371/journal.pone.0114693] [PMID: 25490402]

[38] Chang AL, McKeague M, Liang JC, Smolke CD. Kinetic and equilibrium binding characterization of aptamers to small molecules using a label-free, sensitive, and scalable platform. Anal Chem 2014; 86(7): 3273-8.
[http://dx.doi.org/10.1021/ac5001527] [PMID: 24548121]

[39] Lin PH, Chen RH, Lee CH, Chang Y, Chen CS, Chen WY. Studies of the binding mechanism between aptamers and thrombin by circular dichroism, surface plasmon resonance and isothermal titration calorimetry. Colloids Surf B Biointerfaces 2011; 88(2): 552-8.
[http://dx.doi.org/10.1016/j.colsurfb.2011.07.032] [PMID: 21885262]

[40] Zhu Z, Ravelet C, Perrier S, Guieu V, Fiore E, Peyrin E. Single-stranded DNA binding protein-assisted fluorescence polarization aptamer assay for detection of small molecules. Anal Chem 2012; 84(16): 7203-11.
[http://dx.doi.org/10.1021/ac301552e] [PMID: 22793528]

[41] Sypabekova M, Bekmurzayeva A, Wang R, Li Y, Nogues C, Kanayeva D. Selection, characterization, and application of DNA aptamers for detection of Mycobacterium tuberculosis secreted protein MPT64. Tuberculosis (Edinb) 2017; 104: 70-8.
[http://dx.doi.org/10.1016/j.tube.2017.03.004] [PMID: 28454652]

[42] García-Recio EM, Pinto-Díez C, Pérez-Morgado MI, *et al.* Characterization of MNK1b DNA Aptamers That Inhibit Proliferation in MDA-MB231 Breast Cancer Cells. Mol Ther Nucleic Acids

2016; 5(1): e275.
[http://dx.doi.org/10.1038/mtna.2015.50] [PMID: 26730812]

[43]   Stoltenburg R, Krafčiková P, Víglaský V, Strehlitz B. G-quadruplex aptamer targeting Protein A and its capability to detect Staphylococcus aureus demonstrated by ELONA. Scientific reports 2016; 6(2016): 33812.

[44]   Yan X, Gao X, Zhang Z. Isolation and characterization of 2′-amino-modified RNA aptamers for human TNFalpha. Genomics Proteomics Bioinformatics 2004; 2(1): 32-42.
[http://dx.doi.org/10.1016/S1672-0229(04)02005-4] [PMID: 15629041]

[45]   Wang MS, Reed SM. Direct visualization of electrophoretic mobility shift assays using nanoparticle-aptamer conjugates. Electrophoresis 2012; 33(2): 348-51.
[http://dx.doi.org/10.1002/elps.201100308] [PMID: 22170687]

[46]   Alhadrami HA, Chinnappan R, Eissa S, Rahamn AA, Zourob M. High affinity truncated DNA aptamers for the development of fluorescence based progesterone biosensors. Anal Biochem 2017; 525: 78-84.
[http://dx.doi.org/10.1016/j.ab.2017.02.014] [PMID: 28237255]

[47]   Ohuchi S. Cell-SELEX Technology. Biores Open Access 2012; 1(6): 265-72.
[http://dx.doi.org/10.1089/biores.2012.0253] [PMID: 23515081]

[48]   Hong KL, Sooter LJ. Single-stranded DNA aptamers against pathogens and toxins: Identification and biosensing applications. Biomed Res Int 2015; 2015: 1-31.

[49]   Bruno JG. Predicting the uncertain future of aptamer-based diagnostics and therapeutics. Molecules 2015; 20(4): 6866-87.
[http://dx.doi.org/10.3390/molecules20046866] [PMID: 25913927]

[50]   Davydova A, Vorobjeva M, Pyshnyi D, Altman S, Vlassov V, Venyaminova A. Aptamers against pathogenic microorganisms. Crit Rev Microbiol 2016; 42(6): 847-65.
[http://dx.doi.org/10.3109/1040841X.2015.1070115] [PMID: 26258445]

[51]   Vivekananda J, Salgado C, Millenbaugh NJ. DNA aptamers as a novel approach to neutralize Staphylococcus aureus α-toxin. Biochem Biophys Res Commun 2014; 444(3): 433-8.
[http://dx.doi.org/10.1016/j.bbrc.2014.01.076] [PMID: 24472539]

[52]   Vivekananda J, Millenbaugh N. Aptamer drug for detoxification of *Staphylococcus aureus* alpha-toxin. US Pat 9,217,134 2015

[53]   Bruno JG, Kiel JL. Use of magnetic beads in selection and detection of biotoxin aptamers by electrochemiluminescence and enzymatic methods. Biotechniques 2002; 32(1): 178-180, 182-183.
[PMID: 11808691]

[54]   DeGrasse JA. A single-stranded DNA aptamer that selectively binds to Staphylococcus aureus enterotoxin B. PLoS One 2012; 7(3): e33410.
[http://dx.doi.org/10.1371/journal.pone.0033410] [PMID: 22438927]

[55]   Wang K, Gan L, Jiang L, *et al.* Neutralization of staphylococcal enterotoxin B by an aptamer antagonist. Antimicrob Agents Chemother 2015; 59(4): 2072-7.
[http://dx.doi.org/10.1128/AAC.04414-14] [PMID: 25624325]

[56]   Purschke WG, Radtke F, Kleinjung F, Klussmann S. A DNA Spiegelmer to staphylococcal enterotoxin B. Nucleic Acids Res 2003; 31(12): 3027-32.
[http://dx.doi.org/10.1093/nar/gkg413] [PMID: 12799428]

[57]   Wu S, Duan N, Gu H, *et al.* A review of the methods for detection of *Staphylococcus aureus* enterotoxins. Toxins (Basel) 2016; 8(7): 1-20.
[http://dx.doi.org/10.3390/toxins8070176] [PMID: 27348003]

[58]   Zhou D, Xie G, Cao X, Chen X, Zhang X, Chen H. Colorimetric determination of staphylococcal enterotoxin B *via* DNAzyme-guided growth of gold nanoparticles. Mikrochim Acta 2016; 183(10):

2753-60.
[http://dx.doi.org/10.1007/s00604-016-1919-z]

[59]   Hedayati Ch M, Amani J, Sedighian H, *et al.* Isolation of a new ssDNA aptamer against staphylococcal enterotoxin B based on CNBr-activated sepharose-4B affinity chromatography. J Mol Recognit 2016; 29(9): 436-45.
[http://dx.doi.org/10.1002/jmr.2542] [PMID: 27091327]

[60]   Huang Y, Chen X, Duan N, *et al.* Selection and characterization of DNA aptamers against Staphylococcus aureus enterotoxin C1. Food Chem 2015; 166: 623-9.
[http://dx.doi.org/10.1016/j.foodchem.2014.06.039] [PMID: 25053102]

[61]   Ochsner UA, Katilius E, Janjic N. Detection of Clostridium difficile toxins A, B and binary toxin with slow off-rate modified aptamers. Diagn Microbiol Infect Dis 2013; 76(3): 278-85.
[http://dx.doi.org/10.1016/j.diagmicrobio.2013.03.029] [PMID: 23680240]

[62]   Hong KL, Maher E, Williams RM, Sooter LJ. *In vitro* selection of a single-stranded DNA molecular recognition element against Clostridium difficile toxin B and sensitive detection in human fecal matter. J Nucleic Acids 2015; 2015: 808495.
[http://dx.doi.org/10.1155/2015/808495] [PMID: 25734010]

[63]   Gold L, Ayers D, Bertino J, Bock C, Bock A, Brody EN, *et al.* Aptamer-based multiplexed proteomic technology for biomarker discovery. Gelain F, editor. PLoS One. 2010;5(12):e15004.

[64]   Ruscito A, DeRosa MC. Small-molecule binding aptamers: Selection strategies, characterization, and applications. Front Chem 2016; 4(14): 14.
[PMID: 27242994]

[65]   Gawande BN, Rohloff JC, Carter JD, *et al.* Selection of DNA aptamers with two modified bases. Proc Natl Acad Sci USA 2017; 114(11): 2898-903.
[http://dx.doi.org/10.1073/pnas.1615475114] [PMID: 28265062]

[66]   Voth DE, Ballard JD. Clostridium difficile toxins: mechanism of action and role in disease. Clin Microbiol Rev 2005; 18(2): 247-63.
[http://dx.doi.org/10.1128/CMR.18.2.247-263.2005] [PMID: 15831824]

[67]   Kuijper EJ, Coignard B, Tüll P. Emergence of Clostridium difficile-associated disease in North America and Europe. Clin Microbiol Infect 2006; 12 (Suppl. 6): 2-18.
[http://dx.doi.org/10.1111/j.1469-0691.2006.01580.x] [PMID: 16965399]

[68]   Luo P, Liu Y, Xia Y, Xu H, Xie G. Aptamer biosensor for sensitive detection of toxin A of Clostridium difficile using gold nanoparticles synthesized by Bacillus stearothermophilus. Biosens Bioelectron 2014; 54: 217-21.
[http://dx.doi.org/10.1016/j.bios.2013.11.013] [PMID: 24287407]

[69]   Ren S, Shin H, Gedi V, Dua P. Selection of DNA aptamers against botulinum neurotoxin E for development of fluorescent aptasensor. Bull Korean 2017; 38(3): 324-8.
[http://dx.doi.org/10.1002/bkcs.11085]

[70]   Rossetto O, Pirazzini M, Montecucco C. Botulinum neurotoxins: genetic, structural and mechanistic insights. Nat Rev Microbiol 2014; 12(8): 535-49.
[http://dx.doi.org/10.1038/nrmicro3295] [PMID: 24975322]

[71]   Tok JB, Fischer NO. Single microbead SELEX for efficient ssDNA aptamer generation against botulinum neurotoxin. Chem Commun (Camb) 2008; (16): 1883-5.
[http://dx.doi.org/10.1039/b717936g] [PMID: 18401506]

[72]   Bruno JG, Richarte AM, Carrillo MP, Edge A. An aptamer beacon responsive to botulinum toxins. Biosens Bioelectron 2012; 31(1): 240-3.
[http://dx.doi.org/10.1016/j.bios.2011.10.024] [PMID: 22061266]

[73]   Chang TW, Janardhanan P, Mello CM, Singh BR, Cai S. Selection of RNA Aptamers Against Botulinum Neurotoxin Type A Light Chain Through a Non-Radioactive Approach. Appl Biochem

Biotechnol 2016; 180(1): 10-25.
[http://dx.doi.org/10.1007/s12010-016-2081-0] [PMID: 27085355]

[74] Challa S, Tzipori S, Sheoran A. Selective evolution of ligands by exponential enrichment to identify RNA aptamers against shiga toxins. J Nucleic Acids 2014; 2014

[75] Bruno J, Richarte A. Aptamer-quantum dot lateral flow test strip development for rapid and sensitive detection of pathogenic Escherichia coli *via* intimin, O157-specific LPS and Shiga toxin. Curr Bionanotechnol 2015; 1(2): 80-6.
[http://dx.doi.org/10.2174/2213529402999160502115500]

[76] McKeague M, Velu R, Hill K, Bardóczy V, Mészáros T, DeRosa MC. Selection and characterization of a novel DNA aptamer for label-free fluorescence biosensing of ochratoxin A. Toxins (Basel) 2014; 6(8): 2435-52.
[http://dx.doi.org/10.3390/toxins6082435] [PMID: 25153252]

[77] Vasilescu A, Marty J. Aptasensors, an analytical solution for mycotoxins detection. Compr Anal Chem 2017; 77: 101-46.
[http://dx.doi.org/10.1016/bs.coac.2017.05.006]

[78] Goldblatt L, Ed. Aflatoxin: scientific background, control, and implications. Elsevier 2012.

[79] Ma X, Wang W, Chen X, Xia Y, Wu S, Duan N, *et al.* Selection, identification, and application of Aflatoxin B1 aptamer. Eur Food Res Technol 2014; 238(6): 919-25.
[http://dx.doi.org/10.1007/s00217-014-2176-1]

[80] Setlem K, Mondal B, Ramlal S, Kingston J. Immuno affinity SELEX for simple, rapid, and cost-effective aptamer enrichment and identification against aflatoxin B1. Front Microbiol 2016; 7(DEC): 1909.
[PMID: 27990137]

[81] Shum KT, Lui EL, Wong SC, *et al.* Aptamer-mediated inhibition of Mycobacterium tuberculosis polyphosphate kinase 2. Biochemistry 2011; 50(15): 3261-71.
[http://dx.doi.org/10.1021/bi2001455] [PMID: 21381755]

[82] Ngubane NA, Gresh L, Pym A, Rubin EJ, Khati M. Selection of RNA aptamers against the M. tuberculosis EsxG protein using surface plasmon resonance-based SELEX. Biochem Biophys Res Commun 2014; 449(1): 114-9.
[http://dx.doi.org/10.1016/j.bbrc.2014.04.163] [PMID: 24813997]

[83] Qin L, Zheng R, Ma Z, *et al.* The selection and application of ssDNA aptamers against MPT64 protein in Mycobacterium tuberculosis. Clin Chem Lab Med 2009; 47(4): 405-11.
[http://dx.doi.org/10.1515/CCLM.2009.097] [PMID: 19284297]

[84] Rotherham LS, Maserumule C, Dheda K, Theron J, Khati M. Selection and application of ssDNA aptamers to detect active TB from sputum samples. PLoS One 2012; 7(10): e46862.
[http://dx.doi.org/10.1371/journal.pone.0046862] [PMID: 23056492]

[85] Tang XL, Zhou YX, Wu SM, Pan Q, Xia B, Zhang XL. CFP10 and ESAT6 aptamers as effective Mycobacterial antigen diagnostic reagents. J Infect 2014; 69(6): 569-80.
[http://dx.doi.org/10.1016/j.jinf.2014.05.015] [PMID: 24968239]

[86] Bruno JG, Carrillo MP, Phillips T, Andrews CJ. A novel screening method for competitive FRET-aptamers applied to E. coli assay development. J Fluoresc 2010; 20(6): 1211-23.
[http://dx.doi.org/10.1007/s10895-010-0670-9] [PMID: 20443050]

[87] Queirós RB, Gouveia C, Fernandes JR, Jorge PA. Evanescent wave DNA-aptamer biosensor based on long period gratings for the specific recognition of E. coli outer membrane proteins. Biosens Bioelectron 2014; 62: 227-33.
[http://dx.doi.org/10.1016/j.bios.2014.06.062] [PMID: 25016253]

[88] Queirós RB, De-Los-Santos-Álvarez N, Noronha JP, Sales MG. A label-free DNA aptamer-based impedance biosensor for the detection of E. coli outer membrane proteins. Sens Actuators B Chem

2013; 181: 766-72.
[http://dx.doi.org/10.1016/j.snb.2013.01.062]

[89]   Rudenko N, Abbasova S, Grishin E. Production and characterization of the monoclonal antibodies to Bacillus anthracis protective antigen. Russ J Bioorganic 2011; 37(3): 316-21.
[http://dx.doi.org/10.1134/S1068162011030162]

[90]   Cella LN, Sanchez P, Zhong W, Myung NV, Chen W, Mulchandani A. Nano aptasensor for protective antigen toxin of anthrax. Anal Chem 2010; 82(5): 2042-7.
[http://dx.doi.org/10.1021/ac902791q] [PMID: 20136122]

[91]   Oh BN, Lee S, Park H-Y, Baeg J-O, Yoon M-Y, Kim J. Sensitive fluorescence assay of anthrax protective antigen with two new DNA aptamers and their binding properties. Analyst (Lond) 2011; 136(16): 3384-8.
[http://dx.doi.org/10.1039/c0an00978d] [PMID: 21743920]

[92]   Biondi E, Lane JD, Das D, *et al.* Laboratory evolution of artificially expanded DNA gives redesignable aptamers that target the toxic form of anthrax protective antigen. Nucleic Acids Res 2016; 44(20): 9565-77.
[PMID: 27701076]

[93]   Ryabko A, Kozyr A, Kolesnikov A, Marin M. DNA aptamers blocking activity of anthrax lethal toxin. FASEB J 2016; 30(1): 138.

[94]   Cossart P, Pizarro-Cerdá J, Lecuit M. Invasion of mammalian cells by Listeria monocytogenes: functional mimicry to subvert cellular functions. Trends Cell Biol 2003; 13(1): 23-31.
[http://dx.doi.org/10.1016/S0962-8924(02)00006-5] [PMID: 12480337]

[95]   Ohk SH, Koo OK, Sen T, Yamamoto CM, Bhunia AK. Antibody-aptamer functionalized fibre-optic biosensor for specific detection of Listeria monocytogenes from food. J Appl Microbiol 2010; 109(3): 808-17.
[http://dx.doi.org/10.1111/j.1365-2672.2010.04709.x] [PMID: 20337767]

[96]   Yamamoto C, Sen T. Nucleic acid ligands capable of binding to internalin B or internalin A. US Pat 7,838,242 2010

[97]   Yamamoto C, Sen T. Aptamers that bind to Listeria surface proteins. US Pat 7,645,582

[98]   Zhang XL, Tsui IS, Yip CM, *et al.* Salmonella enterica serovar typhi uses type IVB pili to enter human intestinal epithelial cells. Infect Immun 2000; 68(6): 3067-73.
[http://dx.doi.org/10.1128/IAI.68.6.3067-3073.2000] [PMID: 10816445]

[99]   Pan Q, Zhang XL, Wu HY, *et al.* Aptamers that preferentially bind type IVB pili and inhibit human monocytic-cell invasion by Salmonella enterica serovar typhi. Antimicrob Agents Chemother 2005; 49(10): 4052-60.
[http://dx.doi.org/10.1128/AAC.49.10.4052-4060.2005] [PMID: 16189080]

[100]   Hawver LA, Jung SA, Ng W-L. Specificity and complexity in bacterial quorum-sensing systems. Shen A, editor. FEMS Microbiol Rev. 2016;40(5):738–52.

[101]   Miller MB, Bassler BL. Quorum sensing in bacteria. Annu Rev Microbiol 2001; 55(1): 165-99.
[http://dx.doi.org/10.1146/annurev.micro.55.1.165] [PMID: 11544353]

[102]   de Kievit TR, Iglewski BH. Bacterial quorum sensing in pathogenic relationships. Infect Immun 2000; 68(9): 4839-49.
[http://dx.doi.org/10.1128/IAI.68.9.4839-4849.2000] [PMID: 10948095]

[103]   Ventola CL. The antibiotic resistance crisis: part 1: causes and threats. P&T 2015; 40(4): 277-83.
[PMID: 25859123]

[104]   Smith RS, Iglewski BH. Pseudomonas aeruginosa quorum sensing as a potential antimicrobial target. J Clin Invest 2003; 112(10): 1460-5.
[http://dx.doi.org/10.1172/JCI200320364] [PMID: 14617745]

[105] Zhao ZG, Yu YM, Xu BY, Yan SS, Xu JF, Liu F, *et al.* Screening and anti-virulent study of N-acyl homoserine lactones DNA aptamers against Pseudomonas aeruginosa quorum sensing. Biotechnol Bioprocess Eng; BBE 2013; 18(2): 406-12.
[http://dx.doi.org/10.1007/s12257-012-0556-6]

[106] Ochsner UA, Green LS, Gold L, Janjic N. Systematic selection of modified aptamer pairs for diagnostic sandwich assays. Biotechniques 2014; 56(3): 125-128, 130, 132-133.
[http://dx.doi.org/10.2144/000114134] [PMID: 24641476]

[107] Jorge A.; Penner, Gregory. Determination of ochratoxin A with a DNA aptamer. J Agric Food Chem 2008; 56(22): 10456-61.
[http://dx.doi.org/10.1021/jf801957h] [PMID: 18983163]

[108] Pozmogova GE, Zaitseva MA, Smirnov IP, Shvachko AG, Murina MA, Sergeenko VI. Anticoagulant effects of thioanalogs of thrombin-binding DNA-aptamer and their stability in the plasma. Bull Exp Biol Med 2010; 150(2): 180-4.
[http://dx.doi.org/10.1007/s10517-010-1099-5] [PMID: 21240367]

[109] Jensen KB, Atkinson BL, Willis MC, Koch TH, Gold L. Using *in vitro* selection to direct the covalent attachment of human immunodeficiency virus type 1 Rev protein to high-affinity RNA ligands. Proc Natl Acad Sci USA 1995; 92(26): 12220-4.
[http://dx.doi.org/10.1073/pnas.92.26.12220] [PMID: 8618873]

[110] Escolano JM, Díaz-Durán B, DeMiguel-Ramos M, Olivares J, Geday MA, Iborra E. Selection of aptamers to *Neisseria meningitidis* and *Streptococcus pneumoniae* surface specific proteins and affinity assay using thin film AlN resonators. Sens Actuators B Chem 2017; 246: 591-6.
[http://dx.doi.org/10.1016/j.snb.2017.02.098]

[111] Malyshev DA, Romesberg FE. The expanded genetic alphabet. Angew Chem Int Ed Engl 2015; 54(41): 11930-44.
[http://dx.doi.org/10.1002/anie.201502890] [PMID: 26304162]

[112] Sefah K, Yang Z, Bradley KM, *et al. In vitro* selection with artificial expanded genetic information systems. Proc Natl Acad Sci USA 2014; 111(4): 1449-54.
[http://dx.doi.org/10.1073/pnas.1311778111] [PMID: 24379378]

[113] Kimoto M, Yamashige R, Matsunaga K, Yokoyama S, Hirao I. Generation of high-affinity DNA aptamers using an expanded genetic alphabet. Nat Biotechnol 2013; 31(5): 453-7.
[http://dx.doi.org/10.1038/nbt.2556] [PMID: 23563318]

[114] Lipi F, Chen S, Chakravarthy M, Rakesh S, Veedu RN. *In vitro* evolution of chemically-modified nucleic acid aptamers: Pros and cons, and comprehensive selection strategies. RNA Biol 2016; 13(12): 1232-45.
[http://dx.doi.org/10.1080/15476286.2016.1236173] [PMID: 27715478]

[115] Ulrich H, Magdesian MH, Alves MJ, Colli W. *In vitro* selection of RNA aptamers that bind to cell adhesion receptors of Trypanosoma cruzi and inhibit cell invasion. J Biol Chem 2002; 277(23): 20756-62.
[http://dx.doi.org/10.1074/jbc.M111859200] [PMID: 11919187]

[116] Dey AK, Griffiths C, Lea SM, James W. Structural characterization of an anti-gp120 RNA aptamer that neutralizes R5 strains of HIV-1. RNA 2005; 11(6): 873-84.
[http://dx.doi.org/10.1261/rna.7205405] [PMID: 15923374]

[117] Barfod A, Persson T, Lindh J. *In vitro* selection of RNA aptamers against a conserved region of the Plasmodium falciparum erythrocyte membrane protein 1. Parasitol Res 2009; 105(6): 1557-66.
[http://dx.doi.org/10.1007/s00436-009-1583-x] [PMID: 19693540]

[118] Gopinath SC, Hayashi K, Kumar PK. Aptamer that binds to the gD protein of herpes simplex virus 1 and efficiently inhibits viral entry. J Virol 2012; 86(12): 6732-44.
[http://dx.doi.org/10.1128/JVI.00377-12] [PMID: 22514343]

[119] Wang J, Jiang H, Liu F. *In vitro* selection of novel RNA ligands that bind human cytomegalovirus and block viral infection. RNA 2000; 6(4): 571-83.
[http://dx.doi.org/10.1017/S1355838200992215] [PMID: 10786848]

[120] Homann M, Lorger M, Engstler M, Zacharias M, Göringer HU. Serum-stable RNA aptamers to an invariant surface domain of live African trypanosomes. Comb Chem High Throughput Screen 2006; 9(7): 491-9.
[http://dx.doi.org/10.2174/138620706777935324] [PMID: 16925510]

[121] Bugaut A, Toulmé J-J, Rayner B. SELEX and dynamic combinatorial chemistry interplay for the selection of conjugated RNA aptamers. Org Biomol Chem 2006; 4(22): 4082-8.
[http://dx.doi.org/10.1039/b610890c] [PMID: 17312962]

[122] Alves Ferreira-Bravo I, Cozens C, Holliger P, DeStefano JJ. Selection of 2'-deoxy--'-fluoroarabinonucleotide (FANA) aptamers that bind HIV-1 reverse transcriptase with picomolar affinity. Nucleic Acids Res 2015; 43(20): 9587-99.
[PMID: 26476448]

[123] Sczepanski JT, Joyce GF. Binding of a structured D-RNA molecule by an L-RNA aptamer. J Am Chem Soc 2013; 135(36): 13290-3.
[http://dx.doi.org/10.1021/ja406634g] [PMID: 23977945]

[124] Kaida Y, Fukami K, Matsui T, *et al.* DNA aptamer raised against AGEs blocks the progression of experimental diabetic nephropathy. Diabetes 2013; 62(9): 3241-50.
[http://dx.doi.org/10.2337/db12-1608] [PMID: 23630304]

[125] Matsui T, Higashimoto Y, Nishino Y, Nakamura N, Fukami K, Yamagishi S-I. RAGE-aptamer blocks the development and progression of experimental diabetic nephropathy. Diabetes 2017; 66(6): 1683-95.
[http://dx.doi.org/10.2337/db16-1281] [PMID: 28385802]

[126] Wyatt JR, Vickers TA, Roberson JL, *et al.* Combinatorially selected guanosine-quartet structure is a potent inhibitor of human immunodeficiency virus envelope-mediated cell fusion. Proc Natl Acad Sci USA 1994; 91(4): 1356-60.
[http://dx.doi.org/10.1073/pnas.91.4.1356] [PMID: 7906414]

[127] Sheehan JP, Phan TM. Phosphorothioate oligonucleotides inhibit the intrinsic tenase complex by an allosteric mechanism. Biochemistry 2001; 40(16): 4980-9.
[http://dx.doi.org/10.1021/bi002396x] [PMID: 11305914]

[128] Sheehan JP, Lan HC. Phosphorothioate oligonucleotides inhibit the intrinsic tenase complex. Blood 1998; 92(5): 1617-25.
[PMID: 9716589]

CHAPTER 6

Overcoming Fungal Multidrug Resistance by Natural Compounds Targeting Efflux Pumps

Shweta Singh, Sandeep Hans, Zeeshan Fatima[*] **and Saif Hameed**[*]

Amity Institute of Biotechnology, Amity University Haryana, Gurugram (Manesar)-122413, India

Abstract: Since ages, fungal pathogens are exploiting the human host by causing superficial to deep-seated fungal infections. *Candida albicans,* being the most prevalent pathogen, accounts for approximately 50–60% or more causes of candidiasis in humans leading to alarming mortality worldwide. In spite of significant advances being made in the improvement of antifungal drugs, only limited number of antifungal drugs are currently available and that too are not able to keep pace with the evolution and development of multidrug resistance (MDR) in *C. albicans.* Among the several causes of MDR, overexpression of drug efflux pumps contributes majorly to MDR. Thus, blocking or modulating the function of the drug efflux pumps still represents an attractive approach to combat MDR. The natural sources have the plethora of many promising natural compounds which can efficiently be exploited to improve the antifungal therapeutics. There is a need to unravel the intrinsic studies on natural inhibitors of efflux pumps. This book chapter unfolds the role of such natural compounds that target drug efflux pumps (the major culprits of MDR) thereby having the potential to chemosensitize towards known antifungal drugs.

Keywords: ABC transporters, *Candida*, CaMdr1p, Cdr1p, Efflux pumps, Efflux pump inhibitors, Fluconazole, MDR, MFS transporters, Natural compounds.

INTRODUCTION

The incidences of human fungal infections, particularly pathogenic yeast *Candida albicans* and its related species, acquiring resistance to antifungals have increased at alarming rates and pose grave concern towards its successful therapeutics. Clinical management of fungal diseases is hampered by the emergence of drug resistance by a phenomenon known as multidrug resistance (MDR) in fungi, leading to the elimination of the available drug. An understanding to combat antifungal resistance at the molecular level is indispensable for the development of strategies to combat MDR. Many of the commonly known mechanisms contri-

---
[*] **Corresponding Authors Saif Hameed and Zeeshan Fatima:** Amity Institute of Biotechnology, Amity University Haryana, Gurugram (Manesar)-122413, India; Tel: +91-124-2337015, Ext: 1116; E-mails: saifhameed@yahoo.co.in, drzeeshanfatima@gmail.com

Atta-ur-Rahman & M. Iqbal Choudhary (Eds.)

buting to MDR development include drug cleavage, drug inactivation by chemical modification, drug target alteration (by mutation), decreased penetration, increased efflux, mobile genetic elements. Out of all the mechanisms, overexpression of drug efflux pumps is the leading cause and serves as a gateway for the acquisition of MDR phenotype in *C. albicans*. In fact, in many clinical studies, drug efflux is one of the prominent mechanisms employed to acquire MDR phenotype, as the strains with knock out of efflux pump genes display attenuated virulence and enhanced drug susceptibilities. Therefore inhibiting efflux using efflux pump inhibitors (EPI) would eventually increase the effectual intracellular concentration of drug and chemosensitize *Candida* cells to mitigate MDR. Natural compounds represent a plethora of diverse entities which are yet to be exploited for their maximum benefit. This chapter focuses on the recent developments in search of EPIs of *C. albicans* from natural sources (Fig. **1**) that have gained wide attention to be exploited for efficient therapeutics.

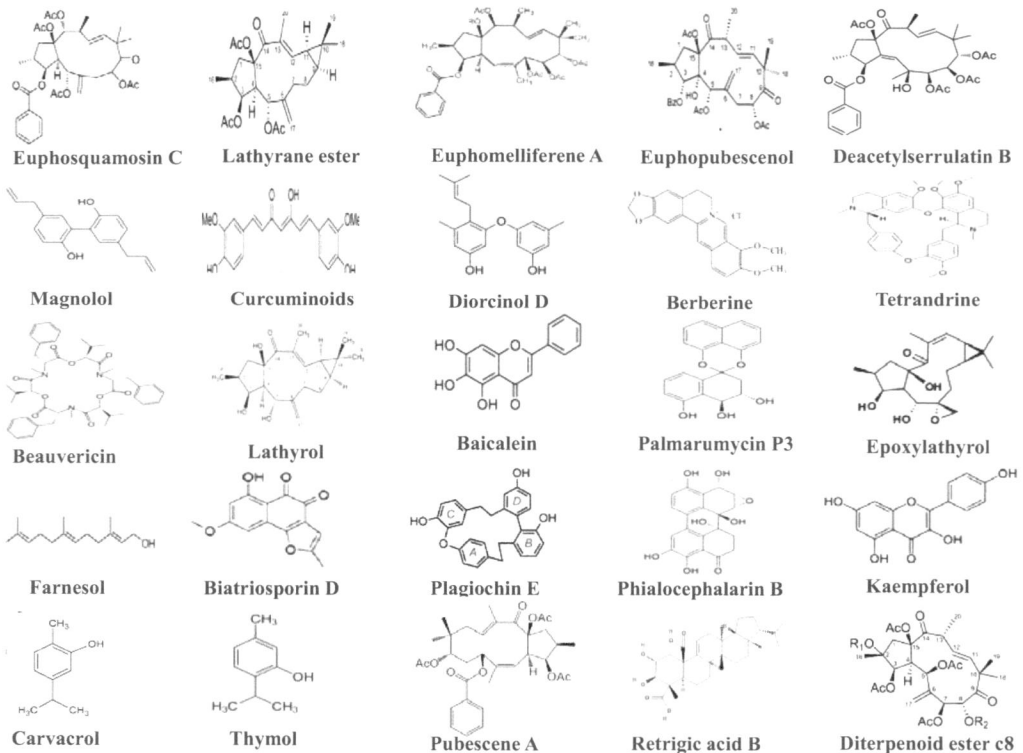

Fig. (1). Chemical structures of the various EPIs showing activity against Efflux pumps.

CANDIDA EFFLUX PUMPS

Majorly, the genes encoding for transporter proteins which cause drug extrusion belong to the classes namely ABC (the ATP-binding cassette) and MFS (major facilitator) superfamilies. The rapid efflux of drugs due to over expression of efflux pumps work as a defense system for the candidal cells to safeguard from lethal concentrations of the drug. The following subsection deals with a brief overview of the two types of efflux pumps known to have implications in MDR acquisition (Fig. **2**).

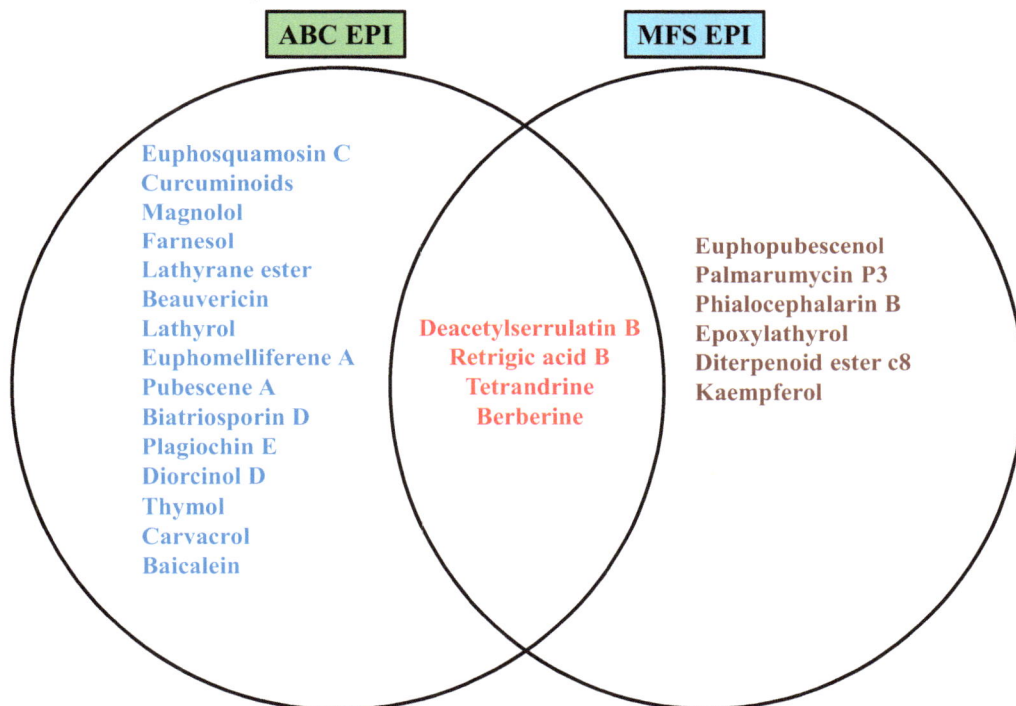

ABC EPI   **MFS EPI**

Euphosquamosin C
Curcuminoids
Magnolol
Farnesol
Lathyrane ester
Beauvericin
Lathyrol
Euphomelliferene A
Pubescene A
Biatriosporin D
Plagiochin E
Diorcinol D
Thymol
Carvacrol
Baicalein

Deacetylserrulatin B
Retrigic acid B
Tetrandrine
Berberine

Euphopubescenol
Palmarumycin P3
Phialocephalarin B
Epoxylathyrol
Diterpenoid ester c8
Kaempferol

Fig. (2). Venn diagram showing EPIs which are common and distinct for ABC and MFS drug transporters.

ABCS TRANSPORTER FAMILY

ABC class of efflux pumps is considered as one of the largest superfamily of *Candida* transporters. There are total 19 putative ABC protein family members found in *C. albicans*. These proteins contain at least one nucleotide binding domain (NBD) which is the energy source for these pumps, and further contains highly conserved motifs such as the Walker A, Walker B, and signature sequences. Most of these proteins also possess the transmembrane domains

(TMDs). The ABC transporter *Candida* drug resistance 1 protein (Cdr1p) is the most prominent player along with Cdr2, among these transporters that enable *Candida* to outplay the arsenal of antifungals encountered [1]. These pump proteins not only efflux the azoles but expel many structurally unrelated compounds. It has been reported that the other homologues of Cdr1 such as Cdr3 and Cdr4 are also present but neither their deletion nor their overexpression causes any change. Structurally Cdr1 is composed of two homologous parts of hydrophilic, cytoplasmic NBD and a TMD which is represented by transmembrane segments (TMS) [2]. The TMS consists of 12 α helical TMS while the NBD consists of α helices and β-sheets. The domains of NBD consist of several protein motifs such as Walker A or P-loop, the Walker B and the ABC signature motif or C-loop [3]. The nonspecific nature of NBD contributes to the host toxicity. The other TMD region contributes to the substrate channel through the membrane. One of the key features of this transporter is the use of ATP for the transfer of drug across the membrane against the concentration gradient. It has been reported that interactions between the intracellular loops (ICL) present in the TMDs and NBDs are crucial for inter-domain interaction and coupling between ATP hydrolysis and substrate transport [4]. The binding of the drug induces the NBDs to hydrolyze ATP which causes conformational changes within the NBD as well as in the TMDs leading the bound drug/ substrate to be effluxed by the transporter [2].

MFS TRANSPORTER FAMILY

In contrast to the ABC families, which are in general multicomponent primary active transporters capable of transporting both small molecules and macromolecules coupled to ATP hydrolysis, the MFS transporters are single-polypeptide secondary carriers capable only of transporting small solutes in response to chemiosmotic ion gradients. It is the largest family of secondary active transporters and involved in the transportation of various molecules like the drugs, peptides, amino acids, organic anions, and intermediates etc. The subfamilies of the MFS consist of six TMS α-helical segments connected through cytoplasmic loops, but they do not have NBD like in ABC transporters [5]. They are defined by a number of TMS segments within the TMD. The key feature which distinguishes it from ABC transporter is the proton antiporters which utilize the energy from electrochemical potential and proton-motive force to translocate the substrate across membranes [3]. In *C. albicans*, a total of 95 putative proteins has been identified computationally, which are clustered into 17 families [4]. Till date, only few MFS transporters namely MDR1, FLU1, NAG3, NAG4, JEN1, ARN1 and NGT1 have been identified and characterized in *C. albicans* out of which only MDR1 and FLU1 are drug efflux pump transporters. The MDR1 transporter protein consists of 12 TMSs which are connected by hydrophilic loops in the cytoplasm. Structurally, the N-terminal (TMS1 to TMS6) of these proteins are involved in proton translocation and C-terminal (TMS 7 to TMS12) are involved in substrate recognition [6, 7]. The DHA family possess a central cytoplasmic loop (CCL) to form a cytosolic domain to connect with the plasma membrane. These CCL connecting TMDs plays very important role in many MFS proteins [8]. It has been reported that there are five motifs namely (D2, A, B, C and G) present in the DHA1 family. Among them, Motif-C, (antiporter motif), plays a crucial role in the drug/H$^+$ antiporter activity of the proteins which belong to both the DHA1 and DHA2 families [9]. The expression of MDR1 is also regulated by different transcription factors, which includes Cph1, Mrr1, Upc2, and Mcm1. These transcription factors are known to regulate the MDR1 expression by binding to elements in the promoter region of MDR1 and confer its overexpression [6]. Another transporter protein FLU1 has been reported in *Candida* cells involved in the drug resistance, where it shows resistance against mycophenolic acid and salivary human antimicrobial peptide histatin 5 [10, 11].

NATURAL EPI TARGETING ABC TRANSPORTERS

Since last decade, there is a rapid increase in search for novel antifungal drugs from natural sources which can overcome MDR. The natural compounds belong to many classes of compounds like terpenoids, alkaloids, phenolic compounds etc. These compounds have their own mechanism of action to cease the fungal growth through which they can work alone or synergistically with the known antifungal drugs. The intrinsic studies have shown that some of the compounds specifically target the efflux pump genes CDR1 and CDR2 or they can also modulate the activity of efflux pump transporters. A recent study by Tran-Nguyen and coworkers [12] on the modulators of Cdr1p efflux pump and their related mechanisms documented many compounds acting as EPIs. The modulation of the efflux pump activity was also reported for jatrophane esters from Euphorbia spp. For instance, euphosquamosin C and deacetylserrulatin B are jatrophane terpenoid and substrate of CaCdr1p thereby affects binding [13]. Moreover, lathyrane ester from latex extracts *E. insularis* was found to be involved in modulation of drug efflux transporter Cdr1p of *C. albicans* [14].

The jatrophane terpenoid namely euphomelliferene A and pubescene A inhibits Cdr1p efflux transporter by binding to the different amino acid residues within the binding pocket of the Cdr1 protein [15]. Curcumin is a natural product from turmeric derived from rhizomes of *Curcuma longa*, known to reverse the drug resistance phenotypes in cancer cells overexpressing ABC transporters. It was demonstrated that curcuminoids have shown modulating activity against Cdr1p efflux pump transporter by binding to the substrate or an allosteric site of Cdr1p [16]. It also acts synergistically with the fluconazole (FLC) which can sensitize the MDR phenotype in clinical isolates of *Candida* [17]. Similarly, Biatriosporin D which is a hepaketides extracted from Endolichenic Fungus *Biatriospora spp* can work synergistically with FLC and also have effect on efflux pump depicted by flow cytometry using the Rhodamine 123 accumulation. It also inhibits the efflux by reducing the transcriptional expression of CDR1 and CDR2 [18]. Plagiochin E, a derived bisbibenzyl compound which belongs to the phenolic family, extracted from liverwort plant *Marchantia polymorpha* L, is known to reverse the FLC resistance relating to efflux pump by downregulation of CDR1 and also works mutually with the FLC [19]. Diorcinol D is an antifungal extracted from lichen endophytic fungus and berberine, an alkaloid used in traditional Chinese medicine retards the activity of efflux pump by downregulating the expression of CDR1 [20, 21]. It also inhibits the activity of efflux pump transporter Cdr1p along with the additive effect with FLC [22]. Beauvericin, a cyclic depsipeptide, extracted from *Fusarium spp* reduces the activity of efflux pump transporters Cdr1p and CaCdr2, by inhibition of substrate binding site at the TMDs [23]. A recent study by Monico A and coworkers [24] demonstrated that lathyrol derivatives can also modulate the activity of Cdr1p efflux pump transporters. The monoterpenes namely thymol and carvacrol, the main components of thyme oil, also reverse the azole resistance by inhibiting the expression of CDR1 and CDR2 by 70-90% [25]. Magnolol is a lignan which is derived from the bark of *Magnolia officinalis* and used as traditional medicine. It has known antifungal properties against *Candida albicans, Microsporium gypseum, Epidermophyton floccosum, Aspergillus niger, Trichophyton mentagrophytes Cryptococcus neoformans*. The expression of CDR1 was downregulated in the presence of magnolol, with inhibition in the binding of substrates into the substrate-binding site(s) at the TMDs along with its combined effort with the FLC in azole-resistant strains of *C. albicans*. The other proposed mechanism could be the alteration in the composition of lipid raft of Cdr1p which displaces its position on the plasma membrane [26]. In a study by Chang W and coworkers [27], the expression of CDR1 was found transcriptionally downregulated by the action of retigeric acid B, a lichen-derived pentacyclic triterpenoid. The extract from the *Echinophora platyloba* also known as a pasture plant is mainly used for food flavoring in Iran. The composition of extract contains saponin, alkaloid, and flavonoid. They reduce the transcriptional expression of CDR1 and CDR2 in FLC resistance strains of *C. albicans* [28]. The tetrandrine is a bis-benzylisoquinoline alkaloid extracted from the roots of *S. tetrandra*. It can increase the candicidal activity of FLC by decreasing the Cdr1p and Cdr2p efflux. The mechanism underlying its activity is the downregulation of the expression of CDR1 and CDR2 genes which code for Cdr1p and Cdr2p [29]. Generally, farnesol which is a quorum sensing molecule is the precursor in the sterol synthesis in *C. albicans*. It is well known for its action on biofilm development and morphological transition, mitochondrial dysfunction, ROS generation leading to apoptosis resulting in cell death [30]. It has been shown to function as a specific modulator in the drug extrusion mediated by ABC transporter proteins by inhibiting the substrate binding to the Cdr1p in the TMD without itself acting as a substrate. It also showed synergism with the azoles and polyenes [31].

Natural compounds not only retard the efflux pump activity in *C. albicans* but also in non *albicans* species of *Candida* like *C. glabrata, C. krusei, and C. parapsilosis*. A study demonstrated the effect of baicalein extracted from *Scutellaria baicalensis* showing a reduction in FLC resistance due to downregulation in the expression of efflux pump related genes [32]. The natural compounds also modulate the activity of efflux pumps in concert with different mechanisms. For instance, the study on FLC resistant *C. tropicalis* has shown alliance of berberine with FLC which could lead to ROS generation, inhibition of ergosterol biosynthesis and a decrease in efflux transporter [22]. Another study by Edwina Thomas and coworkers [33] demonstrated that mitochondrial dysfunction could also lead to retardation in efflux pump activity. When CDR1 activity is reduced then the protein is missorted to the vacuole, which in turn indicates that mitochondria exert posttranslational regulation on Cdr1p levels. The effect of these natural compounds have been demonstrated on the clinical isolates of FLC resistant strains [17, 20]

NATURAL EPI TARGETING MFS TRANSPORTERS

Many natural compounds act as EPIs and target the CaMdr1 transporter of *C. albicans* which belongs to MFS superfamily in addition to a CDR1 transporter of ABC superfamily (Fig. **3**). The quinone derivatives namely palmarumycin P3 and phialocephalarin B from *Phialocephala fortinii* (endolichenic fungus) can inhibit the activity CaMdr1p by modulating the transcriptional expression of MDR1 gene and by interacting with the transcription factors like Mrr1 and Cap1 [34]. They can reverse the azole resistance and can function as potent chemosensitizers [20]. The jatrophanes which are EPIs against the Cdr1 transporter have also shown inhibitory activity on Mdr1 transporter. Jatrophanes deacetylserrulatin B extracted from the Iranian spurge *Euphorbia squamosa* are potential EPI of CaMdr1p along with the synergism with FLC [13]. Another Jatrophane diterpenoid euphopubescenol extracted from *Euphorbia pubescens* inhibits the CaMdr1 efflux pump protein by acting as substrate and binding to the protein [15]. The epoxylathyrol jatrophanes showed 85% inhibition by inhibiting the MDR1 efflux activity [24]. The latex extracts include many compounds, and among them one diterpenoid ester from *E. semiperfoliata* downregulate the MDR1 expression by 74% and involved in modulation of Mdr1p activity of *C. albicans* along with the synergism with FLC [14]. Some natural compounds like kaempferol which is

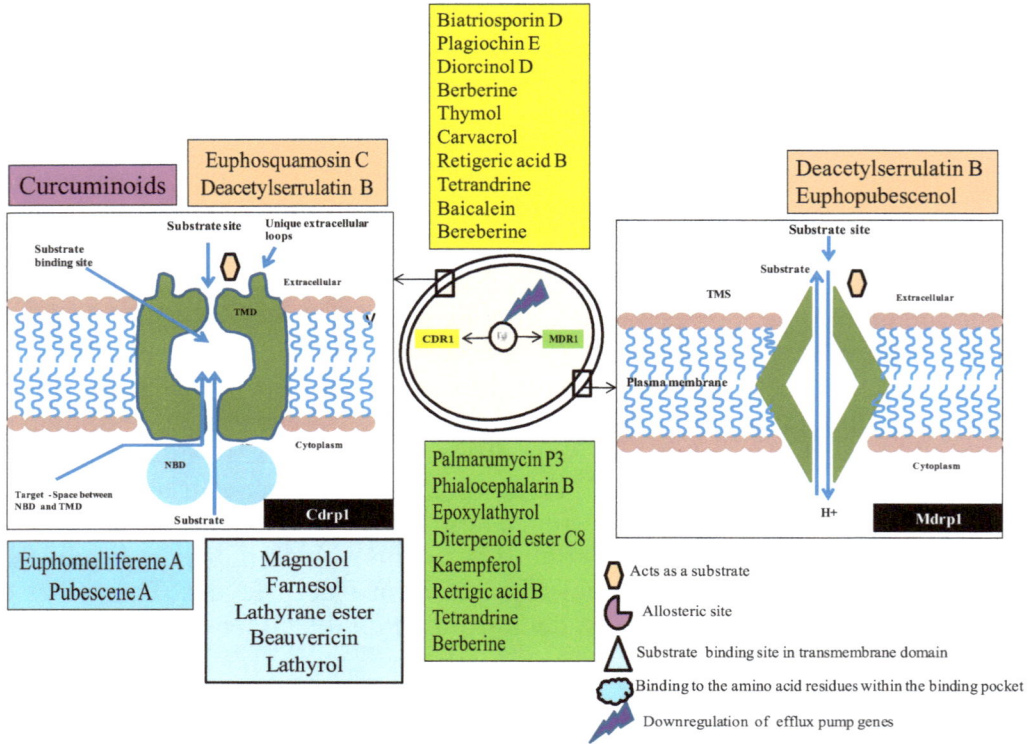

Fig. (3). Schematic representation of various sites of action (denoted by different color keys) of EPIs on Cdr1p and Mdr1p drug efflux pump transporters.

found in many flowers and fruits like Delphinium, Witch-hazel, grapefruit and other plant derived foods can revert the FLC resistance. It is one of the active flavonoids, which has a broad-spectrum anti-inflammatory, antioxidant, and anticancer properties. Among its many functions, it is known to have antibacterial and antifungal properties which have given satisfactory results due to its potential nature. It has been studied that kaempferol decreases the expression of Mdr1 along with the FLC synergism [35]. A pentacyclic triterpenoid isolated from the lichen *Lobaria kurokawa* called as retrigic acid B can significantly reduce the transcriptional expression of MDR1 which codes for CaMdr1p efflux pump transporter [27]. Alkaloid tetrandrine is a known calcium channel blocker, which inhibits the expression of CDR1 and CDR2. It is isolated from *Stephania tetrandra,* a native herbaceous perennial, and other Chinese and Japanese herbs. It helps in reducing the blood pressure by functioning as a vasodilator. It is also used for treating liver disease and has known anti-inflammatory, antiallergenic properties. A study by Hong Zhang and coworkers [29] demonstrated that on treatment with tetrandrine, there is a reduction in transcriptional expression of MDR1 and FLU 1 efflux pump genes. It reverses the azole resistance by inhibiting the overexpression of CaMdr1p and interacting directly with the multidrug transporters. In fact, *in vivo* studies have shown its synergistic nature with FLC. Similarly, berberine-containing Berberis species can synthesize the substances 5'-methoxyhydnocarpin-D (5'-MHC-D) and pheophorbide which can inhibit the transcriptional expression of MDR1 efflux pump [36]. The most active extract of *D. formosa, A. annua, H. canadensis,* are the medicinal herbs used for treating influenza. These have been shown to modulate the MFS efflux pump activity and functions in a collaborative manner with FLC [37]. The clinical isolates of FLC resistant of *C. albicans* were tested and have showed reversal of overexpression of efflux pump [35]. Thus dual mode of action for various EPIs is evident from the fact that most of them along with their action on efflux pumps show synergism with FLC (Fig. **4**).

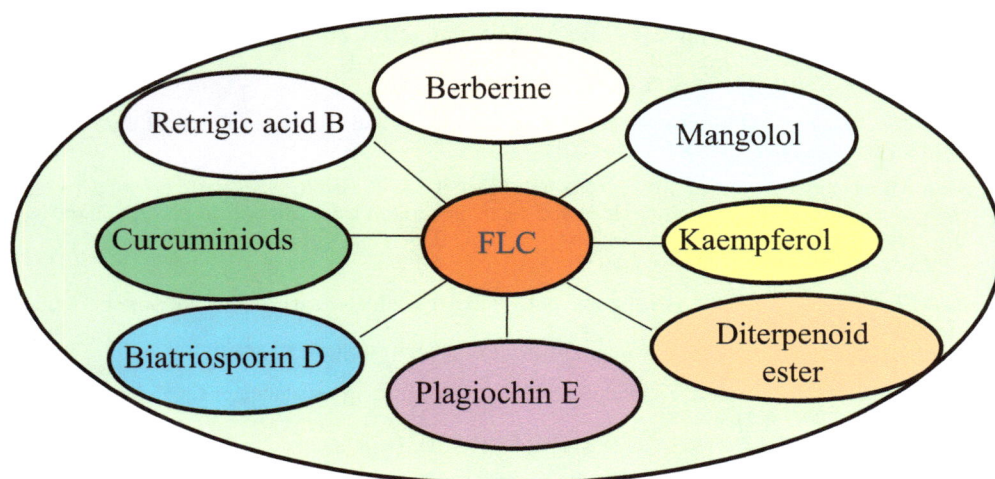

Fig. (4). The EPIs showing synergism with the FLC.

CONCLUSION

Natural compounds have great potential to inhibit the efflux pump activity. They not only reverse the azole resistance but also work synergistically with FLC. Further studies are required for better understanding the mechanisms by which these natural compounds can inhibit or modulate the expressions of CDR1, CDR2, MDR1 and FLU1 efflux pump genes.

CONSENT FOR PUBLICATION

Not applicable.

CONFLICT OF INTEREST

The editor declares no conflict of interest, financial or otherwise.

ACKNOWLEDGEMENTS

Declared none.

REFERENCES

[1]   Gohar AA, Badali H, Shokohi T, Nabili M, Amirrajab N, Moazeni M. Expression patterns of ABC transporter genes in fluconazole-resistant *Candida glabrata.* Mycopathologia 2017; 182(3-4): 273-84. [http://dx.doi.org/10.1007/s11046-016-0074-8] [PMID: 27744635]

[2]   Prasad R, Kapoor K. Multidrug resistance in yeast Candida. Int Rev Cytol 2005; 242(242): 215-48. [PMID: 15598470]

[3]   Holmes AR, Cardno TS, Strouse JJ, *et al.* Targeting efflux pumps to overcome antifungal drug resistance. Future Med Chem 2016; 8(12): 1485-501. [http://dx.doi.org/10.4155/fmc-2016-0050] [PMID: 27463566]

[4]   Shah AH, Prasad R. MFS transporters of Candida species and their role in clinical drug resistance. FEMS Yeast Res 2016; 16(4)

[5]   Shah AH, Banerjee A, Rawal MK, Saxena AK, Mondal AK, Prasad R. ABC transporter Cdr1p harbors charged residues in the intracellular loop and nucleotide-binding domain critical for protein trafficking and drug resistance. FEMS Yeast Res 2015; 15(5): fov036. [http://dx.doi.org/10.1093/femsyr/fov036] [PMID: 26048893]

[6]   Law CJ, Maloney PC, Wang DN. Ins and outs of major facilitator superfamily antiporters. Annu Rev Microbiol 2008; 62(62): 289-305. [http://dx.doi.org/10.1146/annurev.micro.61.080706.093329] [PMID: 18537473]

[7]   Prasad R, Gaur NA, Gaur M, Komath SS. Efflux pumps in drug resistance of Candida. Infect Disord Drug Targets 2006; 6(2): 69-83. [http://dx.doi.org/10.2174/187152606784112164] [PMID: 16789872]

[8]   Xu L, Li Y, Haworth IS, Davies DL. Functional role of the intracellular loop linking transmembrane domains 6 and 7 of the human dipeptide transporter hPEPT1. J Membr Biol 2010; 238(1-3): 43-9. [http://dx.doi.org/10.1007/s00232-010-9317-7] [PMID: 21104182]

[9]   Paulsen IT, Skurray RA. Topology, structure and evolution of two families of proteins involved in antibiotic and antiseptic resistance in eukaryotes and prokaryotes--an analysis. Gene 1993; 124(1): 1-11. [http://dx.doi.org/10.1016/0378-1119(93)90755-R] [PMID: 8440470]

[10]   Calabrese D, Bille J, Sanglard D. A novel multidrug efflux transporter gene of the major facilitator superfamily from *Candida albicans (FLU1)* conferring resistance to fluconazole. Microbiology 2000; 146(Pt 11): 2743-54. [http://dx.doi.org/10.1099/00221287-146-11-2743] [PMID: 11065353]

[11]   Li R, Kumar R, Tati S, Puri S, Edgerton M. *Candida albicans* flu1-mediated efflux of salivary histatin 5 reduces its cytosolic concentration and fungicidal activity. Antimicrob Agents Chemother 2013; 57(4): 1832-9. [http://dx.doi.org/10.1128/AAC.02295-12] [PMID: 23380720]

[12]   Tran-Nguyen VK, Prasad R, Falson P, Boumendjel A. Modulators of the efflux pump cdr1p of *Candida albicans*: Mechanisms of action and chemical features. Curr Med Chem In press [PMID: 28545374]

[13]   Rawal MK, Shokoohinia Y, Chianese G, *et al.* Jatrophanes from *Euphorbia squamosa* as potent inhibitors of *Candida albicans* multidrug transporters. J Nat Prod 2014; 77(12): 2700-6. [http://dx.doi.org/10.1021/np500756z] [PMID: 25437914]

[14]   Esposito M, Nim S, Nothias LF, *et al.* Evaluation of Jatrophane Esters from Euphorbia spp. as Modulators of *Candida albicans* Multidrug Transporters. J Nat Prod 2017; 80(2): 479-87. [http://dx.doi.org/10.1021/acs.jnatprod.6b00090] [PMID: 28106996]

[15]   Nim S, Mónico A, Rawal MK, *et al.* Overcoming multidrug resistance in *Candida albicans*: macrocyclic diterpenes from Euphorbia species as potent inhibitors of drug efflux pumps. Planta Med 2016; 82(13): 1180-5. [http://dx.doi.org/10.1055/s-0042-106169] [PMID: 27145238]

[16]   Sharma M, Manoharlal R, Shukla S, *et al.* Curcumin modulates efflux mediated by yeast ABC multidrug transporters and is synergistic with antifungals. Antimicrob Agents Chemother 2009; 53(8): 3256-65. [http://dx.doi.org/10.1128/AAC.01497-08] [PMID: 19470507]

[17]   Garcia-Gomes AS, Curvelo JA, Soares RM, Ferreira-Pereira A. Curcumin acts synergistically with fluconazole to sensitize a clinical isolate of Candida albicans showing a MDR phenotype. Med Mycol 2012; 50(1): 26-32. [http://dx.doi.org/10.3109/13693786.2011.578156] [PMID: 21539505]

[18]   Zhou YH, Zhang M, Zhu RX, *et al.* Heptaketides from an Endolichenic Fungus Biatriospora sp. and Their Antifungal Activity. J Nat Prod 2016; 79(9): 2149-57. [http://dx.doi.org/10.1021/acs.jnatprod.5b00998] [PMID: 27556953]

[19]   Guo XL, Leng P, Yang Y, Yu LG, Lou HX. Plagiochin E, a botanic-derived phenolic compound, reverses fungal resistance to fluconazole relating to the efflux pump. J Appl Microbiol 2008; 104(3): 831-8. [http://dx.doi.org/10.1111/j.1365-2672.2007.03617.x] [PMID: 18194250]

[20]   Li Y. Chang W1, Zhang M1, Li X1, Jiao Y1, Lou H. Synergistic and drug-resistant reversing effects of diorcinol D combined with fluconazole against *Candida albicans*. FEMS Yeast Res 2015; 15(2) [http://dx.doi.org/10.1093/femsyr/fov001]

[21]   Shao J, Shi G, Wang T, Wu D, Wang C. Antiproliferation of berberine in combination with fluconazole from the perspectives of reactive oxygen species, ergosterol and drug efflux in a fluconazole-resistant *Candida tropicalis* isolate. Front Microbiol 2016; 7: 1516. [http://dx.doi.org/10.3389/fmicb.2016.01516] [PMID: 27721812]

[22]   Li DD, Xu Y, Zhang DZ, *et al.* Fluconazole assists berberine to kill fluconazole-resistant *Candida albicans*. Antimicrob Agents Chemother 2013; 57(12): 6016-27. [http://dx.doi.org/10.1128/AAC.00499-13] [PMID: 24060867]

[23]   Szczepaniak J, Łukaszewicz M, Krasowska A. Detection of inhibitors of *Candida albicans* Cdr transporters using a diS-C3(3) fluorescence. Front Microbiol 2015; 6: 176. [http://dx.doi.org/10.3389/fmicb.2015.00176] [PMID: 25806026]

[24]   Mónico A, Nim S, Duarte N, *et al.* Lathyrol and epoxylathyrol derivatives: Modulation of Cdr1p and Mdr1p drug-efflux transporters of *Candida albicans* in Saccharomyces cerevisiae model. Bioorg Med Chem 2017; 25(13): 3278-84. [http://dx.doi.org/10.1016/j.bmc.2017.04.016] [PMID: 28479022]

[25]   Ahmad A, Khan A, Manzoor N. Reversal of efflux mediated antifungal resistance underlies synergistic activity of two monoterpenes with fluconazole. Eur J Pharm Sci 2013; 48(1-2): 80-6. [http://dx.doi.org/10.1016/j.ejps.2012.09.016] [PMID: 23111348]

[26]   Sun LM, Liao K, Liang S, Yu PH, Wang DY. Synergistic activity of magnolol with azoles and its possible antifungal mechanism against *Candida albicans*. J Appl Microbiol 2015; 118(4): 826-38.
[http://dx.doi.org/10.1111/jam.12737] [PMID: 25641229]

[27]   Chang W, Li Y, Zhang L, Cheng A, Liu Y, Lou H. Retigeric acid B enhances the efficacy of azoles combating the virulence and biofilm formation of *Candida albicans*. Biol Pharm Bull 2012; 35(10): 1794-801.
[http://dx.doi.org/10.1248/bpb.b12-00511] [PMID: 22863995]

[28]   Khajeh E, Hosseini Shokouh SJ, Rajabibazl M, *et al.* Antifungal effect of *Echinophora platyloba* on expression of CDR1 and CDR2 genes in fluconazole-resistant *Candida albicans*. Br J Biomed Sci 2016; 73(1): 44-8.
[http://dx.doi.org/10.1080/09674845.2016.1155269] [PMID: 27182677]

[29]   Zhang H, Gao A, Li F, Zhang G, Ho HI, Liao W. Mechanism of action of tetrandrine, a natural inhibitor of *Candida albicans* drug efflux pumps. Yakugaku Zasshi 2009; 129(5): 623-30.
[http://dx.doi.org/10.1248/yakushi.129.623] [PMID: 19420894]

[30]   Shirtliff ME, Krom BP, Meijering RA, *et al.* Farnesol-induced apoptosis in *Candida albicans*. Antimicrob Agents Chemother 2009; 53(6): 2392-401.
[http://dx.doi.org/10.1128/AAC.01551-08] [PMID: 19364863]

[31]   Sharma M, Prasad R. The quorum-sensing molecule farnesol is a modulator of drug efflux mediated by ABC multidrug transporters and synergizes with drugs in Candida albicans. Antimicrob Agents Chemother 2011; 55(10): 4834-43.
[http://dx.doi.org/10.1128/AAC.00344-11] [PMID: 21768514]

[32]   Tsang PW, Chau KY, Yang HP. Baicalein exhibits inhibitory effect on the energy-dependent efflux pump activity in non-albicans Candida fungi. J Chemother 2015; 27(1): 61-2.
[http://dx.doi.org/10.1179/1973947814Y.0000000177] [PMID: 24548098]

[33]   Thomas E, Roman E, Claypool S, Manzoor N, Pla J, Panwar SL. Mitochondria influence CDR1 efflux pump activity, Hog1-mediated oxidative stress pathway, iron homeostasis, and ergosterol levels in *Candida albicans*. Antimicrob Agents Chemother 2013; 57(11): 5580-99.
[http://dx.doi.org/10.1128/AAC.00889-13] [PMID: 23979757]

[34]   Xie F, Chang W, Zhang M, *et al.* Quinone derivatives isolated from the endolichenic fungus Phialocephala fortinii are Mdr1 modulators that combat azole resistance in *Candida albicans*. Sci Rep 2016; 6: 33687.
[http://dx.doi.org/10.1038/srep33687] [PMID: 27650180]

[35]   Shao J, Zhang M, Wang T, Li Y, Wang C. The roles of CDR1, CDR2, and MDR1 in kaempferol-induced suppression with fluconazole-resistant *Candida albicans*. Pharm Biol 2016; 54(6): 984-92.
[http://dx.doi.org/10.3109/13880209.2015.1091483] [PMID: 26459663]

[36]   Musumeci R, Speciale A, Costanzo R, *et al.* Berberis aetnensis C. Presl. extracts: antimicrobial properties and interaction with ciprofloxacin. Int J Antimicrob Agents 2003; 22(1): 48-53.
[http://dx.doi.org/10.1016/S0924-8579(03)00085-2] [PMID: 12842327]

[37]   Kolaczkowski M, Kolaczkowska A, Stermitz FR. Modulation of the antifungal activity of new medicinal plant extracts active on *Candida glabrata* by the major transporters and regulators of the pleiotropic drug-resistance network in *Saccharomyces cerevisiae*. Microb Drug Resist 2009; 15(1): 11-7.
[http://dx.doi.org/10.1089/mdr.2009.0854] [PMID: 19216644]

CHAPTER 7

The Infections and Hydrogen Sulfide

Ravinder R. Gaddam, Piyush Jha and **Madhav Bhatia***

Department of Pathology and Biomedical Science, University of Otago-Christchurch, Christchurch, New Zealand

Abstract: There is a growing interest in "medical gases" for their role in infection. Hydrogen sulfide (H_2S) is a physiological gaseous mediator that has been recognized as an important signalling molecule to regulate infections. The role of H_2S in different infections such as viruses (paramyxoviruses), bacteria (*Mycobacterium tuberculosis*), mycoplasma (*Mycoplasma fermentans*) and fungi (*Aspergillus niger*) as well as in conditions like sepsis and malaria and in antibiotic resistance is being actively investigated because of its therapeutic potential. As we do not have definitive therapeutic agents such as antimicrobials or vaccines against many pathogenic agents, the immuno-regulatory and microbial properties of H_2S make it an ideal candidate for the treatment of infectious diseases. Therefore, understanding the mechanisms underlying H_2S-mediated regulation of different infectious diseases would help in developing H_2S-based drugs as therapeutic molecules. A description of recent understanding of H_2S role in different infections is presented in this chapter.

Keywords: Antibiotic resistance, Hydrogen sulfide, Infection, Malaria, Sepsis.

INTRODUCTION

Hydrogen sulfide (H_2S) is a colorless, water-soluble, flammable gas with a characteristic smell of rotten eggs. It has traditionally been considered a highly toxic gas and environmental hazard; however, in recent years the physiological importance of H_2S has been recognized [1].

Endogenously, H_2S is synthesized through mainly two pathways: enzymatic and non-enzymatic. Cystathionine-γ-lyase (CSE) and cystathionine-β-synthase (CBS) are two main enzymes of an enzymatic pathway that produce H_2S using sulfur amino acids such as homocysteine and L-cysteine during their metabolism. Pyridoxal-5'-phosphate (PLP), an active form of vitamin B6, acts as a co-factor for both CSE and CBS in the process of H_2S generation. Although CSE and CBS expression is widely distributed in different cells and tissues, CSE is the major

---

* **Corresponding author Madhav Bhatia:** Department of Pathology and Biomedical Science, University of Otago, Christchurch, 2 Riccarton Avenue, P.O. Box 4345, Christchurch 8140, New Zealand; Tel: 64 3 378 6238; Fax: 64 3 364 0009; E-mail: madhav.bhatia@otago.ac.nz

Atta-ur-Rahman & M. Iqbal Choudhary (Eds.)

H_2S-synthesizing enzyme in vasculature and peripheral organs, whereas CBS is highly localized in the central nervous system. In addition to CSE and CBS, 3-mercaptopyruvate sulfurtransferase (3-MST), along with cysteine aminotransferase (CAT), partially synthesizes H_2S from L-cysteine both in peripheral organs and the central nervous system. Recent investigation has revealed that D-amino acid oxidase (DAO), along with 3-MST, produce H_2S in the cerebellum and kidney [2].

Stored forms of sulfur are alternative sources of the H_2S pool, releasing free H_2S through non-enzymatic pathways; however, this pathway is physiologically less significant. Two forms of sulfur stores have been identified: bound sulfane-sulfur and acid-labile sulfur. Presence of reductants or reducing conditions and acidic conditions (low pH) make bound sulfane-sulfur (*e.g.* protein persulfide and polysulfides) and acid-labile sulfur (*e.g.* iron-sulfur clusters) to release free H_2S, respectively (Fig. **1**).

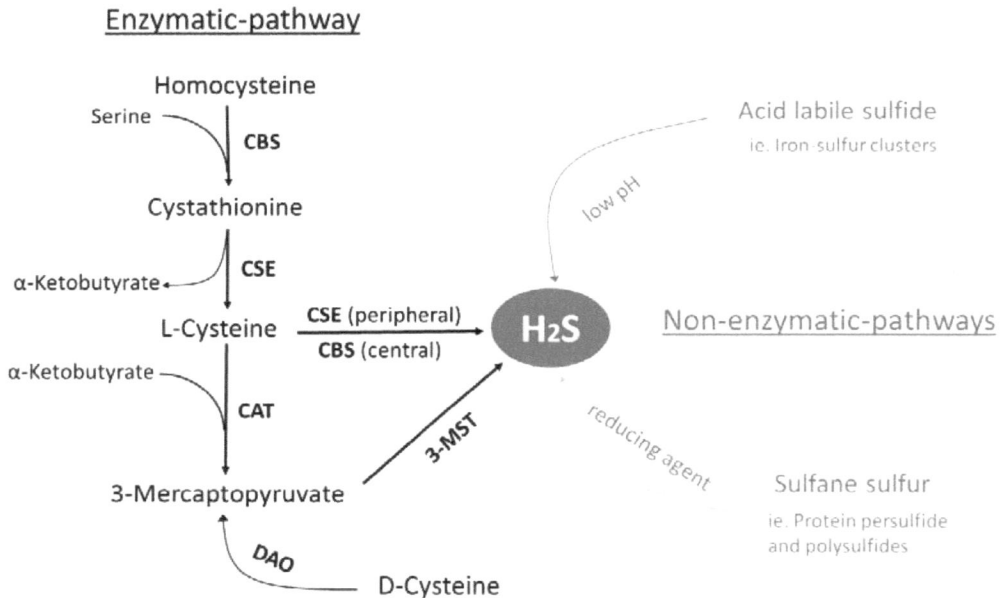

Fig. (**1**). **Schematic representation of mammalian endogenous H_2S generation through enzymatic and non-enzymatic pathways.** CSE: cystathionine-γ-lyase; CBS: cystathionine-β-synthase; 3-MST: 3-mercaptopyruvate sulfurtransferase; CAT: cysteine aminotransferase; DAO: D-amino oxidase.

Gut-microbiota is also a very good source of H_2S produced from different sources. For example, resident microbes of the colon, particularly sulfate-reducing bacteria, generate H_2S through the dissimilarity sulfate reduction (DSR) pathway. Alternatively, microbes of different genera such as *Helicobacter, Salmonella,*

Streptococcus, Enterobacter and *Fusobacterium* generate H_2S through cysteine desulfhydrase by utilizing L-cysteine as a substrate [3].

The type of biological activity of H_2S mainly depends on the availability of H_2S at the site of action. There is still little unanimity on endogenous levels of H_2S availability for different physiological actions. This is due to the difficulty in accurately measuring H_2S in a biological solution. Numerous analyses over the years have reported plasma or blood sulfide concentrations are typically between 30 and 300 μmol/L, thus supporting the biological studies.

H_2S AND VIRAL INFECTIONS

H_2S has antiviral and immunoregulatory properties. It modulates viral replication and regulates proinflammatory gene expression [4]. Recent investigations by Li *et al.* uncovered a protective role of H_2S against paramyxovirus infections such as human metapneumovirus (hMPV), respiratory syncytial virus (RSV) and Nipah Virus (NiV) by modulating viral replication and immune response both *in vitro* and *in vivo* [5]. Airway epithelial cells (AECs) infected with RSV display a decrease in H_2S synthesis by decreased expression of CSE and enhanced degradation of H_2S. Inhibition of H_2S generation using CSE inhibitor DL-propargylglycine (PAG) in RSV-infected AECs and mice deficient in the CSE gene infected with RSV results in enhanced viral replication and cytokine and chemokine production in AECs and decreased disease severity in mice [5, 6]. These results together suggest that RSV infection is associated with imbalanced cellular H_2S homeostasis.

On the other hand, treatment of RSV-, hMPV- and NiV-infected AECs with slow H_2S releasing donor GYY4137 inhibited viral replication and reduced proinflammatory cytokine and chemokine production, suggesting that H_2S has a broad inhibitory effect against different paramyxovirus infections. Administration of GYY4137 repressed RSV replication without affecting viral transcription and the translation process, indicating that H_2S may affect signalling pathways other than those involved in mRNA and protein synthesis, such as viral assembly or release [4, 5]. Another study by Ivanciuc *et al.* demonstrated that RSV infected mice treated with GYY4137 showed a decrease in viral replication and improved clinical parameters of lung dysfunction. The protective role of GYY4137 may be due to a reduction in virus-induced lung cellular infiltrates and subsequent production of proinflammatory mediators. In addition to its anti-inflammatory and anti-viral activity, H_2S has anti-oxidative properties that reduce oxidative cell damage caused by virus infection. These results support an important modulatory role of H_2S in cellular antioxidant pathway in the course of RSV infection [6].

Overall, the results of previous research indicate that H_2S has potential antiviral and anti-inflammatory activity, signifying a novel pharmacologic approach for ameliorating virus-induced lung disease. However, the mechanisms by which H_2S modulates viral-induced cellular signalling and defining the contribution of H_2S-generating enzyme (CSE) in cellular anti-viral and anti-inflammatory activity remain to be elucidated.

H_2S AND BACTERIAL INFECTIONS

There is growing evidence for the role of H_2S in different bacterial diseases. Therefore, understanding the mechanism of H_2S mediated regulation of bacterial infections is essential for developing new therapeutic approaches based on H_2S donors and inhibitors.

The impacts of H_2S on *Mycobacterium tuberculosis* (Mtb) infection and tuberculosis (TB) disease in humans are not well known. Regardless of the physiochemical properties of H_2S, its established immunomodulatory role may facilitate the potential role of this gas mediator in TB. Since the major H_2S synthesizing enzymes CSE and CBS are important in alveolarization and functioning of the lungs (the primary organ of Mtb infection), it is reasonable to assume that Mtb may have mechanisms for sensing and responding to H_2S [7 - 9].

Alternatively, H_2S plays a role in mitochondrial respiration by targeting cytochrome c oxidase [10]. Mtb is known to exhibit immense respiratory flexibility, which is crucial for maintaining an intracellular pathogenic lifestyle [11, 12]. NADH dehydrogenase I and aa3-type cytochrome c oxidase are two proton-pumping complexes in the Mtb that are required for growth and oxygen production, respectively. Mtb also expresses cytochrome b oxidase, an alternative terminal oxidase for the loss in activity of the bc1-aa3 complex [13]. Recent Mtb infection studies on CBS knockout mice (CBS[+/-]) have shown decreased bacillary burden and lung tissue damage due to a reduced Th2 cytokine response in CBS[+/-] mice [14]. Research findings from this study suggest that H_2S is a modulator of Mtb bioenergetics and contribute to Mtb latency and TB disease.

Collectively, the importance of H_2S in Mtb infection is poorly understood. Previous research has presented a range of views on the role of H_2S in Mtb infection. Therefore, further studies will be of significant interest regarding the nature of the role of H_2S in Mtb infection and pathogenesis of TB.

H_2S AND MYCOPLASMA INFECTION

Mycoplasmas are the smallest and simplest organized prokaryotic organisms capable of self-reproduction. Unlike other bacteria, mycoplasma do not have a cell wall, but a simple plasma membrane composed of sterols [14]. Mycoplasma is used as a bacterial model of acute infection [15]. Recent research has revealed the protective role of H_2S against inflammation and oxidative stress during *Mycoplasma fermentans* infection. Upon treatment with H_2S, primary macrophages and human monocytic cell line (U937) infected with *M. fermentans,* showed decrease in monocyte chemoattractant protein-1 (MCP-1) levels and NF-κB activation and translocation into nucleus [16]. Another study demonstrated that a mycoplasma-infected U937 cell line showed an increase in Nrf2 expression, leading to an increased production of antioxidant or detoxificant enzymes such as heme oxygenase 1 (HO-1), peroxiredoxin (Prdx) and superoxide dismutase 1 (SOD1) and decreased levels of ROS. This effect was enhanced by treatment with H_2S donors NaHS and GYY4137 [17]. These results together suggest that H_2S has anti-inflammatory and antioxidant effects by modulating NF-κB and Nrf2 signalling pathways during *M. fermentans* infection. However, further investigations are required to determine whether specific components of NF-κB and Nrf2 pathways are directly regulated by H_2S. Results from a recent study suggested S-sulfhydration of the cysteine residues of NF-κB by H_2S accountable for its anti-apoptotic effects [18]. Also, it has been shown that H_2S induces changes in cysteine residues in Kaep1, resulting in the release of Nrf2 [19]. Therefore, understanding how H_2S mediates S-sulfhydration and subsequent NF-κB or Nrf2 signalling during mycoplasma infection is crucial.

Another mycoplasma*, M. pneumoniae* is primarily an atypical pneumonia causing organism. In addition, it causes auto-immune disorders, debilitating mucositis, epidermal dermatopathies and chronic diseases such as arthritis and asthma [20 - 22]. Recent research identified H_2S as a potential virulence factor of *M. pneumoniae*. It has shown that H_2S produced by HapE, an unusual bifunctional cysteine desulfurase/desulfhydrase enzyme, in *M. pneumoniae* has haemolytic activity [23]; however, the mechanisms are yet to be investigated.

H_2S AND SEPSIS

Sepsis is a dysregulated host response to infection and leads to life-threatening organ dysfunction. Despite advances in care, it remains a challenging global health problem and the number of reports on sepsis incidence are increasing. The precise role of H_2S in inflammation during sepsis is still unclear: in fact, it can have both pro- or anti-inflammatory roles in the pathogenesis of sepsis and septic shock. Several studies have confirmed the proinflammatory role of H_2S in lipopolysaccharide (LPS)-induced endotoxemia and cecal-ligation and puncture (CLP)-induced sepsis. Significant increases in CSE expression and activity and H_2S production are associated with increased leukocyte infiltration, inflammatory response and organ damage following LPS-induced endotoxemia and CLP-induced sepsis [24 - 29]. H$_2$S donor NaHS aggravated sepsis-induced leukocyte infiltration and organ damage, whereas these effects were reduced when treated with PAG [27, 30, 31]. In recent years, our group has shown that silencing the CSE gene with siRNA protects against inflammatory response and liver and lung damage through a mechanism involving a decrease in activation of ERK1/2 and NF-κB p65 and subsequent production of cytokines and chemokines following CLP-induced sepsis; this also occurs in mice deficient in the CSE gene [31, 32]. Similarly, a clinical study has shown that patients with sepsis showed higher plasma H$_2$S levels compared to non-septic patients [33]. These results together suggest the proinflammatory role of H$_2$S in sepsis.

On the other hand, the anti-inflammatory and protective role of H$_2$S has also been reported. For example, H$_2$S donors such as GYY4137 and S-diclofenac have showed protection against LPS-induced endotoxemia by decreased infiltration of leukocytes into tissues, cytokines and eicosanoids generation and NF-κB activation [34]. In addition, H$_2$S produced anti-inflammatory effects through the inhibition of iNOS and p38 MAPK signalling pathways in LPS-stimulated astrocytes and microglia. Also, NaHS and another H$_2$S donor, Lawesson's reagent, improved migration of neutrophils and increased survival rates in CLP-induced sepsis; the mechanism of this action included activation of K$_{ATP}$ channels [35]. In the similar way, another study of CLP-induced sepsis reported that NaHS treatment increased survival rates in mice by inhibition of the C/EBP homologous protein 10 (CHOP) [36].

Together, previous studies have reported the inflammatory role of H$_2$S in sepsis. It has been shown to have both pro- and anti-inflammatory roles in different animal models of sepsis. The discrepancies in H$_2$S effects in different studies seem to be due to the use of different H$_2$S inhibitors and donors and their dosage regime, route of administration and duration of the study model.

H$_2$S AND ANTIBACTERIAL RESISTANCE

Understanding underlying mechanisms of antimicrobial resistance (AMR) will help in designing effective treatment approaches against different human pathogens. Research has shown that H$_2$S protects bacteria against antibiotic-induced oxidative stress by maintaining redox homeostasis through alternative oxidases and antioxidants. It has also shown that inhibition of H$_2$S synthesis reversed antibiotic resistance, whereas exposure to H$_2$S-releasing drugs restored drug tolerance in multidrug resistant (MDR) bacteria of patient origin. In addition, bacterial-derived H$_2$S is involved in antibiotic tolerance through cytoprotective actions against antibiotic-induced oxidative stress. Inactivation of H$_2$S synthesizing enzymes CBS, CSE and 3-MST in different bacterial pathogens

(*Pseudomonas aeruginosa, Staphylococcus aureus, Bacillus anthracis and Escherichia coli*) caused these pathogens to become more sensitive to antibiotics [37]. As endogenous H_2S reduces the efficacy of clinically-used antibiotics, targeting this gas mediator should potentially be considered as an augmentation therapy against a wide-range of pathogenic organisms. Bacterial CSE, CBS and 3-MST are substantially different compared to their mammalian counter-parts suggesting there is the possibility of designing specific inhibitors to target these enzymes [38]. For example, Nudler *et al.* demonstrated similar cytoprotective effects of H_2S produced by CBS, CSE and 3-MST in prokaryote bacteria as in mammalian cells. In four clinically relevant and evolutionarily distant pathogenic species of bacteria, all three enzymes were demonstrated to produce H_2S. The overexpression of 3-MST increases spectinomycin resistance, whereas the chemical inhibition of CSE, CBS or 3-MST renders bacteria more sensitive to antibiotics. NaHS suppresses the antibiotic sensitivity of CSE-, CBS- and 3-MST-deficient bacteria. These observations suggest that endogenously produced H_2S enhances the resistance of bacteria to antibiotics and that designing specific inhibitors against H_2S-synthesizing bacterial enzymes may enhance the effect of antibiotics against different types of pathogens [39].

H_2S AND FUNGAL INFECTIONS

Previous research has shown the inhibitory role of H_2S against fungal infections. H_2S donor NaHS has decreased post-harvest decay in fruits caused by *Aspergillus niger* and *Penicillium italicum*. When exposed to H_2S under *in vitro* conditions, fungal growth was inhibited at different stages of the life cycle (spore germination and elongation) and induced abnormal mycelial contractions and growth were shown. The mechanisms include decreased intracellular reactive oxygen species by H_2S, mainly due to decreased catalase (CAT) and superoxide dismutase (SOD). In addition, the growth of *Candida albicans, Saccharomyces cerevisiae* and *Rhizopusoryzae* was inhibited by H_2S. Together, these results indicate the potential role of H_2S against fungal infections, helping to reduce postharvest decay and spoilage of food by microbe propagation [40].

H_2S AND PROTOZOAL INFECTION - MALARIA

Cerebral malaria (CM) is a complex cerebrovascular disease caused by *Plasmodium falciparum* infection. *In vitro* research has shown that H_2S is a potential inhibitor of *P. falciparum* growth and metabolism. H_2S releasing drugs such as NaHS and GYY4137 showed a dose-dependent inhibition of *P. falciparum* proliferation and metabolism. The observed effects of H_2S may be associated with inhibition of cytochrome c oxidase in mitochondria. In addition, HS^- may partially contribute to parasite stress *via* protein modification associated with changes in cellular redox balance [41]. Another study by Jiang *et al.* explored the association between H_2S levels and experimental cerebral malaria (ECM). Results from this study showed that ECM was associated with reduced bioavailability of brain H_2S due to a decreased expression of brain CBS. Mice administered with NaHS showed decreased blood brain barrier destruction, secretion of IL-18, MMP-9 and serum CD40 and afforded protection against ECM [42]. These results together suggest that H_2S is one of the critical mediators of CM pathogenesis and therapeutic approaches based on H_2S would benefit against CM.

CONCLUSION

In conclusion, although previous research has shown the importance of H_2S in different types of infections and inflammation associated with infections (Table 1), there is still a large scientific gap concerning the mechanisms through which H_2S plays its crucial role in regulating different types of infections. Though recent reports support the possibility of exploring the role of H_2S during infections, these studies are limited by a number of factors in their understanding of the precise role of H_2S in infectious diseases. Future research on H_2S in infections using better study approaches will help in understanding and developing H_2S-based therapeutic molecules to control infections.

Table 1. The role of H_2S in different infections.

Type of Infection	Testing System	Treatment or Approach	Type of H_2S Activity	Reference
Viral infections	*In vitro (HEp-2 cells)*	H_2S donor GYY4137	Inhibits viral replication and assembly or release	[5]
Bacterial (*Mtb)* infections	*In vivo* (mouse model)	CBS $^{+/-}$ mice	H_2S modulates bioenergetics of Mtb	[14]
Mycoplasma infection	*In vitro (U937 cells)*	H_2S donors NaHS and GYY4137	Anti-inflammatory activity	[16]
Fungal infections	*In vitro (postharvest fruits)*	H_2S donors NaHS and GYY4137	Anti-fungal activity	[39]
Protozoal (Malaria) infection	*In vitro (P. falciparum*-infected human erythrocytes*); in vivo* (mouse model)	H_2S donors NaHS and GYY4137	Inhibits *P. falciparum* growth and metabolism	[40]
Sepsis	*In-vivo (CHOP$^{-/-}$* mice)	H_2S donor NaHS	Anti-inflammatory	[36]
Antibiotic resistance	*In-vitro: pathogenic species*	H_2S donor NaHS	Suppresses antibiotic sensitivity	[39]

CONSENT FOR PUBLICATION

Not applicable.

CONFLICT OF INTEREST

The authors declare no conflict of interest, financial or otherwise.

ACKNOWLEDGEMENTS

Declared none.

REFERENCES

[1]   Calvert JW, Coetzee WA, Lefer DJ. Novel insights into hydrogen sulfide-mediated cytoprotection. Antioxid Redox Signal 2010; 12(10): 1203-17.
        [http://dx.doi.org/10.1089/ars.2009.2882] [PMID: 19769484]

[2]   Kimura H. The physiological role of hydrogen sulfide and beyond. Nitric Oxide 2014; 41: 4-10.
        [http://dx.doi.org/10.1016/j.niox.2014.01.002] [PMID: 24491257]

[3]   Singh SB, Lin HC. Hydrogen sulfide in physiology and diseases of the digestive tract. Microorganisms 2015; 3(4): 866-89.
        [http://dx.doi.org/10.3390/microorganisms3040866] [PMID: 27682122]

[4]   Bazhanov N, Escaffre O, Freiberg AN, Garofalo RP, Casola A. Broad-range antiviral activity of hydrogen sulfide against highly pathogenic RNA viruses. Sci Rep 2017; 7: 41029.
        [http://dx.doi.org/10.1038/srep41029] [PMID: 28106111]

[5]   Li H, Ma Y, Escaffre O, *et al.* Role of hydrogen sulfide in paramyxovirus infections. J Virol 2015; 89(10): 5557-68.
        [http://dx.doi.org/10.1128/JVI.00264-15] [PMID: 25740991]

[6]   Ivanciuc T, Sbrana E, Ansar M, *et al.* Hydrogen sulfide is an antiviral and anti-inflammatory endogenous gasotransmitter in the airways: role in respiratory syncytial virus infection. Am J Respir Cell Mol Biol 2016; 55(5): 684-96.
        [http://dx.doi.org/10.1165/rcmb.2015-0385OC] [PMID: 27314446]

[7]   Madurga A, Golec A, Pozarska A, *et al.* The H_2S-generating enzymes cystathionine β-synthase and cystathionine γ-lyase play a role in vascular development during normal lung alveolarization. Am J Physiol Lung Cell Mol Physiol 2015; 309(7): L710-24.
        [http://dx.doi.org/10.1152/ajplung.00134.2015] [PMID: 26232299]

[8]   Miles EW, Kraus JP. Cystathionine beta-synthase: structure, function, regulation, and location of homocystinuria-causing mutations. J Biol Chem 2004; 279(29): 29871-4.
        [http://dx.doi.org/10.1074/jbc.R400005200] [PMID: 15087459]

[9]   Pan LL, Liu XH, Gong QH, Yang HB, Zhu YZ. Role of cystathionine γ-lyase/hydrogen sulfide pathway in cardiovascular disease: a novel therapeutic strategy? Antioxid Redox Signal 2012; 17(1): 106-18.
        [http://dx.doi.org/10.1089/ars.2011.4349] [PMID: 22017202]

[10]   Cooper CE, Brown GC. The inhibition of mitochondrial cytochrome oxidase by the gases carbon monoxide, nitric oxide, hydrogen cyanide and hydrogen sulfide: chemical mechanism and physiological significance. J Bioenerg Biomembr 2008; 40(5): 533-9.
        [http://dx.doi.org/10.1007/s10863-008-9166-6] [PMID: 18839291]

[11]   Loebel RO, Shorr E, Richardson HB. The influence of adverse conditions upon the respiratory metabolism and growth of human tubercle bacilli. J Bacteriol 1933; 26(2): 167-200.

[PMID: 16559650]

[12]   Arora K, Ochoa-Montaño B, Tsang PS, *et al.* Respiratory flexibility in response to inhibition of cytochrome C oxidase in Mycobacterium tuberculosis. Antimicrob Agents Chemother 2014; 58: 6962-5.
       [http://dx.doi.org/10.1128/AAC.03486-14] [PMID: 25155596]

[13]   Rao SP, Alonso S, Rand L, Dick T, Pethe K. The protonmotive force is required for maintaining ATP homeostasis and viability of hypoxic, nonreplicating Mycobacterium tuberculosis. Proc Natl Acad Sci USA 2008; 105: 11945-50.
       [http://dx.doi.org/10.1073/pnas.0711697105] [PMID: 18697942]

[14]   Saini V, Stein A, Chinta KC, *et al.* Hydrogen sulfide alters M. tuberculosis bioenergetics and promotes tuberculosis disease. Free Radic Biol Med 2015; 87: 141.
       [http://dx.doi.org/10.1016/j.freeradbiomed.2015.10.365]

[15]   Razin S. Peculiar properties of mycoplasmas: the smallest self-replicating prokaryotes. FEMS Microbiol Lett 1992; 100: 423-31.
       [http://dx.doi.org/10.1111/j.1574-6968.1992.tb05735.x] [PMID: 1478475]

[16]   Benedetti F, Davinelli S, Krishnan S, *et al.* Sulfur compounds block MCP-1 production by Mycoplasma fermentans-infected macrophages through NF-κB inhibition. J Transl Med 2014; 12: 145.
       [http://dx.doi.org/10.1186/1479-5876-12-145] [PMID: 24886588]

[17]   Benedetti F, Curreli S, Krishnan S, *et al.* Anti-inflammatory effects of H_2S during acute bacterial infection: a review. J Transl Med 2017; 15: 100.
       [http://dx.doi.org/10.1186/s12967-017-1206-8] [PMID: 28490346]

[18]   Sen N, Paul BD, Gadalla MM, *et al.* Hydrogen sulfide-linked sulfhydration of NF-κB mediates its antiapoptotic actions. Mol Cell 2012; 45: 13-24.
       [http://dx.doi.org/10.1016/j.molcel.2011.10.021] [PMID: 22244329]

[19]   Hourihan JM, Kenna JG, Hayes JD. The gasotransmitter hydrogen sulfide induces nrf2-target genes by inactivating the keap1 ubiquitin ligase substrate adaptor through formation of a disulfide bond between cys-226 and cys-613. Antioxid Redox Signal 2013; 19: 465-81.
       [http://dx.doi.org/10.1089/ars.2012.4944] [PMID: 23145493]

[20]   Atkinson TP, Balish MF, Waites KB. Epidemiology, clinical manifestations, pathogenesis and laboratory detection of Mycoplasma pneumoniae infections. FEMS Microbiol Rev 2008; 32: 956-73.
       [http://dx.doi.org/10.1111/j.1574-6976.2008.00129.x] [PMID: 18754792]

[21]   Waites KB, Balish MF, Atkinson TP. New insights into the pathogenesis and detection of Mycoplasma pneumoniae infections. Future Microbiol 2008; 3: 635-48.
       [http://dx.doi.org/10.2217/17460913.3.6.635] [PMID: 19072181]

[22]   Vujic I, Shroff A, Grzelka M, *et al.* Mycoplasma pneumoniae-associated mucositis-case report and systematic review of literature. J Eur Acad Dermatol Venereol 2015; 29: 595-8.
       [http://dx.doi.org/10.1111/jdv.12392] [PMID: 24665876]

[23]   Großhennig S, Ischebeck T, Gibhardt J, Busse J, Feussner I, Stülke J. Hydrogen sulfide is a novel potential virulence factor of Mycoplasma pneumoniae: characterization of the unusual cysteine desulfurase/desulfhydrase HapE. Mol Microbiol 2016; 100: 42-54.
       [http://dx.doi.org/10.1111/mmi.13300] [PMID: 26711628]

[24]   Collin M, Anuar FB, Murch O, Bhatia M, Moore PK, Thiemermann C. Inhibition of endogenous hydrogen sulfide formation reduces the organ injury caused by endotoxemia. Br J Pharmacol 2005; 146: 498-505.
       [http://dx.doi.org/10.1038/sj.bjp.0706367] [PMID: 16100527]

[25]   Li L, Bhatia M, Zhu YZ, *et al.* Hydrogen sulfide is a novel mediator of lipopolysaccharide-induced inflammation in the mouse. FASEB J 2005; 19: 1196-8.

[http://dx.doi.org/10.1096/fj.04-3583fje] [PMID: 15863703]

[26]   Ahmad A, Gero D, Olah G, *et al.* Effect of lipopolysaccharide (LPS)-induced endotoxemia in mice genetically deficient in either one of the three major hydrogen-sulfide producing enzymes. FASEB J 2016; 30: 127-38.

[27]   Zhang H, Zhi L, Moochhala SM, Moore PK, Bhatia M. Endogenous hydrogen sulfide regulates leukocyte trafficking in cecal ligation and puncture-induced sepsis. J Leukoc Biol 2007; 82: 894-905.
         [http://dx.doi.org/10.1189/jlb.0407237] [PMID: 17599903]

[28]   Zhang H, Zhi L, Moore PK, Bhatia M. Role of hydrogen sulfide in cecal ligation and puncture-induced sepsis in the mouse. Am J Physiol Lung Cell Mol Physiol 2006; 290: L1193-201.
         [http://dx.doi.org/10.1152/ajplung.00489.2005] [PMID: 16428267]

[29]   Zanardo RC, Brancaleone V, Distrutti E, Fiorucci S, Cirino G, Wallace JL. Hydrogen sulfide is an endogenous modulator of leukocyte-mediated inflammation. FASEB J 2006; 20: 2118-20.
         [http://dx.doi.org/10.1096/fj.06-6270fje] [PMID: 16912151]

[30]   Zhang H, Moochhala SM, Bhatia M. Endogenous hydrogen sulfide regulates inflammatory response by activating the ERK pathway in polymicrobial sepsis. J Immunol 2008; 181: 4320-31.
         [http://dx.doi.org/10.4049/jimmunol.181.6.4320] [PMID: 18768890]

[31]   Badiei A, Chambers ST, Gaddam RR, Bhatia M. Cystathionine-γ-lyase gene silencing with siRNA in monocytes/ macrophages attenuates inflammation in cecal ligation and puncture-induced sepsis in the mouse. J Biosci 2016; 41: 87-95.
         [http://dx.doi.org/10.1007/s12038-016-9598-9] [PMID: 26949091]

[32]   Gaddam RR, Fraser R, Badiei A, *et al.* Cystathionine-γ-lyase gene deletion protects mice against inflammation and liver sieve injury following polymicrobial sepsis. PLoS One 2016; 11(8): e0160521.
         [http://dx.doi.org/10.1371/journal.pone.0160521] [PMID: 27518439]

[33]   Gaddam RR, Chambers S, Murdoch D, Shaw G, Bhatia M. Circulating levels of hydrogen sulfide and substance P in patients with sepsis. J Infect 2017; 75: 293-300.
         [http://dx.doi.org/10.1016/j.jinf.2017.07.005] [PMID: 28760413]

[34]   Ekundi-Valentim E, Santos KT, Camargo EA, *et al.* Differing effects of exogenous and endogenous hydrogen sulphide in carrageenan-induced knee joint synovitis in the rat. Br J Pharmacol 2010; 159: 1463-74.
         [http://dx.doi.org/10.1111/j.1476-5381.2010.00640.x] [PMID: 20136840]

[35]   Spiller F, Orrico MI, Nascimento DC, *et al.* Hydrogen sulfide improves neutrophil migration and survival in sepsis *via* K^+_{ATP} channel activation. Am J Respir Crit Care Med 2010; 182: 360-8.
         [http://dx.doi.org/10.1164/rccm.200907-1145OC] [PMID: 20339148]

[36]   Ferlito M, Wang Q, Fulton WB, *et al.* Hydrogen sulfide [corrected] increases survival during sepsis: protective effect of CHOP inhibition. J Immunol 2014; 192: 1806-14.
         [http://dx.doi.org/10.4049/jimmunol.1300835] [PMID: 24403532]

[37]   Chen YH, Yao WZ, Gao JZ, Geng B, Wang PP, Tang CS. Serum hydrogen sulfide as a novel marker predicting bacterial involvement in patients with community-acquired lower respiratory tract infections. Respirology 2009; 14: 746-52.
         [http://dx.doi.org/10.1111/j.1440-1843.2009.01550.x] [PMID: 19659653]

[38]   Kimura H. Production and physiological effects of hydrogen sulfide. Antioxid Redox Signal 2014; 20(5): 783-93.
         [http://dx.doi.org/10.1089/ars.2013.5309] [PMID: 23581969]

[39]   Shatalin K, Shatalina E, Mironov A, Nudler E. H₂S: a universal defense against antibiotics in bacteria. Science 2011; 334: 986-90.
         [http://dx.doi.org/10.1126/science.1209855] [PMID: 22096201]

[40]   Fu LH, Hu KD, Hu LY, *et al.* An antifungal role of hydrogen sulfide on the postharvest pathogens *Aspergillus niger* and *Penicillium italicum*. PLoS One 2014; 9: e104206.

[http://dx.doi.org/10.1371/journal.pone.0104206] [PMID: 25101960]

[41]   DellaValle B, Staalsoe T, Kurtzhals JA, Hempel C. Investigation of hydrogen sulfide gas as a treatment against P. falciparum, murine cerebral malaria, and the importance of thiolation state in the development of cerebral malaria. PLoS One 2013; 8(3): e59271.
[http://dx.doi.org/10.1371/journal.pone.0059271] [PMID: 23555646]

[42]   Jiang P, Xu Z, Xiao B, *et al.* Hydrogen sulfide protects against the development of experimental cerebral malaria in a C57BL/6 mouse model. Mol Med Reports 2017; 16: 2045.: 2050.

SUBJECT INDEX

Atta-ur-Rahman & M. Iqbal Choudhary (Eds.)
All rights reserved-© 2018 Bentham Science Publishers

U

Ubiquitin-proteasome pathway (UPP) 45 47, 55
Unfolded protein response (UPR) 45, 47, 54, 55

V

Viral 59, 62, 63 64, 65, 67 70, 71, 72, 263, 268
   infection 63, 67, 70, 71, 263
   production 59, 62
   replication 62, 64, 65, 70, 72, 263, 268
Virtual screening 153, 154, 155, 172, 176, 177, 178, 187, 188, 189, 194, 196, 197, 199, 200, 201, 202, 203
   structure-based 199, 202

Virulence factors 27, 117, 132, 223, 227, 232, 233

W

Weighted holistic invariant molecular (WHIM) 191
West Nile virus (WNV) 45, 46, 71

Y

Yellow fever virus (YFV) 45, 46

Z

Zingiberaceae 102, 103, 104, 122, 123

www.ingramcontent.com/pod-product-compliance
Lightning Source LLC
Chambersburg PA
CBHW050815220326
41598CB00006B/220